FOOD *for* FITNESS

How to ~~eat~~ ... ~~ance~~ ...dition

...ean

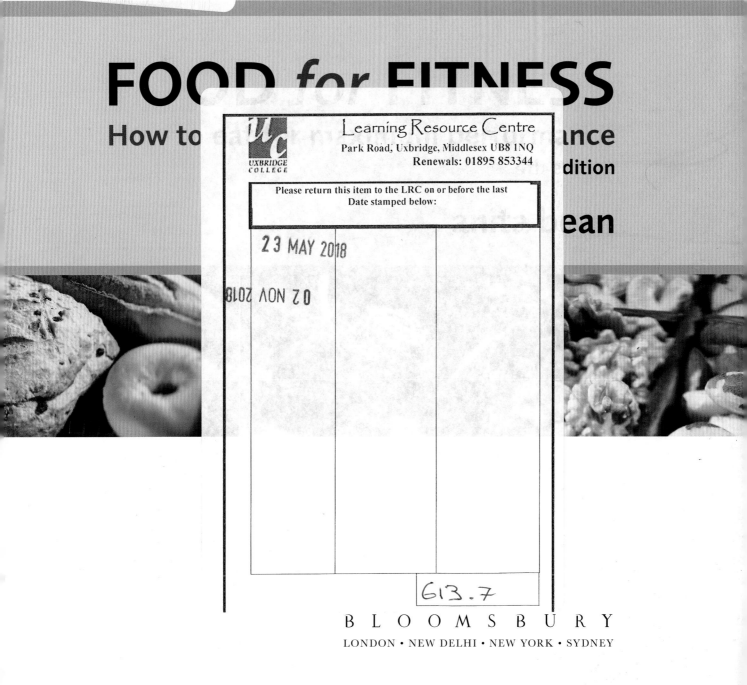

BLOOMSBURY

LONDON · NEW DELHI · NEW YORK · SYDNEY

Note
While every effort has been made to ensure that the content of this book is as technically accurate and as sound as possible, neither the author nor the publishers can accept responsibility for any injury or loss sustained as a result of the use of this material.

Published by Bloomsbury Publishing Plc
50 Bedford Square
London WC1B 3DP
www.bloomsbury.com

Fourth edition 2014
Third edition 2007, reprinted 2009
Second edition 2002
First edition 1998, reprinted 1999

Copyright © 1998, 2002, 2008 and 2014 Anita Bean
ISBN (print): 978-1-4729-0199-6
ISBN (epub): 978-1-4729-0282-5
ISBN (epdf): 978-1-4729-0283-2

A CIP catalogue record for this book is available from the British Library.

Acknowledgements
Cover photograph © Getty Images; author photo © Tom Croft
Inside photographs: All images © Shutterstock with the exception of p. 69 Naturasports/Shutterstock.com; p. 73 © Radu Razvan/Shutterstock.com; p. 134 Daniel Goodings/Shutterstock.com; p. 137 © Maxisport/Shutterstock.com; p. 149 © ostill/Shutterstock.com; p. 173 © Shamleen/Shutterstock.com; p. 187 Francesco Carucci/Shutterstock.com; p. 196 Naturasports/Shutterstock.com; pp. 1, 48, 100, 120, 121, 122, 139, 141, 145, 159, 194, 210 and 217 © Getty Images
Commissioning Editor: Charlotte Croft
Editor: Sarah Cole
Design: James Watson

This book is produced using paper that is made from wood grown in managed, sustainable forests. It is natural, renewable and recyclable. The logging and manufacturing processes conform to the environmental regulations of the country of origin

Typeset in 9.5pt on 13pt Myriad Pro by Margaret Brain, Wisbech, Cambs
Printed and bound in China by C&C Offset Printing Co
10 9 8 7 6 5 4 3

CONTENTS

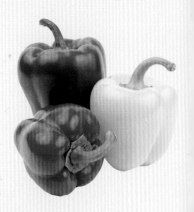

FOREWORD

I am a great believer in an active lifestyle. I know from first hand experience that diet plays a very big part in any fitness programme as well as sporting success. When I was training for the Olympics, I would eat a lot of food – a typical week would include more than twenty hours in the pool as well as ten in the gym – so I was always hungry. But, to be the best in my sport, I made sure that I ate a lot of the right foods, as well as trained very hard. I won an Olympic silver medal, double Commonwealth gold, competed in three Olympics in three decades, as well as set 200 British records. I now work for the BBC as a presenter on swimming among other things.

Although I no longer compete, I am still committed to a fitness regime. These days I basically exercise to stay in shape – regularly working out in my home gym, skiing, walking the dog and playing with my kids – but I still pay attention to what I eat. I don't diet, I've tried them, they don't work for me, I just eat healthily, balancing what I eat with my activity needs. When I eat well, I have more energy and I perform a lot better too. It's simple really, calories in equals calories out – or you put on weight!

I've known Anita for several years and always shared her practical approach to nutrition. I welcome this book, it combines the best of nutrition knowledge with fitness training and an active lifestyle. It gives you clear no-nonsense advice about what to eat, how much to eat and when to eat. There are hundreds of useful facts and tips to help you put together a healthy eating plan, whether you are working out for fitness or in serious training for competitions. I'm sure that you will find this book useful and a great investment in your well-being.

Sharron Davies MBE
Olympic Swimming Champion

INTRODUCTION

If you are reading this, then you have just taken a big step towards improving your fitness. If you're already an accomplished athlete, this book will help you reach the next level. If you're new to fitness, then this book will give you a head start and you'll begin reaping the benefits straight away.

Getting your nutrition right is perhaps more important than the training you do if you want to maximise your fitness. After all, performance starts with fuelling, not training! Correct nutrition will enable you to train harder and more effectively, recover quicker, miss fewer sessions through illness, injury or fatigue, and gain a competitive edge. Without it, you will not be making the most of your training.

In this 4th edition of *Food For Fitness*, you will learn how to fuel your training programme effectively, how to time your nutritional intake for fastest results, what the best recovery foods are, and which supplements really work. You'll also discover how to achieve your ideal weight, how to gain muscle, lose fat and create the perfect diet for your fitness programme or sport. You'll find core eating plans for runners, cyclists, swimmers, triathletes, and team players, as well as eating strategies for competitions that will help you achieve your best performance.

This 4th edition represents the most up-to-date advice on nutrition for sport and exercise. Since the publication of the 3rd edition of *Food For Fitness*, there have been hundreds of new studies and scientific discoveries that have changed the dietary advice I give to athletes, particularly on topics such as carbohydrate requirements, fat and sugar. There's also been a shift in the scientific consensus on hydration, nutrient timing and protein intake. I've incorporated the latest science into this new edition, giving you all the most cutting-edge information on nutrition and fitness at your fingertips.

I'm a firm believer in evidence-based advice so in this book, you'll find that all the facts are supported by referenced sources at the end of each chapter. I've endeavoured to present current, useful and practical advice to help you improve your performance, not personal opinions, anecdotes or cherry-picked evidence to promote a personal view. I should point out that I don't sell products or supplements so you can be assured that the advice in this book is unbiased and scientifically-based. By demystifying the hype and hearsay, this book will save you time, effort and money – you won't be eating foods or supplements that you don't need.

Over the years, I've had the privilege of working with many athletes in different sports and have learnt that nutrition really can make a big difference to everyone's performance, whether a newcomer, club athlete or Olympian. But that can only happen when the individual has the means to put the theory (about nutrients) into practice (daily diet). In other words, you need to know exactly what meals and snacks to eat! And in Part 3 I've devised over 50 delicious fitness recipes for breakfasts, main meals and snacks. They're all quick and simple to make, healthy, inexpensive and best of all require minimal cooking skills!

Good luck and happy cooking and training!

Anita Bean
2014

ACKNOWLEDGEMENTS

My gratitude extends, as ever, to my husband for his patience during the writing of this book. I am forever thankful for my two daughters, Chloe and Lucy, who not only provide me with unending inspiration, but also faithfully feedback on my recipes and menus. My thanks also extend to the terrific editorial team at Bloomsbury, especially Charlotte Croft for her vision and insight and to Sarah Cole for her sheer hard work.

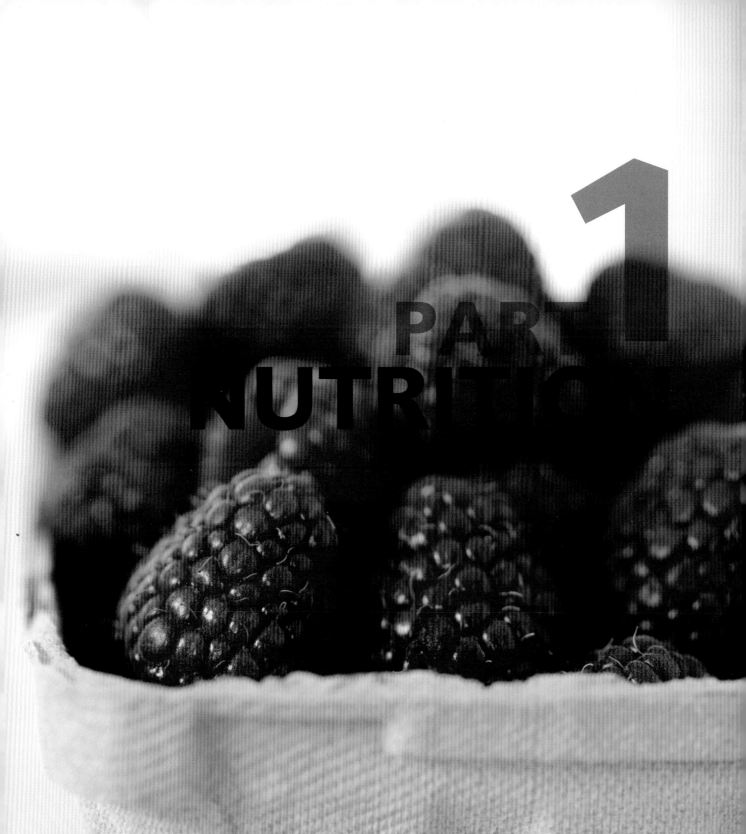

PART 1
NUTRITION

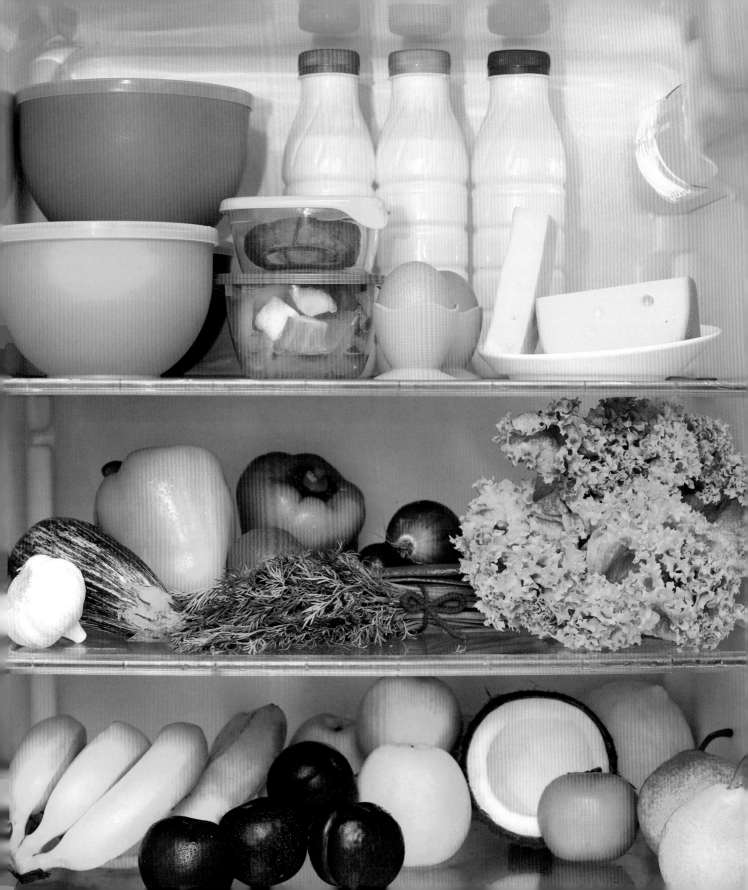

1 NUTRITION ESSENTIALS

Your diet not only affects your health but also your performance. It affects how energetic you feel, your stamina, your strength and your power. It is undoubtedly the biggest factor when it comes to body weight and body composition, both of which are critical for peak performance (as well as health). What, how much, and when you eat can also make a crucial difference to your ability to recover after exercise as well as your performance in competition. So, whether you're exercising for fitness or training for competitions, eating a healthy diet and maintaining proper hydration will help improve your performance, keep you healthy and promote fast recovery.

Exactly what should you eat then? Well, there's no 'ideal diet' that's right for everyone but a good place to start when it comes to designing your daily diet are the guidelines developed by the International Olympic Committee (IOC, 2011) and the ACSM (Rodrigues *et al.*, 2009). These form the basis of the nutrition advice in this chapter. However, your exact calorie and nutritional needs will depend on your weight, size, age, daily calorie expenditure, individual metabolism, training programme and even such factors as the temperature and humidity. To help you make the healthiest food choices, here are the essential facts about nutrition for sport and exercise.

1. Energy (calories)

Where do I get energy?

You get energy from four components in food and drink: carbohydrate, fat, protein and (though not strictly a nutrient) alcohol. Each of these provides different amounts of energy. 1 g provides approximately:

protein	4 kcal (17 kJ)	alcohol	7 kcal (29 kJ)
carbohydrate	4 kcal (17 kJ)	fat	9 kcal (38 kJ)

These fuels are broken down in your body and transformed via various biochemical pathways into a compound called adenosine triphosphate (ATP). Energy is produced when one of the phosphate molecules splits off, leaving adenosine diphosphate (ADP). This energy can then be used to fuel your muscles.

How many calories do I need?

You can estimate your daily calorie needs by working out your basal metabolic rate (BMR) and multiplying it by your physical activity level.

Your BMR is the number of calories you burn at rest over 24 hours maintaining essential functions such as respiration, digestion and brain function. BMR accounts for 60–75 per cent of the calories you burn daily.

Step 1: Estimate your basal metabolic rate (BMR)

(A) Quick method: As a rule of thumb, BMR uses 11 calories for every 0.5 kg of a woman's body weight, and 12 calories for every 0.5 kg of a man's body weight.

Women: BMR = weight in kg x 2 x 11 (alternatively weight in pounds x 11)
Men: BMR = weight in kg x 2 x 12 (alternatively weight in pounds x 12)
Example: BMR for a 60 kg woman = 60 x 2 x 11 x 1,320 kcal.

(B) Longer method: For a more accurate estimation of your BMR, use the following equations or an online calculator (http://www.bmi-calculator.net/bmr-calcuator/)

TABLE 1.1 WEIGHT CALCULATIONS

Age	Men	Women
10–18 years	*(weight in kg x 17.5) + 651*	*(weight in kg x 12.2) + 746*
18–30 years	*(weight in kg x 15.3) + 679*	*(weight in kg x 14.7) + 479*
31–60 years	*(weight in kg x 11.6) + 879*	*(weight in kg x 8.7) + 829*
60+ years	*(weight in kg x 13.5) + 487*	*(weight in kg x 10.5) + 596*

Example: BMR for a 60 kg woman aged 31–60 years =
(60 x 8.7) + 829 = 1,351 kcal.

Step 2: Estimate your physical activity level (PAL)

Your physical activity level (PAL) is the ratio of your overall daily energy expenditure to your BMR. It's a rough measure of your lifestyle activity.

Mostly inactive or sedentary (mainly sitting)	1.2
Fairly active (include walking and exercise 1–2 x weekly)	1.3
Moderately active (exercise 2–3 x weekly)	1.4
Active (exercise hard more than 3 x weekly)	1.5
Very active (exercise hard daily)	1.7

Step 3: Multiply your BMR by your PAL to work out your daily calorie needs

BMR x PAL

Example: Daily energy needs for an active 60 kg woman = 1,351 x 1.5 =2,027 kcal.

That's roughly how many calories you burn a day to maintain your weight, assuming you have an 'average' body composition. If you have higher than average muscle mass, add 150 calories.

To lose weight, reduce your daily calorie intake by 15 per cent or multiply the figure above (maintenance calorie needs) by 0.85. This will produce a fat loss of about 0.5 kg per week.

Example: Daily energy needs for an active 60 kg woman to lose weight =
2,027 x 0.85 = 1,723 kcal.

To gain weight, increase your daily calorie intake by 20 per cent or multiply the figure above (maintenance calorie needs) by 1.2. In conjunction with a resistance training programme, expect a weight gain of 0.25–0.5 kg per month.

Example: Daily energy needs for an active 60 kg woman to gain weight =
2,027 x 1.2 = 2,432 kcal.

2. Carbohydrate

Why do I need carbohydrate?

Strictly speaking, there is no physiological need for carbohydrate (or 'carbs'); your body could get by with energy derived from fats and protein – provided you didn't exercise! Carbohydrate are an important fuel for muscles – almost all types of activities rely on carbohydrate (glucose) for energy. Perhaps the only exception is a single all-out lift in the gym or a single jump. But sprinting, running, jogging, swimming, cycling, walking, playing football … they all use carbohydrate to a greater or lesser degree. The longer and harder you exercise, the more carbohydrate you burn.

So, the main purpose of carbohydrate is to fuel the muscles. It's also the preferred fuel for the brain, nervous system and heart, which use about 130 g daily, although it is possible to survive on less than this, perhaps as little as 50 g. That's because the body can make glucose from protein in a process called gluconeogenesis. If you eat less than this amount (this is not recommended for athletes), then your body will go into a state of ketosis. This means that fats are converted into ketone bodies in the liver, which can then be used by the brain for fuel instead of glucose. However, they cannot provide fuel for the muscles, which is why low-carbohydrate diets are not generally advised for athletes.

Can I over-consume carbohydrate?

The carbohydrate in your food is converted into glycogen and stored in your liver and muscles. However, these stores are relatively small – you can store only about 100 g (equivalent to 400 calories) in the liver and 400 g (or 1,600 calories) in the muscles. Once your glycogen stores are 'full', then your body will convert any excess carbohydrate to fat. So, while it is important to refill your glycogen stores

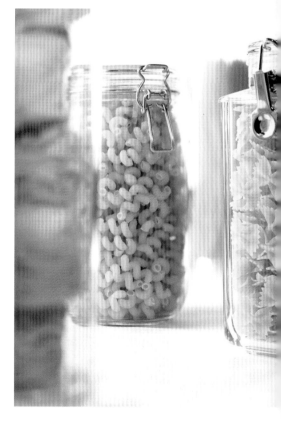

after working out, you should be careful not to over-consume carbohydrate. More carbohydrate does not equal more energy. Just as over-filling the fuel tank in your car won't make it go faster, over-consuming carbohydrate won't improve your performance. Excess carbohydrate can mean excess fat weight, which will almost certainly hinder your performance.

Can I eat too little carbohydrate?

On the other hand, consuming a low-carbohydrate diet or exercising with low glycogen stores can result in early fatigue, reduced stamina and poor performance, particularly for high-intensity endurance activities lasting longer than an hour. If you eat too little carbohydrate after training, your recovery will be impaired and, over time, you may develop symptoms of overtraining. Therefore, it's important that you plan your carbohydrate intake around your training sessions carefully to avoid weight gain as well as under-performance.

How much carbohydrate do I need?

A high-carbohydrate diet has long been the cornerstone of nutrition advice for all regular exercisers. However, scientific thinking around how much carbohydrate you need has shifted since the publication of the 3rd edition of *Food for Fitness* in favour of a higher fat intake and lower-carbohydrate intake, particularly for those trying to lose weight.

Previously, sports scientists recommended that everyone should get around 60 per cent of their calories from carbohydrate. However this doesn't take account of different exercise modes (endurance or anaerobic), body weights or training volumes. One size doesn't fit all! The quantity of carbohydrate you should eat depends on your goals (e.g. to lose, maintain or gain weight), how much exercise you do, the type and intensity of your activity and your body weight. Also, for most people, the amount of activity you do varies from day to day, so you will need to vary your carbohydrate intake accordingly. For instance, on days when you are more active, you should eat more carbohydrate; conversely, on rest days or when you do a lighter workout, you should eat less carbohydrate.

As a rule of thumb, the longer and harder you train, the more carbohydrate you need to fuel your muscles (Rodrigues *et al.*, 2009; IOC, 2011). The Australian Institute of Sport recommend that those who do relatively low-intensity exercise, such as brisk walking, slow jogging or skill-based workouts, consume 3–5 g carbohydrate/kg of body weight daily (Burke, L., 2007; Burke *et al.*, 2011). If you do moderate-intensity training, such as cycling, swimming or running, for an hour a day, then you should aim to consume 5–7 g/kg of body weight daily. Doing moderate- to high-intensity training up to 3 hours a day increases your

HOW CAN I TELL IF I AM EATING TOO MUCH OR TOO LITTLE CARBOHYDRATE?

A good guide as to whether you are eating enough carbohydrate is how energetic you feel during your workouts. If you feel easily fatigued but haven't changed the amount of rest and sleep you get, nor increased your training volume, this may suggest low glycogen levels and an insufficient carbohydrate intake. Upping your carbohydrate intake by an extra 50–100 g daily should restore glycogen levels and stave off fatigue. However, over-eating carbohydrate won't increase your energy levels. Instead, you may feel 'heavy' and, ironically, more lethargic. Once your glycogen stores are filled, excess carbohydrate is converted into fat so you may notice that you put on weight. Try to listen to your body and you'll soon find the balance between too little and too much carbohydrate.

requirement to 7–10 g/kg body weight, while training more than 4 hours daily would push your requirement to the upper end of that range, 10–12 g/kg of body weight. In practice, around 5 g/kg should be more than adequate for most people training 1–2 hours a day. Even if you're lifting heavy weights, this level will be more than enough to fuel a typical workout. Only elite endurance athletes who are in very heavy training need more than 7 g/kg on a daily basis. Table 1.2 gives guidelines for daily carbohydrate intake for different body types and duration of training programmes.

For example, a 60 kg person training at a moderate intensity for 1 hour a day would need approximately (5 x 60)–(7 x 60) or 300–420 g carbohydrate. However, this is only a guideline and you should adjust this according to your specific training goals, how active you are during the rest of the day, and how you feel during and after training. For example, if you want to lose weight, you should eat less than this amount.

Table 1.3 gives the carbohydrate content of various foods but you can also get an idea of your carbohydrate intake by checking the labels of foods or using the free online database (http://www.food-database.co.uk/) for the amounts of carbohydrate in various foods.

TABLE 1.2 HOW MUCH CARBOHYDRATE DO I NEED?

Activity level	Recommended carbohydrate intake g/kg body weight/day	Carbohydrate/day for a 50 kg person	Carbohydrate/day for a 60 kg person	Carbohydrate/day for a 70 kg person
Very light training (low-intensity or skill-based exercise)	3–5 g	150–250 g	180–300 g	210–350 g
Moderate-intensity training (approx 1 hour/day)	5–7 g	250–350 g	300–420 g	350–490 g
Moderate- to high-intensity training (1–3 hours/day)	7–10 g	350–500 g	420–600 g	490–700 g
Very high-intensity training (>4 hours/day)	10–12 g	500–600 g	600–720 g	700–840 g

Source: Burke, L., 2007; Burke *et al.*, 2011.

Low-carbohydrate high-fat diets for athletes?

A few scientists have challenged the conventional high carbohydrate dogma and suggested that athletes can perform as well or better on a low carbohydrate, high-fat (LCHF) diet. The theory is that by restricting carbohydrate, you force your

TABLE 1.3 THE CARBOHYDRATE CONTENT OF DIFFERENT FOODS

Food	Energy (kcal)	Carbohydrate (g)
Apples (one, 100 g)	47	12
Baked beans (200 g)	162	30
Bananas (one, 100 g)	95	23
Biscuits (one, 15 g)	70	10
Bran flakes (40 g)	132	29
Bread (1 slice, 35 g)	80	15
Cereal bar (one, 30 g)	140	18
Flapjacks (one, 70 g)	345	44
Jam or honey (15 g)	40	10
Milk, semi-skimmed (300 ml)	138	14
Oatcakes (one, 13 g)	54	8
Orange juice (200 ml)	72	18
Pasta (85 g raw weight)	196	64
Pitta bread (one, 60 g)	160	34
Porridge (200 g)	166	23
Potatoes (200 g)	150	34
Rice (85 g raw weight)	303	69
Roll (one, 50 g)	120	22
Shreddies (40 g)	138	31
Sweetcorn (80 g)	89	16
Weetabix (two, 40 g)	141	30
Yoghurt (1 pot, 150 g)	117	21

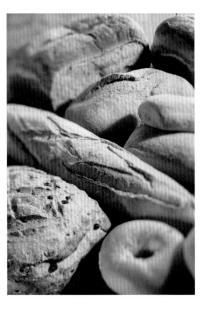

muscles to burn more calories from fat and less from carbs during exercise, thus 'sparing' valuable glycogen stores and allowing you to exercise longer before experiencing fatigue.

A LCHF may suit those looking to lose weight or those with type 2 diabetes or insulin resistance (when your cells are less sensitive to insulin so cannot process carbohydrate into fuel efficiently) **while doing mainly low to moderate intensity training** (e.g. jogging or 'easy pace' running or cycling). However, a LCHF diet will not support high intensity training. That's because you need carbohydrate to fuel exercise above 65% VO_2max (lactate threshold). If you try to perform high-intensity endurance exercise with low glycogen stores, you'll quickly find that exercise feels considerably harder, your pace will drop and you'll fatigue earlier. This is not recommended!

IS SUGAR ADDICTIVE OR TOXIC?

A few scientists believe that sugar is addictive, acting on the brain in a similar way to alcohol and nicotine (Lustig, 2013). However, there is no scientific evidence to support this (Benton, 2009) and a consensus report from European researchers concluded that no single food or ingredient causes addiction (Neurofast, 2013). Equally, it is far-fetched to call sugar a toxin – the majority of studies linking sugar with disease have been done with rodents (not humans) fed up to 300g fructose a day.

There is little evidence that LCHF diets improve athletic performance. Only one study, carried out in 1983 at the University of Connecticut, concluded that LCHF diets do not reduce endurance performance but it involved just five subjects, only one of whom actually improved their performance and the rest either reduced their performance or remained unchanged (Phinney *et al.*, 1983). A more recent study with competitive mountain bikers found those who followed a LCHF diet actually experienced a drop in power and performance at high exercise intensities (Zajac *et al.*, 2014).

When it comes to weight loss, the evidence from large meta-analyses suggests LCHF diets are overall no worse or better than low fat diets for weight loss (Pagoto & Appelhans, 2013; Hu *et al.*, 2012, Johnston *et al.*, 2006). What matters most is achieving a calorie deficit and then being able to sustain the diet long term.

1. Performance

When it comes to performance, sugar can be useful for maintaining blood glucose concentrations during intense training sessions or events lasting more than 60 minutes when the muscles may run low on glycogen and need extra fuel quickly. In these scenarios, consuming sugar (say, in the form of a banana, gel, dried fruit, a sports drink, or a cereal bar) would help you continue exercising longer and/or maintain your intensity, i.e. perform to your potential. However, it would be unnecessary for shorter sessions. Sugar may also be beneficial for refuelling muscles during the 2-hour period after exercise particularly if you plan to train again within 12 hours and require rapid refuelling (*see* page 10).

But eating more sugar won't necessarily make you feel more energetic or 'give you more energy'. In fact, the opposite holds true – if you consume too much or get the timing wrong (Burke *et al.*, 1998; Wu and Williams, 2006). If you eat too much before exercising or your body produces too much insulin after eating sugar, then you may be left with lower blood glucose levels than before. This rebound effect can make you feel tired, weak and lightheaded. It is 'safer' to eat a low-GI meal 2–4 hours before exercise or consume only small amounts of sugar (e.g. a banana) if you need an energy boost before exercise.

2. Health

The main problem with sugar is that it causes tooth decay. Indeed, studies have shown that athletes who consume lots of sports drinks and gels experience significant tooth decay and erosion (Needleman *et al.*, 2015). These products are high in sugar and if you take frequent sips of sports

IS SUGAR GOOD OR BAD FOR ATHLETES?

Sugar is a carbohydrate, which means it is an energy source for the body. It can be used to fuel muscles during exercise; convert into glycogen; or turn into fat. The dilemma for athletes is knowing when sugar may be useful for performance or when it may be harmful for health.

Q&A

How much sugar is 'safe' to eat?

The Scientific Advisory Committee on Nutrition (SACN) in the UK recommends you should get no more than 5 per cent of your daily calories from added sugars, which equates to about 25 g for the average person consuming 2,000 calories a day. This is similar to the US guidelines which recommend no more than 25 g for women and 38 g for men (Johnson *et al.*, 2009). To put that into perspective, one 330 ml can of coke contains 35 g of sugar while a Kit Kat contains 23 g of sugar.

The GDA that appears on food labels is 120 g for men and 90 g for women, but these figures are confusing as they include both naturally occurring (e.g. fruit and milk) and added sugars. Some scientists believe the GDA is set too high (Malhotra, 2013).

drinks you are effectively bathing your teeth in sugar for prolonged periods. Gels and energy bars can be particularly damaging due to the sticky nature of these products.

Another problem is that sugar makes food and drink more palatable and therefore easy to over-consume. Although sugar is not uniquely fattening, it can contribute towards an overconsumption of calories, especially when combined with lots of fat in the form of cakes, chocolates, biscuits and snacks. Rather than satisfy hunger, sugar can sometimes make us want to eat more! Although high intakes have been linked with obesity and type 2 diabetes, the main contributor to these diseases is excess calories rather than sugar itself.

On balance, athletes and regular exercisers need not be over-concerned about sugar. Small amounts are unlikely to do you any harm and provided you time your sugar intake around exercise, it may even aid your performance. Ideally, opt for sources that also provide other nutrients, for example bananas and other fruit. While fruit juice and smoothies contain more vitamins, they contain a similar amount of sugar to soft drinks (around 10 g/100 ml), which is rapidly absorbed, meaning they are not necessarily a healthier option. Here are some general rules:

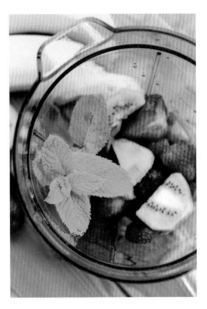

- During training sessions lasting more than 60 minutes, consuming squash, diluted fruit juice and sports drinks, bananas, dried fruit or cereal bars will help fuel tiring muscles and improve your endurance.

- After intense exercise lasting more than 60 minutes, you'll need carbohydrate to re-stock your glycogen, so sugar in flavoured milk, yoghurt, milkshakes or bars can be useful.

- At other times, if you want something sweet, opt for foods that contain fibre (to mitigate the rise in blood glucose) and other nutrients: fresh fruit, dried fruit, yoghurt, dried fruit and nut bars, or granola bars.

- Drink water or milk as a rule, although other unsweetened drinks such as tea and coffee also count towards hydration.

Simple or complex carbohydrate?

Carbohydrates are traditionally classified as simple (mono- or disaccharides) or complex (polysaccharides) according to the number of sugar units in the molecules. But this tells you very little about their effect on your body and your blood glucose level. Nowadays, carbohydrate are more commonly categorised according to their glycaemic index (GI).

What is the glycaemic index (GI)?

The GI was developed by David Jenkins in 1982. He discovered that, contrary to popular belief, many starchy foods affected blood glucose levels quite dramatically, while some sugary foods had little effect.

The GI is a ranking of foods from 0 to 100 based on their immediate effect on blood sugar levels. It's a measure of how quickly the food turns into glucose in the bloodstream. To make a fair comparison, all foods are ranked against a reference food, normally glucose, and are tested in equivalent carbohydrate amounts. Glucose has a GI score of 100.

High-GI foods cause a rapid rise in blood glucose levels and have a GI number above 70 (glucose has the highest score at 100). They include starchy foods such as potatoes, cornflakes, white bread and white rice as well as sugary foods such as soft drinks, biscuits and sweets.

Foods classed as low-GI foods fall below 55 and produce a slower and smaller rise in blood glucose levels. They include beans, lentils, coarse-grain breads, muesli, fruit and dairy products. Moderate-GI foods such as porridge, rice and sweet potatoes have a GI between 55 and 70.

Protein-rich foods such as meat, fish, chicken and eggs and pure fats such as oils, butter and margarine contain no carbohydrate so these foods have no GI value. But adding these foods to meals will slow the digestion and absorption of carbohydrate from the gut, and thus reduce the GI of the entire meal. Cooking and ripening (of fruits) tends to increase the GI value.

So which carbohydrate when?

You can use the GI value of foods to help you plan what to eat and drink around your training session or competition. In general, high-GI foods and drinks are useful during moderate- to high-intensity exercise lasting longer than an hour. As they are digested rapidly, they help maintain blood glucose levels and provide readily available fuel for your muscles. Similarly, after exercise, high-GI foods and drinks will help restore muscle glycogen stores faster, particularly when combined with protein in a ratio of approximately 3 to 1 (*see* page 49). Before exercise, it is best to consume a low-GI meal about 2–4 hours beforehand as this will provide a more sustained rise in blood glucose. Alternatively, a high-GI snack consumed about 30 minutes before exercise will help maintain blood glucose longer during your workout (there's more about this in Chapter 2).

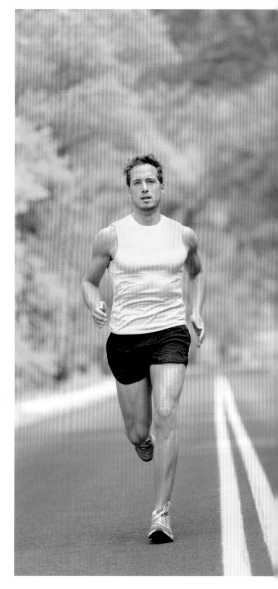

In a nutshell:

Focus on low- or moderate-GI foods for your day-to-day meals. These help regulate blood glucose and insulin levels, promote glycogen recovery between training sessions, keep your energy levels constant, and also lower your risk of developing type 2 diabetes, obesity and cardiovascular disease (all of which are associated with high insulin levels). If you want to eat high-GI foods, eat them with fats and protein to lower the GI of the meal.

Eat high-GI foods or drinks immediately before, during (if exercising for more than an hour) and immediately after training. These help raise blood glucose quickly so can help increase endurance and speed recovery.

Table 1.4 provides a quick guide to foods with a high, moderate and low GI.

TABLE 1.4 THE GLYCAEMIC INDEX (GI) OF FOODS

Low GI (< 55)					
Peanuts	14	Spaghetti	38	Carrots	47
Fructose	19	Apples	38	Bulgur wheat	48
Cherries	22	Tinned peaches (in fruit juice)	39	Peas	48
Grapefruit	25	Pear	38	Baked beans	48
Lentils (red)	26	Yoghurt drink	38	Muesli	49
Whole milk	27	Protein bar	38	Boiled potato	50
Chick peas	28	Plum	39	Rye bread	50
Red kidney beans	28	Apple juice	40	Mango	51
Lentils (green/brown)	30	Strawberries	40	Strawberry jam	51
Butter beans	31	All-Bran	42	Banana	52
Apricot (dried)	31	Orange	42	Orange juice	52
Meal replacement bar	31	Peach	42	Kiwi fruit	53
Skimmed milk	32	Milk chocoate	43	Buckwheat	54
Protein shake	32	Muffin, apple	44	Sweetcorn	54
Fruit yoghurt , fruit (low-fat)	32	Sponge cake	46	Crisps	54
Chocolate milk	34	Grapes	46	Muesli (Alpen)	55
Custard	35	Pineapple juice	46	Honey	55
Plain low-fat yoghurt	36	Macaroni	47	Brown rice	55
Moderate GI (56–69)					
Potato – boiled, old	56	Apricots	57	Digestive biscuits	59
Sultanas	56	Porridge	58	Pineapple	59
Energy bar	56	Basmatic rice	58	Pizza	60
Pitta bread	57	Squash (diluted)	58	Ice cream	61

Sweet potato	61	Raisins	64	Croissant	67
Muesli bar	61	Couscous	65	Sucrose	68
Tortillas/corn chips	63	Cantaloupe melon	65	Weetabix	74
White rice	64	Mars bar	65	Shredded wheat	75
Shortbread	64	Instant porridge	66		

High GI (>70)

White bread	70	Cheerios	74	Cornflakes	81
Millet	71	Bran flakes	74	Rice Krispies	82
Wholemeal bread	71	Mashed potato	74	Baked potato	85
Bagel	72	Chips	75	French baguette	95
Breakfast cereal bar (crunchy nut cornflakes)	72	Rice cakes	78	Lucozade	95
Watermelon	72	Gatorade	78		

Source: Adapted with permission from the *American Journal of Clinical Nutrition,* © *Am J Clin Nutr American Society for Nutrition (Foster-Powell et al., 2002).*

What is the glycaemic load?

While GI is a very useful concept, it's not the sole predictor of the effects of eating a particular food. That is because blood glucose response is also determined by the amount of food eaten. The glycaemic load (GL) gives you a more accurate idea of how a food behaves in your body. Unlike GI, it takes account of the portion size (i.e. the number of carbohydrate you are eating), so can be regarded as a measure of both the quantity and quality of the carbohydrate.

It is calculated as follows:

GL = (GI x carbohydrate per portion) ÷ 100

One unit of GL is roughly equivalent to the glycaemic effect of 1 g of glucose.

An example for watermelon:

GL = (72 × 6) x 100 = 4.3

	GI value	GL value	Daily GL total
Low	0–55	0–10	0–80
Medium	56–70	11–19	80–120
High	71–100	> 20	>120

For optimal glycogen storage and minimal fat storage, aim to achieve a small or moderate glycaemic load – eat little and often, avoid overloading on carbohydrate, and stick to balanced combinations of carbohydrate, protein and fat.

LOW-GI EATING AT A GLANCE

Essentially, a low-GI diet comprises balanced amounts of carbohydrate with a low GI as well as lean protein and fats. Low-GI foods include:

Fresh fruit

The more acidic the fruit, the lower the GI. Apples, pears, oranges, grapefruit, peaches, nectarines, plums and apricots have the lowest GI values while tropical fruits such as pineapple, papaya and watermelon have higher values. However, as average portion size is small, the GL (*see* page 15) would be low.

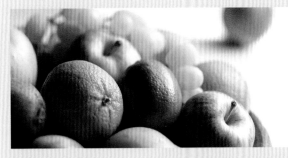

Fresh vegetables

Most vegetables have a very low carbohydrate content and don't have a GI value (you would need to eat enormous amounts to get a significant rise in blood glucose). The exception is potatoes, which have a high GI. For a lower-GI meal, eat them with protein and/or fat, e.g. with butter and beans, cheese or tuna.

Low-GI starchy vegetables

These include sweetcorn (GI 46–48), sweet potato (GI 46), and yam (GI 37).

Low-GI breads

These include stoneground wholemeal bread (not ordinary wholemeal bread), fruit or malt loaf, wholegrain bread with lots of grainy bits, breads containing barley, rye, oats, soy and cracked wheat or those containing sunflower seeds or linseeds, chapati and pitta breads (unleavened), pumpernickel (rye kernel) bread, and sourdough bread.

Low-GI breakfast cereals

These include porridge, muesli and other oat- or rye-based cereals, and high-bran cereals (e.g. All-Bran).

Low-GI grains

These include bulgur wheat, noodles, oats, pasta, basmati rice (not ordinary brown or white rice).

Low-GI beans and lentils

These include chickpeas, red kidney beans, baked beans, cannellini beans, mung beans, black-eyed beans, butter beans, split peas and lentils.

Low-GI nuts and seeds

Nuts include almonds, brazils, cashews, hazelnuts, pine nuts, pistachios and peanuts. Seeds include sunflower, sesame, flax and pumpkin seeds.

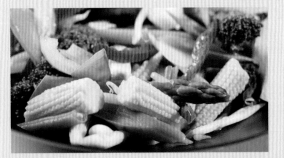

Fish, lean meat, poultry and eggs

These contain no carbohydrate and have no GI value.

Low-fat dairy products

Milk, cheese and yoghurt are important for their calcium and protein content. Opt for lower-fat versions where possible.

Which is best – GI or GL?

A major problem with the GI is that it doesn't take account of portion size, and so it can create a falsely bad impression of a food. For example, watermelon with a GI of 72 – classified as a high-GI food – is off the menu on a low-GI diet. However, an average slice (120 g/4.2 oz) provides only 6 g of carbohydrate – not enough to raise your blood glucose level significantly. You would need to eat 720 g of watermelon to obtain 50 g of carbohydrate – the amount used in the GI test.

Another drawback is that some high-fat foods have a low GI, which gives it a falsely favourable impression. For example, crisps have a lower GI (54) than baked potatoes (85). But they are easy to over-eat because they are not very filling.

Can GI help weight loss?

Foods with a low GI are generally more nutritious than higher-GI foods, but to lose weight you still have to consume fewer calories than you burn. In theory, a low-GI diet should be filling and satisfying because many foods with a low GI are high in fibre and take longer to digest, thus helping to curb your appetite. In practice, it's quite easy to unwittingly load up on calories. Muesli (GI 49), boiled potatoes (GI 50), spaghetti (GI 48) and sponge cake (GI 46) are all low-GI foods, but are also relatively high in calories. Even milk chocolate has low GI (43), but provides as many as 240 calories (1,004 kJ) per 45 g bar!

There have been no long-term studies, but of the short-term studies to date only about half have found that low-GI foods reduce hunger, increase satiety (feelings of fullness) or reduce overall food intake. No difference in satiety or food intake was found in the remaining half. A study published in the *American Journal of Clinical Nutrition* in 2004 found that weight loss on a low-GI diet was no different to that on a high-GI diet (Sloth, 2004). Clearly, you still have to keep a rein on portion sizes and reduce carbohydrate.

3. Fibre

Why do you need fibre?

Fibre is the term used to describe the complex carbohydrate found in plants that are resistant to digestion. There are two kinds of fibre – insoluble and soluble. Most plant foods contain both, but proportions vary. Good sources of insoluble fibre include whole grains, such as wholegrain bread, pasta and rice and vegetables. These help to speed the passage of food through your gut, and prevent constipation and bowel problems. Soluble fibre, found in oats, beans, lentils, nuts, fruit and vegetables, reduces LDL cholesterol levels and helps control blood glucose levels by slowing glucose absorption. High-fibre foods are beneficial for weight loss as they fill you up and promote satiety.

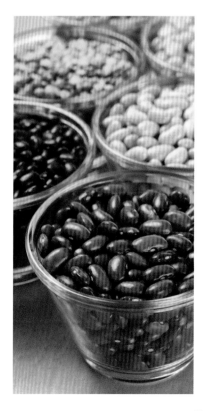

BENEFITS OF A HIGH-FIBRE DIET

✔ **Helps maintain bowel health**

A high-fibre diet may lower your risk of developing haemorrhoids and small pouches in your colon (diverticular disease) and also bowel cancer. Low-fibre intakes can lead to slow transit times (the time taken for food to pass through the gut) and often result in constipation.

✔ **Lowers cholesterol levels**

Soluble fibre found in beans, lentils, oats, fruit and vegetables may help lower total and LDL blood cholesterol levels. Studies have also shown that fibre may have other heart-health benefits, such as reducing blood pressure and inflammation.

✔ **Helps control blood sugar levels**

Fibre, particularly soluble fibre, can slow the absorption of glucose and help improve blood glucose control. A healthy diet that includes insoluble fibre may also reduce the risk of developing type 2 diabetes.

✔ **Helps weight control**

Fibre-rich foods are especially beneficial for weight control as they are more filling and take longer to digest in your stomach. A study of almost 3,000 adults in the USA showed that over ten years the people eating the most fibre gained less weight than those with the lowest intake of fibre. Fibre also increases a food's 'chewing time' so that your body has time to register that you are no longer hungry. This will make you less likely to over-eat and help you feel full for longer.

✔ **Reduces cancer risk**

In countries with traditionally high-fibre diets, diseases such as bowel cancer, diabetes and coronary heart disease are much less common than in the West. However, scientists are unclear as to whether these benefits are due to fibre itself or to other nutrients found naturally in fibre-rich foods. The European Prospective Investigation into Cancer and Nutrition (EPIC) study of 519, 978 individuals, recruited from ten European countries, found that in populations with low average intake of dietary fibre, an approximate doubling of total fibre intake from foods could reduce the risk of colorectal cancer by 40 per cent.

How much do you need?

The UK Scientific Advisory Committee recommends 30g of fibre a day. The average intake in the UK is around 18g/ day, which is considerably less than the recommended level. This can be achieved by including more wholegrains, fruit, vegetables, beans and lentils.

4. Protein

Protein is made up of amino acids joined together in a chain. The body makes some of these amino acids; however, there are some that it cannot make and that therefore need to be consumed in the diet. These are called essential amino acids, of which there are nine (there are 20 in total).

Why do I need protein?

Protein is a structural component of the body needed for growth, formation and repair of all body cells, including muscle, bone, skin, hair and organs. It is also needed for making enzymes, hormones and antibodies. Along with this, the body can also use protein as a fuel.

How much protein do I need?

The Recommended Daily Amount (RDA) for the general population is 0.75 g/kg of body weight a day. For example, for a 70 kg person the amount would be 53 g.

Regular exercisers need more protein than inactive people – around 50 to 100 per cent more than the dietary guidelines for the general public – to repair damaged muscle cells after intense exercise, as well as to build new muscle cells. You'll need 1.3–1.8 g of protein/kg of body weight daily, depending on your sport and how hard and how long you train (Phillips and Van Loon, 2011; Rodriques *et al.*, 2009; Phillips, 2007). If you do mostly endurance activities, such as running, aim to consume 1.2–1.4 g protein/kg of body weight a day. That's 84–98 g daily for a 70 kg person. If you include regular strength and power activities such as weight training in your programme, aim for 1.4–1.8 g/kg of body weight a day. This is 98–126 g daily for a 70 kg person.

Adolescent athletes will need extra protein to account for growth and development as well as the exercise-related requirement. Scientists estimate that they need around 1.2–1.4 g/kg of body weight (Boisseau *et al.*, 2007). That's 72–84 g for a 60 kg athlete.

What happens if you get too little or too much protein?

Skimping on protein occasionally isn't a problem as the body can adapt to low intakes in the short term by recycling amino acids (rather than excreting them). But, in the long term, eating too little protein can cause fatigue and slow recovery after workouts. It can also result in a loss of muscle tissue and strength.

Consuming more protein than you need is unlikely to be a problem provided it isn't excessive. Excess protein is broken down and partly excreted (in the form of urea) and the rest of the molecule used as a fuel source. Contrary to popular belief, excess protein isn't harmful. It doesn't cause liver or kidney damage in healthy people, nor does it cause dehydration or bone mineral loss. On the other hand, extra protein won't give you any performance benefits either. Studies have demonstrated that eating more than you need for daily repair does not result in additional muscle growth, strength, stamina or speed.

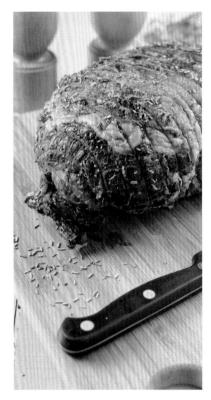

Does protein help with appetite control?

Protein plays an important role in appetite control. It is more satiating than carbohydrate or fat, so is particularly important for those wishing to lose or maintain weight without sacrificing muscle. When you consume protein, gut hormones are released that signal to the appetite control centre in the brain that you are satiated, so you stop eating. Also, specific amino acids from the breakdown of protein (namely, leucine) acts on the hypothalamus region of the brain to reduce hunger (Davidenko *et al.*, 2013).

Studies have shown that consuming a high-protein breakfast improves appetite control and stops food cravings later in the day (Leidy *et al.*, 2011). In one UK study, those who ate eggs for breakfast felt more satisfied and went on to eat fewer calories in the day than those who ate a high-carbohydrate breakfast of cereal or croissants (Fallaize *et al.*, 2012).

In practice, you should include around 20 g protein in each meal, equivalent to about 85–100 g meat or fish or 600 ml milk (Rodrigues *et al.*, 2009). Eating a carbohydrate-rich meal lacking in protein (e.g. a jam sandwich) means you will feel hungry soon after eating. Avoid this by adding some protein (e.g. eggs, meat or cheese) and reducing your carbohydrate portion (e.g. bread).

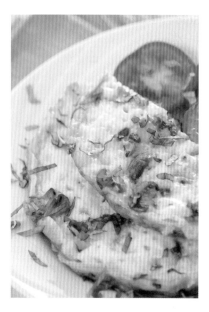

How should I get my daily protein needs?

Different protein sources come with other nutrients (e.g. milk gives you calcium and oily fish gives you omega-3s) so it is a good idea to eat a mix of foods high in protein. That way you will get a good balance of amino acids as well as a wider range of other nutrients such as fibre, vitamins, minerals and carbohydrate. Table 1.5 (overleaf) gives the protein content of various foods, but you can also get an idea of your protein intake by checking the labels of foods or using the free online database: http://www.food-database.co.uk/ for the amounts of protein in foods.

Animal sources such as poultry, fish, meat, dairy products and eggs generally have a higher biological value (BV) than plant sources such as tofu, Quorn™, beans, lentils, nuts and cereals. That is, they contain higher levels of amino acids in a form that is readily digested.

When should I have protein?

You should distribute your protein intake evenly throughout the day, aiming to have about 20g of protein in one sitting. Your body can only fully utilise a limited amount at a time, so avoid eating excessive amounts in one meal. It will still get absorbed but won't necessarily increase muscle synthesis.

Studies suggest that consuming 20 g protein immediately after exercise will maximise muscle repair and promote a more anabolic hormonal environment. The type of protein eaten after exercise is important – proteins that contain all 9 essential amino acids (such as milk) are considered optimal for recovery.

TABLE 1.5 THE PROTEIN CONTENT OF VARIOUS FOODS

Food	Protein (g)	Food	Protein (g)
Meat and fish		**Beans and lentils**	
Beef sirloin steak (85 g)	21 g	Baked beans (200 g)	10 g
Chicken or turkey breast (125 g)	36 g	Lentils (150 g cooked)	13 g
Fish, e.g. salmon or haddock	30 g	Red kidney beans (150 g, cooked)	10 g
fillet (150 g)	24 g	Chickpeas (150 g, cooked)	11 g
Tuna, canned in brine (100 g)		**Soya and Quorn™ products**	
Dairy products		Soy milk (600 ml)	20 g
1 slice (40 g) Cheddar cheese	10 g	Tofu burger (60 g)	5 g
600 ml milk	21 g	Quorn™ burger (50 g)	6 g
Low-fat plain yoghurt (150 g)	7 g	**Grains and cereals**	
Greek plain yoghurt (150 g)	10 g	Wholemeal bread (2 slices, 80 g)	7 g
3 eggs (size 3)	21 g	Wholegrain rice (180 g, cooked)	5 g
Nuts and seeds		Wholegrain spaghetti (180 g, cooked)	9 g
Peanuts (50 g)	12 g	Quinoa (180 g, uncooked)	8 g
Cashews (50 g)	9 g	**Protein supplements**	
Almonds (50 g)	11 g	Whey protein powder (25 g)	20 g*
Peanut butter (20 g)	5 g	Meal replacement powder (25 g)	13 g*
Pumpkin seeds (25 g)	6 g	1 nutrition (sports) bar (60 g)	21 g*

*Values may vary depending on brand

Amino acids in protein explained

Proteins are made up of 20 amino acids, of which 9 are 'essential', meaning they can't be made by the body, so must be provided by the food and drink you consume. The 9 essential amino acids that your body can't make itself are:

- Histidine
- Isoleucine
- Leucine
- Lysine
- Methionine
- Phenylalanine
- Threonine
- Tryptophan
- Valine

All 9 of these essential amino acids have to be present for your body to use food proteins properly. Animal protein sources, as well as soya, contain a good balance of these essential amino acids. But not all proteins are equal – some don't have enough of all the essential amino acids to satisfy your body's needs. These include plant proteins such as beans, lentils, grains and nuts. The general rule is to combine plant proteins to make a full complement of amino acids (e.g. beans on toast, lentils and rice, peanut butter with bread). The 'non-essential amino acids' are listed below. They are made by the body from essential amino acids or in the normal breakdown of proteins:

- Alanine
- Glutamic acid
- Cysteine
- Proline
- Asparagine
- Serine
- Glutamine
- Tyrosine
- Aspartic acid
- Arginine
- Glycine

5. Fat

Why do you need fat?

Fat is not only a fuel for the body, but is also crucial for health. It is made up of fatty acids, which are essential components of every membrane of every cell in your body. Without fatty acids, membranes would not function properly. Fat is also needed to absorb and transport the fat-soluble vitamins A, D, E and K in the bloodstream, and is a source of the essential omega-3 and omega-6 polyunsaturated fatty acids.

Fat itself may be high in calories, but that doesn't mean it's more likely to make you fat. In fact, quite the opposite is true. Fat is satiating, which means it gives the body the feeling of being full and therefore satisfies your appetite. By contrast, reduced-fat and low-fat foods are more likely to be fattening as these foods are not satiating. Without fat (and fibre) in the mix, you are left hungry soon after eating, seek out more food, thus setting up a vicious cycle of over-eating.

How much fat?

The IOC makes no specific recommendations for fat although the ACSM suggests athletes follow the fat guidelines for the general population (20–35 per cent of energy). Since the publication of the 3rd edition of this book, new evidence about fat, obesity and health has emerged and previous advice to limit dietary fat is less certain. UK national dietary guidelines were first issued in 1984 by the Department of Health, based on studies (namely Ancel Keys's Seven Countries study) that suggested heart disease was caused by eating too much fat (Keys, 1980). Since then the link between total fat and heart disease has been proven to be weak. Diets containing moderate amounts of fat (such as the traditional

THE IMPORTANCE OF FAT

- Essential for cell membrane functionality
- Plays a crucial role in the absorption and transportation of essential vitamins
- Eaten with fibre, it helps you stay fuller for longer

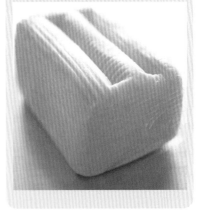

Mediterranean diet) may be more effective than low fat diets for protecting against heart disease, stroke and type 2 diabetes (Estruch et al, 2013). In fact, researchers today generally don't think the total amount of fat you eat has much effect on obesity and heart health. Instead it's the **type** of fat you eat that matters. Artificial trans fats appear to raise cardiovascular risk whereas unsaturated fats lower the risk. Saturated fats fall somewhere in between.

Does fat make you fat?

Despite a reduction in population fat intakes over the past 30 years, obesity has risen 10-fold and in 2011 (the last available figures at the time of publication) was 26 per cent for women and 24 per cent for men. The proportion of people either obese or overweight was 58 per cent for women and 65 per cent for men. Similarly, type 2 diabetes rates have risen dramatically from 800,000 in 1980 to 3 million in 2013.

So why have obesity and diabetes rates been rising? It's unlikely to be due to people eating more fat as intakes have fallen slightly. It's more likely to be due to an increase in total calorie intake as well as declining activity. One of the problems is that people have been cutting fat and replacing it with highly processed refined carbohydrates. Such a diet is not satiating and can result in overconsumption of calories. Worse, eating a highcarbohydrate, low-fat diet increases blood triglyceride (fat) levels and makes a heart attack just as (or more) likely as eating a highfat diet (Astrup *et al.*, 2010; Volek and Forsythe, 2005).

The different types of fats

When we refer to saturated, monounsaturated or poly-unsaturated fats, we're referring to the number of double bonds in the fatty acid molecules:

- Saturated fats contain no double bonds.
- Monounsaturated fats contain one double bond.
- Polyunsaturated fats contain two or more double bonds.

TRAIN LOW, COMPETE HIGH

Sports scientists first developed the 'train low, compete high' protocol in 2005 for athletes looking for a performance edge. The idea is that doing some of your training sessions with low glycogen stores teaches the body to become a better fat-burning machine. Over time, 'training low' increases the number of mitochondria and fat-burning enzymes in your muscle cells, allowing you to burn more fat and less carbohydrate. Theoretically, this should improve your endurance and, ultimately, your performance.

The problem is that training with low glycogen stores for a long period can hamper the muscles' ability to use carbohydrate during high intensity exercise, which would be a disadvantage for most competitive events! (Burke, 2010). At race-pace you need carbohydrate. While a LCHF diet may increase the muscles' adaptive response and reduce the reliance on carbohydrate during exercise there is no clear evidence that this strategy enhances performance.

Some elite athletes are experimenting with a newer strategy called 'carbohydrate periodisation'; performing low-intensity sessions with low glycogen stores, and high-intensity sessions with high glycogen stores. The idea is that matching your carbohydrate intake to your training sessions, improves your 'metabolic flexibility' i.e., your muscles' ability to switch between burning fat and carbohydrate, as well as your body composition and performance.

Saturated fats

Saturated fats are found in all fats, but higher amounts are present in animal fats and products made with palm oil or palm kernel oil. Main sources include:

- Meat
- Butter
- Coconut oil
- Palm oil and palm kernel oil ('vegetable fat')
- Milk, cheese and yoghurt
- Lard
- Egg yolks
- Margarine, spreads, biscuits, cakes, desserts, . etc. made with palm or palm kernel oil

Does saturated fat cause heart disease?

The idea that saturated fat was bad for you first began in the 1950s, when scientists thought that this type of fat raised levels of LDL (low-density lipoproteins) ('bad') cholesterol, which in turn caused atherosclerosis and heart disease. Since then, new studies have shown that the link between saturated fat and heart disease risk is not as clear cut as once thought (Chowdhury et al, 2014; de Oliveira Otto *et al.*, 2012; German *et al.*, 2009). While it is true that saturated fat increases blood cholesterol levels, scientists are not certain how this affects cardiovascular risk. Some studies show that saturated fats increase the risk, while others do not.

The current consensus is that you should replace some of the saturated fat in your diet with unsaturated fat. These healthy fats raise HDL and lower LDL levels. They also improve the ratio of total cholesterol to 'good' HDL cholesterol, lowering the risk of cardiovascular disease. A 2012 review of studies from the Cochrane Collaboration found that people who did this for at least two years reduced their risk of heart attacks, angina and stroke by 14 per cent (Hooper *et al.*, 2012). In practice, this means trimming the fat from meat, eating less processed meat (such as sausages, bacon and salami), and cutting out fatty processed foods (such as biscuits, cakes, pastries and pies). But you don't have to eliminate saturated fats from your diet completely. New research suggests that the saturated fats found in dairy products, butter, meat and eggs not only raise LDL cholesterol but they also raise levels of 'good' HDL (highdensity lipoproteins) cholesterol, so the overall effect on cardiovascular disease risk is neutral (Mensink, 2003; Toth, 2005).

THE ROLE OF SATURATED FATS

- Structure and functioning of cell membranes
- Source of energy for the heart
- Helps the bones take up calcium
- Protects the liver from the effects of alcohol
- Surfactant in lungs (protects from asthma) composed of saturated fatty acids
- Signalling messengers for hormone manufacture
- Proper functioning of the immune system

LDL AND HDL CHOLESTEROL EXPLAINED

Around 70 per cent of the cholesterol in your blood is carried on low *density lipoproteins (LDL)*. These carry cholesterol from the liver to body cells, where the cells take as much cholesterol as they need. There are two types of LDL:

- Small dense LDL that sticks to arteries and causes atherosclerosis (narrowing of the arteries)
- Large LDL, which is harmless and does not cause atherosclerosis

Saturated fats only raise the large LDL, not the small LDL, which means that they do not raise heart disease risk. It is the trans fats (see below) that increase the harmful small LDL. The remaining cholesterol in your blood is carried on *high density lipoproteins (HDL)*. This 'good' HDL picks up and removes excess cholesterol back to the liver for elimination from the body.

Trans fats

Trans fats are the harmful fats. Although tiny amounts occur naturally in meat and dairy products, most are formed artificially during the commercial process of hydrogenation when vegetable oils are converted into hardened hydrogenated fats. Hydrogen gas is pumped under very high pressure into polyunsaturated vegetable oil, which straightens out the fatty acid molecules and packs them closer together, making them hard like lard.

Nowadays trans fats are found in fewer foods but are still used in some takeaway and fast foods and by some manufacturers to make pastries and biscuits crispy, cakes moist and fillings creamy, and many processed foods last longer. However they increase blood levels of the small LDL cholesterol ('harmful' cholesterol) while lowering HDL ('good') cholesterol, which increases your risk of heart disease. They may also encourage fat deposition around your middle and increase the risk of diabetes (Ascherio and Willett, 1997; Mensink and Katan, 1990; Lopez-Garcia *et al.*, 2005).

How much trans fat is safe?

The World Health Organization (WHO) recommend an intake less than 1 per cent of energy, and the UK Department of Health recommends no more than 2 per cent – roughly 5 g/day. As trans fats are found naturally in meat and milk fat, a zero intake would be impractical. The food industry has voluntarily reduced the use of hydrogenated fats and so current average intakes are below the UK recommendation. It is still worth checking food labels for hydrogenated and partially hydrogenated fat as they may be found in some (not all) fast foods and takeaways, pies, pastries and bakery items, margarines, cereal bars and chocolate.

Monounsaturated fats

Monounsaturated fats lower harmful LDL cholesterol levels without affecting 'good' HDL and can cut your heart disease and cancer risk. Main sources include:

- Olive oil
- Rapeseed oil
- Avocados
- Nuts
- Peanut butter
- Seeds
- Mayonnaise made with olive oil

BUTTER VS. MARGARINE

For a long time butter was a no-no as it was believed to increase your risk of heart disease, while margarine was thought to be the healthier option. But now the thinking has reversed and butter may, in fact, be better for you than many margarines. For a start, it's an all-natural product as it's made from cream, whereas margarine is artificial, being made from refined oils and additives. Secondly, the saturated fats in butter aren't quite as bad for the heart as once thought.

But that doesn't mean you should start **adding** butter to your diet. Butter is still high in calories so keep portions small. Olive and rapeseed oils are healthier options than butter as they lower LDL and raise HDL cholesterol.

Spreads made with olive oil are perhaps a healthier option as they contain high levels of heart-healthy monounsaturated fats. As a bonus, they're also slightly lower in calories and fat than butter or margarine.

Eating a diet that is moderate in total fat but rich in monounsaturated fats (such as the traditional Mediterranean diet) is thought to be healthier than low-fat diets, reducing the risk of heart disease and stroke. For example, a large-scale clinical trial (the PREDIMED study) found that those eating a Mediterranean-style diet that included large amounts of olive oil or nuts cut their risk of suffering a heart attack or stroke by 30 per cent compared with those following a conventional low-fat diet (Estruch *et al.*, 2013).

Polyunsaturated fats

Main sources of polyunsaturated fats include vegetable and seed oils:

- Sunflower oil
- Corn oil
- Safflower oil
- Sunflower oil margarine
- Nuts and seeds

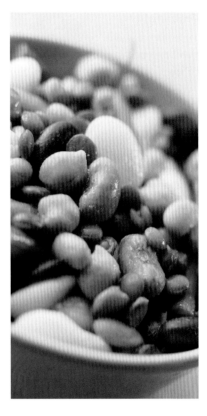

Two types of polyunsaturated fats – the omega-3 and omega-6 fatty acids – are called essential fatty acids, meaning that you need them in your diet because the body cannot produce them. Both are extremely important for maintaining the correct structure of cell membranes in the body.

Omega-3 fats

Omega-3 fatty acids include the short-chain fatty acid alpha-linolenic acid (ALA) found in plant sources (such as walnuts and rapeseed oil), and the long-chain fatty acids eicosapentanoic acid (EPA) and docosahexanoic acid (DHA), both found only in fish oils. Once consumed, the body converts ALA (albeit not very efficiently) to EPA and DHA, the two kinds of omega-3 fatty acids that can be more readily harnessed and used by the body.

They are necessary for proper functioning of the brain, regulating hormones, for the immune system and blood flow. Omega-3 fatty acids protect against heart disease and stroke and, according to recent research, may also help improve brain function, prevent Alzheimer's disease, treat depression, and help improve the behaviour of children with dyslexia, dyspraxia and ADHD. For regular exercisers, omega-3s increase the delivery of oxygen to muscles, and improve aerobic capacity and endurance. They also help to speed up recovery and reduce inflammation and joint stiffness.

You only need small amounts of omega-3 fatty acids to keep yourself healthy. Recommended intakes vary, but the UK government recommends 450–900 mg of the long-chain EPA and DHA per day, which can be met with one portion (140 g) of oily fish per week or 1 tbsp daily of an omega-3-rich oil. (The omega-3 content of various foods is shown in Table 1.6.)

Main sources include:

- Oily fish, such as sardines, mackerel, salmon, fresh (not tinned) tuna, trout, herring
- Walnuts and walnut oil
- Pumpkin seeds and pumpkin seed oil
- Flaxseeds and flaxseed oil
- Dark green leafy vegetables
- Rapeseed oil
- Omega-3-enriched eggs

Omega-6 fats

Omega-6 fatty acids include linolenic acid and gamma linolenic acid (GLA) and are more widely found in foods than omega-3s. For this reason, most people currently eat too much omega-6 in relation to omega-3, which results in an imbalance of prostaglandins (hormone-like chemicals responsible for controlling blood clotting, inflammation and the immune system). It is thought that the average diet used to contain a ratio of 1 to 1, but over the last 100 years or so this has increased to 10 to1 or even 20 to 1 due to an increased intake of processed foods.

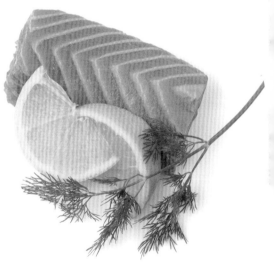

Excessive levels of omega-6 (or a deficiency of omega-3) can lead to a pro-inflammatory state, which has been linked to a number of conditions including cardiovascular disease, arthritis, stroke and cancer. Inflammation is the body's natural response to injury and infection and should be a temporary self-protection response. However, it can become a chronic condition and is thought to be an underlying factor in many diseases.

Omega-6 EFAs are generally pro-inflammatory while Omega-3 EFAs are generally anti-inflammatory in nature, but it's the overall balance or ratio of these fatty acids that's important. In other words, a lower ratio of omega-6 to omega-3 is beneficial, as it can decrease the risk of a number of health conditions.

Recommended intakes are still up for debate, but because omega-6 is abundant in most people's diets, getting enough isn't a problem. In fact, most of us get more than we need.

Sources include most vegetables oils, margarine and products containing them:

- Soya oil
- Corn oil
- Safflower oil
- Sunflower oil
- Peanut or groundnut oil
- Sesame oil

How can I get the balance right between omega-3 and omega-6?
To help redress the balance, limit your intake of processed and deep-fried foods, and use oils that are rich in monounsaturated fats, such as olive oil and rapeseed oil instead of omega-6-rich vegetable and seed oils such as corn oil and sunflower oil.

Aim for one portion of oily fish per week, include omega-3-enriched eggs, or try a fish oil supplement. Studies have also suggested that animal products from grass-fed animals are richer in omega-3 than those from grain-fed animals, so buying free-range or grass-fed animal products may be beneficial.

Which fats are best for cooking?

It is best to avoid polyunsaturated oils (such as corn and sunflower oils) for frying or cooking as they are unstable at high temperatures, which means they can oxidise (i.e. react with oxygen to form free radicals) and produce harmful chemicals called aldehydes. Opt instead for light (non-extra virgin) olive oil and rapeseed oil, which are rich in monounsaturated fats and thus more stable. Coconut oil has become increasingly popular due to it's potential to raise levels of HDL cholesterol. However, it is very high in saturated fat (90%), which means it also raises levels of LDL cholesterol. Thus, its overall effect on heart health is not known.

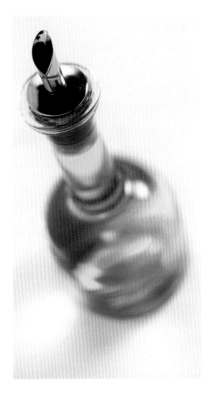

TABLE 1.6 SOURCES OF OMEGA-3 FATTY ACIDS

Food	Omega-3 fatty acids: g/100 g	Portion size	Omega-3 fatty acids: g/portion
Salmon	2.5 g	100 g	2.5 g
Mackerel	2.8 g	160 g	4.5 g
Sardines, tinned	2.0 g	100 g	2.0 g
Trout	1.3 g	230 g	2.9 g
Tuna, canned in oil, drained	1.1 g	100 g	1.1 g
Cod liver oil	24 g	1 tsp (5 ml)	1.2 g
Flaxseed oil	57 g	1 tbsp (15 ml)	8.0 g
Flaxseeds, ground	16 g	1 tbsp (24 g)	3.8 g
Rapeseed oil	9.6 g	1 tbsp (15 ml)	1.3 g
Walnuts	7.5 g	1 tbsp (28 g)	2.6 g
Walnut oil	11.5 g	1 tbsp (15 ml)	1.6 g

Peanuts	0.4 g	Handful (50 g)	0.2 g
Broccoli	1.3 g	3 tbsp (125 g)	1.3 g
Pumpkin seeds	8.5 g	2 tbsp (25 g)	2.1 g
Omega-3 eggs		1 egg	0.7 g
Typical omega-3 supplement		8 capsules	0.5 g

6. Vitamins and minerals

Vitamins and minerals are substances that are needed in tiny amounts to enable your body to work properly and prevent illness. Getting the right balance of vitamins and minerals will also help your performance.

Vitamins support the immune system, help the brain function properly, and aid the conversion of food into energy. They are important for healthy skin and hair, controlling growth and balancing hormones. The Vitamins B and C must be provided daily by the diet, as they cannot be stored.

Minerals are needed for structural and regulatory functions, including bone strength, haemoglobin manufacture, fluid balance and muscle contraction.

How much?

Table 1.7 on pages 29–30 summarises the exercise-related functions, best food sources, and requirements of 14 key vitamins and minerals. But regular exercise places additional demands on your body, and your requirement for many vitamins and minerals is likely to be higher than the RDAs (recommended daily amount) for the general population. Failure to meet your RDAs may leave you lacking in energy and susceptible to minor infections and illnesses.

What are RDAs?

The recommended daily amounts (RDAs) listed on food and supplement labels are estimates of nutrient requirements set by the EU and designed to cover the needs of the majority of a population. The amounts are intended to prevent deficiency symptoms, allow for a little storage, as well as covering differences in needs from one person to the next. They are not targets; rather, they are guides to help you check that your body is getting a minimum amount of nutrients. They do not take into account the increased requirements for athletes or regular exercisers.

Do I need vitamin supplements?

While a healthy diet should provide all the nutrients you need, many people *don't* eat the healthiest diet so a multivitamin may be an inexpensive insurance policy.

COULD YOU BENEFIT FROM SUPPLEMENTS?

- You regularly skip meals, and therefore you are more likely to eat foods that are low in vitamins and minerals.
- You don't eat the recommended minimum five portions of fruit and vegetables daily. These foods are rich in vitamins, minerals and antioxidants.
- You have a food intolerance or allergy. It may be harder to get some of the nutrients you need.
- You are a vegan. It's more difficult (though not impossible) to get enough vitamin B12, calcium and iron from a plant-based diet.
- You are pregnant. Take a supplement containing 0.4 mg of folic acid and follow the advice of your midwife or doctor.

Q&A

Why is vitamin D good for athletes?

Vitamin D is well known for its role in bone health, but recent research suggests it may provide protection from osteoporosis, hypertension, cancer, heart disease, type 2 diabetes, asthma and several autoimmune diseases. It may also play a role in muscle metabolism and performance too. Sunlight (UVB light) is the major source but when this isn't available, then dietary sources become more important. The problem is that Vitamin D is found in relatively few foods: oily fish, eggs, butter and fortified cereals and margarine, so it is not possible to meet your requirements from diet alone. It is believed that 60 per cent of adults in the UK are deficient. Several studies suggest that vitamin D deficiency is widespread among athletes too, particularly those who train mainly indoors or get little sun exposure, or do not consume vitamin D-rich foods. According to recent studies a deficiency reduces muscle function and strength and may also increase the risk of stress fractures and illness – all of which will have a detrimental effect on your training and performance (Hamilton, 2011). One study found that athletes with higher vitamin D levels could jump higher, quicker and with greater power than those with low levels (Larson-Meyer and Willis, 2010). Another found that the vitamin increases the size of fast-twitch muscles and muscle strength (Halliday *et al.*, 2011).

How much do you need? There's no RDA in the UK, but the USA recommend intakes of 15μg/day (600IU) and the EU recommend 5 μg/day. You can get this amount from 3 eggs or ½ tsp (2.5 ml) cod liver oil, or 1 tin (100 g) sardines or ½ a tin (50 g) red salmon or 170 g tinned tuna (in oil).

HOW TO KEEP THE VITAMINS IN

- Buy locally grown produce if you can – ideally from farm shops and local markets.
- Buy British if you have a choice – imported produce is usually harvested under-ripe (before it has developed its full vitamin quota) and will have lost much of its nutritional value during its journey to your supermarket.
- Buy unblemished, undamaged fruit and vegetables.
- Prepare fruit and vegetables just before you make them into a salad or cook them. They start to lose nutrients from the moment they are chopped.
- Fruit and vegetables should be eaten unpeeled wherever possible – many vitamins and minerals are concentrated just beneath the skin.
- Use frozen food if fresh is not available as it is nutritionally similar.
- Cut fruit and vegetables into large pieces rather than small, as vitamins are lost from cut surfaces.
- Steam or boil vegetables in only the minimum amount of water.
- When boiling vegetables, add to fast-boiling water and cook as briefly as possible until they are tender-crisp, not soft and mushy. Save the cooking water for soups, stocks and sauces.
- Do not re-heat leftover cooked vegetables – they will have lost most of their nutritional value.

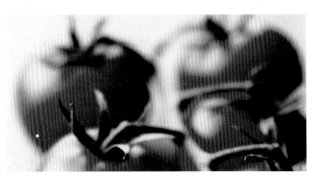

However, getting the recommended daily allowance (RDA) does not mean you are getting the optimal dose of all vitamins, e.g. there is debate about the optimal intake of vitamin D which may be much higher than the RDA.

Supplements should never be regarded as a substitute for food and are far less important for health than the healthy food pattern described in this chapter. Focus instead on eating mostly unprocessed foods: fruits, vegetables, whole grains, nuts, beans, lentils, dairy products, meat, fish and healthy oils. A study published in the *British Journal of Nutrition* reviewed the national dietary surveys in the UK, USA and Europe and concluded that most people do not get enough vitamins in their diet to protect themselves from diseases such as cancer and heart disease, and would benefit from taking a multivitamin supplement (Tresch *et al.*, 2012). The study found that many people are lacking vitamins A, C and E in their diets. As these vitamins are key antioxidant nutrients, this could mean that a large number of the UK population are vulnerable to oxidative damage which is linked to cancer, heart disease, inflammation and accelerated ageing.

Of course, more isn't better and it's important not to take more than the recommended dose. While supplements can help fill some of the gaps in a less than optimal diet, too much can be harmful. When choosing a supplement, check that the levels do not exceed the Safe Upper Limits (see Table 1.7).

WHAT ARE FREE RADICALS?

Free radicals are produced continually as a normal part of cell processes. Even though oxygen is essential for life, it can react with other compounds in the body to produce molecules called free radicals, which are highly reactive and damaging. In small numbers they are not a problem and can actually be beneficial. But excessive free radicals can cause inflammation, damage the arteries and increase the risk of thrombosis, heart disease and cancer. Free radicals are also believed to be partially responsible for post-exercise muscle soreness. The good news is that antioxidants can neutralise them. An antioxidant-rich diet may help protect against these conditions and promote faster recovery after exercise.

TABLE 1.7 A GUIDE TO VITAMINS AND MINERALS

Vitamin/mineral	How much?*	Why is it needed?	Importance for exercise	Best food sources
Vitamin A	*700 µg (men)* *600 µg (women)* *No SUL*** *FSA recommends 1,500 µg max*	*Helps vision in dim light; promotes healthy skin*	*Maintain normal vision and healthy skin*	*Liver, cheese, oily fish, eggs, butter, margarine*
Carotenoids	*No official RNI* *15 mg beta-car-otene suggested* *SUL = 7 mg*	*Vision in dim light; healthy skin; converts into vitamin A*	*As antioxidants, may protect against certain cancers, and reduce muscle soreness. Exercise increases need for antioxidants*	*Intensely coloured fruit and vegetables, e.g. apricots, peppers, tomatoes, mangoes, broccoli*

Vitamin/ mineral	How much?*	Why is it needed?	Importance for exercise	Best food sources
Thiamin	0.4 mg/ 1,000 kcal No SUL mg FSA recommends 100 mg	Converts carbohydrate to energy	To process the extra carbohydrate eaten	Wholemeal bread and cereals; pulses; meat
Riboflavin	1.3 mg (men) 1.1 mg (women) No SUL FSA recommends 40 mg	Converts carbohydrate to energy	To process the extra carbohydrate eaten	Milk and dairy products; meat; eggs
Niacin	6.6 mg/1,000 kcal SUL = 17 mg	Converts carbohydrate to energy	To process the extra carbohydrate eaten	Meat and offal; nuts; milk and dairy products; eggs; wholegrain cereals
Vitamin C	40 mg SUL = 1,000 mg	Healthy connective tissue, bones, teeth, blood vessels, gums and teeth; promotes immune function; helps iron absorption	Exercise increases need for antioxidants; may help reduce free radical damage, protect cell membranes and reduce post-exercise muscle soreness	Fruit and vegetables (e.g. raspberries, blackcurrants, kiwi, oranges, peppers, broccoli, cabbage, tomatoes)
Vitamin D	No UK RNI 5 µg in EU SUL = 50 µg	Aids calcium absorption; bone health; muscle metabolism; immune function	Needed for optimum muscle function and strength; decreases injury and illness risk	Oily fish, liver, eggs, and fortified cereals
Vitamin E	No UK RNI 10 mg in EU SUL = 540 mg	Antioxidant which helps protect against heart disease; promotes normal cell growth and development	Exercise increases need for antioxidants; may help reduce free radical damage, protect cell membranes and reduce post-exercise muscle soreness	Vegetable oils; margarine, oily fish; nuts; seeds; egg yolk; avocado
Calcium	1,000 mg (men) 700 mg (women) SUL = 1,500 mg	Builds bone and teeth; blood clotting; nerve and muscle function	Low oestrogen in female athletes with amenorrhoea, increases bone loss and need for calcium	Milk and dairy products; sardines; dark green leafy vegetables; pulses; nuts and seeds
Iron	8.7 mg (men) 14.8 mg (women) SUL = 17 mg	Formation of red blood cells; oxygen transport; prevents anaemia	Female athletes may need more to compensate for menstrual losses	Meat and offal; wholegrain cereals; fortified breakfast cereals; pulses; green leafy vegetables

Vitamin/ mineral	How much?*	Why is it needed?	Importance for exercise	Best food sources
Zinc	9.5 mg (men) 7.0 mg (women) SUL = 25 mg	Healthy immune system; wound healing; skin; cell growth	Exercise increases need for antioxidants; may help immune function	Eggs; wholegrain cereals; meat; milk and dairy products
Magnesium	300 mg (men) 270 mg (women) SUL = 400 mg	Healthy bones; muscle and nerve function; cell formation	May improve recovery after strength training; increase aerobic capacity	Cereals; fruit; vegetables; milk
Potassium	3,500 mg SUL = 3,700 mg	Fluid balance; muscle and nerve function	May help prevent cramp	Fruit; vegetables; cereals
Selenium	75 µg (men) 60 µg (women) SUL = 350 µg	Antioxidant which helps protect against heart disease and cancer	Exercise increases free radical production	Cereals; vegetables; dairy products; meat; eggs

Notes:

mg = milligrams (1,000 mg = 1 g)

µg = micrograms (1,000 µg = 1 mg)

*The amount needed is given as the Reference Nutrient Intake (RNI, Department of Health, 1991). This is the amount of a nutrient that should cover the needs of 97 per cent of the population. Athletes may need more.

**SUL = Safe Upper Limit recommended by the Expert Group on Vitamins and Minerals, an independent advisory committee to the Food Standards Agency.

7. Phytonutrients

What are they?

Phytonutrients are plant compounds that have particular health benefits. They include plant pigments, found in fruit and vegetables, and plant hormones, found in grains, beans, lentils, soya products and herbs. Many phytonutrients work as antioxidants while others influence enzymes (such as those that block cancer agents). They also:

- Fight cancer
- Reduce inflammation
- Combat free radicals
- Lower cholesterol
- Reduce heart disease risk
- Boost immunity
- Balance gut bacteria
- Fight harmful bacteria and viruses

Best sources?

There are hundreds of types of phytonutrients. To make sure you get enough of them, eat plenty of fruits and vegetables, as well as nuts, beans, lentils and whole grains, ensuring you include as wide a variety as possible. Try to consume a range of different coloured fruit and vegetables. Each colour relates to different phytonutrients in the food, every one having individual health benefits. Orange, yellow and red foods (carrots, apricots and mangoes) get their colour from beta-carotene and other carotenoids, while tomatoes and watermelon are rich in lycopene, a type of carotenoid. Carotenoids are powerful antioxidants. Green foods (broccoli, cabbage, spinach) are rich in magnesium, iron and chlorophyll. Red/purple foods (plums, cherries, red grapes, blackberries, strawberries) get their colour from anthocyanins, which are even more powerful at fighting harmful free radicals than vitamin C. White foods (apples, pears, cauliflower) contain flavanols, which protect against heart disease and cancer.

8. Antioxidants

What are they?

Antioxidant nutrients include various vitamins such as beta-carotene, vitamin C and vitamin E; minerals such as selenium; and phytonutrients. They are found mostly in fruit and vegetables, seed oils, nuts, whole grains, beans and lentils.

Intense exercise raises levels of harmful free radicals. The body generally produces higher levels of antioxidant enzymes in response to regular exercise, but additional antioxidants from food, or supplements, will help strengthen your defences.

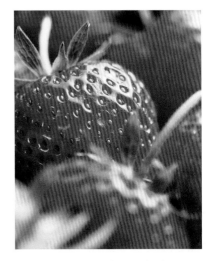

THE ANTIOXIDANT POWER OF FRUIT AND VEGETABLES

Researchers at Tuft's University in Boston, in the USA, compiled a database of 277 foods, ranked according to their ability to combat free radicals. They 'scored' each antioxidant with ORAC (Oxygen Radical Absorbance Capacity), which is a test tube analysis that measures the total antioxidant power of foods and other chemical substances. All of the foods in Table 1.8 will significantly raise the antioxidant levels in your blood – those at the top will have a greater effect than those at the bottom of the table.

TABLE 1.8 THE ANTIOXIDANT CAPACITY OF VARIOUS FOODS

Food	Serving size	Antioxidant capacity/serving size
Small red bean	½ cup dried beans	13,727
Wild blueberry	1 cup	13,427
Red kidney bean	½ cup dried beans	13,259
Pinto bean	½ cup	11,864
Blueberry	1 cup (cultivated berries)	9,019
Cranberry	1 cup (whole berries)	8,983
Artichoke hearts	1 cup, cooked	7,904
Blackberry	1 cup (cultivated berries)	7,701
Prune	½ cup	7,291
Raspberry	1 cup	6,058

Strawberry	1 cup	5,938
Red Delicious apple	1 apple	5,900
Granny Smith apple	1 apple	5,381
Pecan	1 oz (25 g)	5,095
Sweet cherry	1 cup	4,873
Black plum	1 plum	4,844
Russet potato	1, cooked	4,649
Black bean	½ cup dried beans	4,181
Plum	1 plum	4,118
Gala apple	1 apple	3,903

Source: United States Department of Agriculture (2007)

9. Salt

Why do I need salt?

Salt is made of sodium and chloride molecules. There are approximately 2.4 g of sodium in 6 g salt. This means that approximately 40 per cent of salt is sodium. In order to regulate the volume of blood circulating in the body and for the movement of fluid between cells, we need sodium. It also helps cells to absorb nutrients from the blood and muscles to contract. The potassium/sodium balance is absolutely critical to the overall functioning of every cell in the human body. If salt levels fall too low, a condition called hyponatraemia can develop, which can be fatal (*see* page 64).

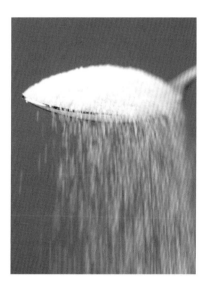

How much salt should I consume?

You need a minimum amount of 575 mg sodium in your diet (equivalent to 1.4 g salt) to be healthy. Going under this level is associated with health problems and a greater risk of death. Eating too much salt can also be harmful – most studies suggest that excess sodium can increase blood pressure.

Currently, the Department of Health and most other medical organisations recommend limiting your daily salt intake to 6 g or 2.4 g sodium. They also advise limiting foods containing more than 1.25 g salt/100 g.

However, the evidence linking salt to heart disease and stroke is weak. A study published in the *American Journal of Hypertension*, which analysed data from over 6,000 people, failed to find an association between lowered salt intake and lowered risk for heart attacks, strokes, or death (Taylor *et al.*, 2011).

Another large-scale study, the International Study of Salt & Blood Pressure (Intersalt), involving 10,000 adults in 32 countries, found no relationship between sodium intake and hypertension. It found only a slight decrease in blood pressure (3–6 mmHg systolic and 0–3mmHg diastolic) when there was a dramatic decrease in salt excretion. Others have found that following a low-salt diet produces only minimal reductions in blood pressure in most people. This may be due to the fact that individuals vary in how they respond to salt.

Should I be worried about salt and blood pressure?

For most people, there is probably no need to be concerned about salt; your kidneys regulate the amount of sodium in your body so if you consume more than you need, then it is excreted in the urine. It will cause just a temporary increase in blood pressure as extra water is drawn into the bloodstream to dilute it. But this soon returns to normal as the sodium is excreted and blood volume returns to normal.

However, some people are more sensitive to sodium than others and generally as you get older your sensitivity to sodium increases. This means excess sodium may cause an above-normal rise in blood pressure. To reduce your risk of developing high blood pressure, you should not only cut salty foods from your diet, but also eat less processed food.

The bottom line is that if you eat mostly unprocessed food you probably won't need to worry too much about salt. As 75 per cent of the salt in most people's diets comes from processed food (e.g. ham, bacon, sausages and burgers, bread, soups, sauces, cheese, ready meals, pizzas, baked beans, breakfast cereals and biscuits), it's virtually impossible to eat a lot of salt if you base your diet on unprocessed foods. Eating less processed foods not only means you'll be getting less salt, but you will also be getting less sugar, refined flour and calories. And it's the latter three factors that cut your risk of obesity, high blood pressure, type 2 diabetes and heart disease.

Do I need extra salt on days when I exercise?

For most types of exercise lasting less than three hours, there is no need to consume extra salt before, during or after exercise. It will not prevent cramps, heat illness or sodium deficiency (Noakes, 2012).

10. Water

Why do I need it?

Of all the nutrients, water is the most important. It makes up more than 60 per cent of your body weight and is vital to all cells. Water is the medium in which

> **TO REDUCE YOUR BLOOD PRESSURE**
>
> - Consume extra fruit, vegetables and dairy products for potassium, magnesium and calcium.
> - Exercise (and lose weight if you need to).
> - Limit your intake of alcohol.

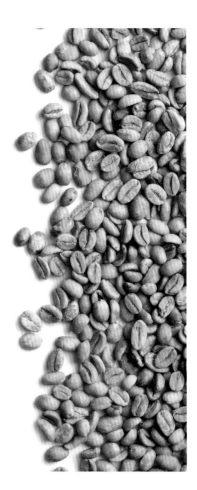

all metabolic reactions take place, including energy production. Fluid acts as a cushion for your nervous system and is a lubricant for your joints and eyes. Blood – another key fluid – carries nutrients and oxygen to the cells and helps rid the body of toxins.

Physical and cognitive performance can suffer when we are poorly hydrated, especially in hot, humid conditions or when exercise is prolonged. Dehydration during exercise can lead to increased heart rate, increased perception of effort, and reduced performance.

How much should I drink each day?

You need to top up your fluid levels frequently because you lose water through sweat, breathing and urine. The European Food Safety Authority recommends an intake of 2.5 litres of water for men and 2.0 litres of water for women per day (Jequier and Constant, 2010). This is supported by the Department of Health, which recommends that we should drink six to eight glasses of fluid per day. An easy way to monitor changes in hydration status is to check the colour of your urine. It should be pale straw colour – anything darker and it shows more fluid is needed.

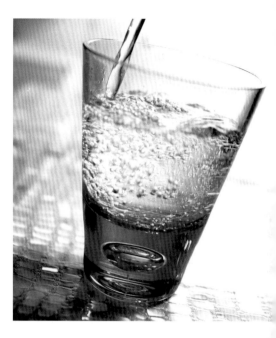

Maintaining normal hydration during exercise helps you work out longer and perform better. The amount you should drink depends on your sweat rate, the duration and intensity of exercise, and the surrounding temperature and humidity (*see* Chapter 3). Dehydration may impair performance, speed and stamina.

As a rule, you should:

■ Begin your exercise session well hydrated.

■ Replenish fluid regularly, especially when sweat rates are high.

■ Be guided by thirst and don't force yourself to drink (this may result in hyponatraemia – low blood sodium levels).

■ Drink water during moderate-intensity activities lasting less than 1 hour.

■ Drink water or isotonic drinks during high-intensity activities lasting more than 1 hour.

■ Rehydrate after exercise – for most activities, water is the best option.

11. Alcohol

What is a safe level of alcohol?

The UK Department of Health advises a maximum of 3 units per day and 14 units per week for women; and a maximum of 4 units per day and 21 units per week for men. One unit is equivalent to 10 ml or 8 g of alcohol, or half a pint of ordinary-strength beer or lager, one small glass (125 ml) of 10 per cent wine, or a single shot (25 ml) of spirits. A standard 175 ml glass of 13 per cent wine contains 2 units.

Is alcohol beneficial or harmful?

Alcohol is a toxin, which means it harms your liver and every cell in your body. It cannot be stored so is broken down by the liver, ultimately yielding ATP (energy). That means that any remaining calories that you have consumed are likely to be converted to fat.

Drinking more than the recommended level of alcohol makes you feel tired and reduces your immunity, making you more susceptible to infections. In the long term it increases the risk of a long list of health conditions: breast, bowel, stomach, throat and mouth cancers, heart disease, and stroke. For every 10 g of alcohol (approximately 1 unit) the risk of breast cancer increases by 7–12 per cent. Too much alcohol also puts you at risk of high blood pressure, infertility and alcohol-related liver disease. Women are more vulnerable to the harmful effects of alcohol than men because they have less water and more fat in their bodies, and their livers do not metabolise alcohol as quickly.

Alcohol in moderation is associated with a lowered heart disease risk, due in part to its ability to increase levels of 'good' HDL cholesterol and reduce blood platelet stickiness. However, most of the research has been carried out on middle-aged men and may not apply to women and younger men. Any heart protective effect is probably small.

In saying this however, there might be other protective effects from red wine, which contains polyphenols, saponins and a compound called resveratrol, all of which can help lower 'bad' LDL cholesterol and protect from heart disease.

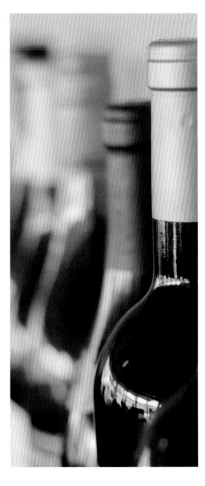

Can alcohol harm performance?

If you've had a drink, it's best to avoid exercising as alcohol will affect your balance, judgement, concentration and level of hydration. All the negative side effects of alcohol fully outweigh any possible benefits it can have. It can reduce your strength, endurance, recovery, aerobic capacity, your ability to metabolise fat and also impair muscle growth.

It causes inflammation in the muscle cells, which prevents muscle repair and, in the long term, can actually damage the cells and result in a loss of functional muscle tissue.

Alcohol also slows muscle recovery and performance by disrupting your sleep. Researchers have found that alcohol reduces sleep duration and increases wakefulness (particularly in the second half of the night). This can reduce your human growth hormone output – which builds muscle – by as much as 70 per cent.

It's no surprise that working out while dehydrated isn't ideal and this not only prolongs muscle recovery (due to decreased blood flow in the muscles), but can also increase the risk of heat-related illness.

It's best to avoid alcohol the night before a competition. Although small amounts are unlikely to do much harm, if you overdo it, alcohol can linger in the blood even after a good night's rest, so avoid drinking altogether. Alcohol's diuretic effect also increases the need to urinate, resulting in the loss of electrolytes.

Similarly, it's not a good idea to quench your thirst with alcoholic drinks after a workout or competition. Chances are exercise will have left you a little dehydrated so drinking alcohol could slow your recovery. Always rehydrate with water – and not alcohol. Furthermore, if you're trying to lose weight, it makes no sense replacing all the calories you've just burned up during exercise with alcoholic drinks.

Moderate drinking (within government guidelines) on non-exercising days probably won't jeopardise your exercise performance (provided you avoid dehydration), but you need to account for the calories it provides. Try to have at least two alcohol-free days a week so you are not putting your liver under constant strain.

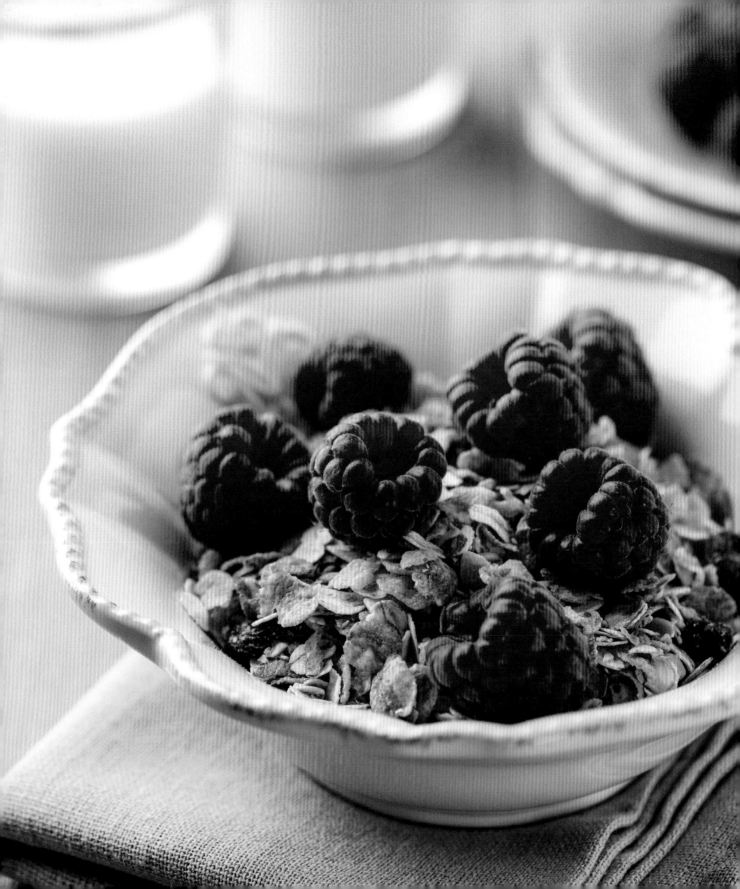

2 NUTRIENT TIMING AND RECOVERY NUTRITION

As important as *what* you eat is *when* you eat. The right fuel at the right time influences how well you feel, perform and recover. It also affects how much body fat, glycogen or even muscle tissue you burn. Get the timing wrong and you may find yourself struggling to complete your planned workout and performing under-par. Even worse, you could end up burning muscle rather than fat as your fuel reserves dip. After a session, good nutrition habits help your body adapt to the stress imposed by exercise, so you become fitter, stronger and faster.

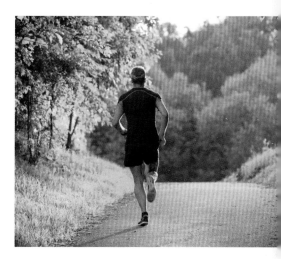

Eating before training

It takes 24 hours to refill muscle glycogen stores, so what you've consumed the previous day matters. For most regular exercisers, a daily diet providing around 3–7 g/kg of carbohydrate (*see* page 7) will ensure full muscle glycogen stores.

The main purpose of your pre-workout meal is to stabilise your blood sugar levels during exercise. It also staves off hunger and minimises the risk of problems such as stitch and hypoglycaemia (low blood sugar levels).

Will training on an empty stomach improve my performance?

If you want to improve performance, then it is *not* advisable to train on an empty stomach.

First, you may feel hungry, lethargic and unmotivated when you haven't eaten for several hours. Eating a light snack a couple of hours before your workout will reduce the temptation to skip your training.

Second, when your brain isn't getting enough fuel you may feel faint, lose concentration and risk injury. You may become lightheaded, weak and shaky – all symptoms of low blood sugar levels – and this will certainly stop you from working out.

Finally, you are more likely to fatigue early if muscle glycogen and blood sugar levels dip too low. According to Italian researchers, exercising in a fasted state may reduce your endurance and encourage your muscles to turn to protein for fuel (Paoli *et al.*, 2011). Just as you wouldn't take your car out on a long journey with little petrol or diesel in the tank, so you can't expect to exercise very hard or very long when you haven't fuelled your body for several hours.

For most activities, eating a pre-exercise meal that includes carbohydrate will help increase your stamina and allow you to train harder for longer (Chryssanthopoulos *et al.*, 2002; Neufer *et al.*, 1987; Sherman *et al.*, 1991; Wright *et al.*, 1991).

When is the best time to eat before exercising?

Ideally, you should aim to have a meal 2–4 hours before a workout. This should leave enough time to partially digest your food although, in practice, the exact timing of your pre-workout meal may depend on your daily schedule. You should feel comfortable – neither full nor hungry.

According to a study at the University of North Carolina, eating a moderately high-carbohydrate, low-fat meal 3 hours before exercise allows you to exercise longer and perform better (Maffucci and McMurray, 2000). Athletes ate a meal either 3 hours or 6 hours before exercising on a treadmill for periods of 30 minutes without breaks; first at moderate intensity, then switching to high intensity, until they couldn't run any further. The athletes ran significantly longer after eating the meal 3 hours before training compared with when they had eaten 6 hours before.

What should I eat before exercise?

In general, opt for a low-GI meal – that is, foods that produce a gradual rise in blood sugar levels (*see* page 11). Low-GI foods help spare muscle glycogen and avoid problems of low blood sugar levels during long training sessions (Thomas *et al.*, 1991).

Low-GI meals may also help you burn more fat and less glycogen during exercise. A 2003 study at Loughborough University found that runners who ate a low-GI meal 3 hours before exercise burned more fat than those who ate a high-GI meal with the same amount of carbohydrate (Wu *et al.*, 2003).

A low-GI meal before exercise also helps improve your endurance capacity. A study found that runners who ate a low-GI meal were able to run 7 minutes longer than those who ate high-GI foods (Wu and Williams,

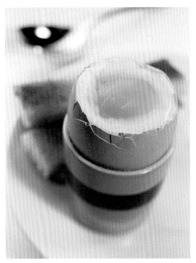

Q&A

How much carbohydrate should I consume before exercise if my training will be longer than an hour?

If your training will be longer than an hour, plan a small carbohydrate-rich snack before the activity. The exact amount you should eat depends on the time interval between eating and training and how hard and long you plan to exercise. You'll need to eat more for longer, harder workouts. In general, you should consume approximately 1 g carbohydrate/kg of body weight 1 hour before exercise, 2 g/kg 2 hours before, and so on. As the time before exercise increases, the amount of carbohydrate will increase. Larger amounts of carbohydrate (3–4 g/kg) are appropriate when more time is available (3 to 4 hours prior).

For longer workouts or endurance events lasting more than 2 hours, you may need to eat a little more than this. The time required for foods to digest depends on the type and quantity of the food consumed. Don't eat a big meal just before a workout otherwise you will feel uncomfortable, sluggish and 'heavy'. Eating a smaller meal and choosing foods lower in fat and fibre will help to reduce the risk of gastrointestinal (GI) discomfort. You should experiment to find the quantity of food that best works for you.

2006). This may be explained by the lower rise in blood glucose and insulin following the low-GI meal, which means the muscles burn less glycogen and glucose and more fat throughout the exercise session.

Ideally a low-GI pre-exercise meal should include protein and fat as well as carbohydrate. Both protein and fat slow the digestion and absorption of carbohydrate and help to produce a slower and more sustained rise in blood glucose. This should help give you longer-lasting energy, and so greater endurance during your workout or event, and therefore produce better performance. Without protein and fat in the mix, you may get a rapid rise in blood glucose, but this will be followed by a rapid return to baseline levels (or even a dip) as insulin levels rise. This can leave you tired and lacking energy during your workout and result in early fatigue. Make sure you also include vegetables and/or fruit in your pre-exercise meal as their high-fibre content will also slow the delivery of carbohydrate to your bloodstream and avoid rapid rises in glucose and insulin.

It's important to get the balance right. If you eat too much carbohydrate and too little protein or fat (e.g. pasta with tomato sauce or a jam sandwich), then you may find yourself hungry and running low on energy halfway through your workout. You need some fat and protein in the mix to promote satiety. They help prevent hunger and allow you to exercise longer without consuming extra carbohydrate. On the other hand, too much fat (e.g. fried burger or sausages and chips) can delay stomach emptying, so you may begin your workout feeling full and heavy. During your workout, digestion is further slowed as more blood is routed to your exercising muscles, so any carbohydrate in your pre-exercise meal are not available as fuel during your session.

The general rules are:

- Eat a meal about 2–4 hours before exercise (if your schedule allows) to maximise your endurance and performance. For example, if your training session starts at 5 p.m., have your low-GI meal between 1 p.m. and 3 p.m.
- For a low-GI meal, include some protein and fat along with some carbohydrate.

Should I eat anything in the hour before exercise?

Fears that eating in the hour before exercise will produce hypoglycaemia are unfounded as the majority of studies have shown this to be untrue (Jeukendrup and Killer, 2010). Some studies have shown an improvement in performance (Sherman *et al.*, 1991) while others have found none (Febbraio *et al.*, 2000). But, on balance, if you need a pre-exercise energy boost, the safest strategy is to consume a small snack as close to the start of your session as possible. That way, you'll get a smaller and more sustained rise in blood glucose (good), a smaller

Q&A

I prefer to train on an empty stomach – should I force myself to eat if I'm not hungry?

Many runners claim they can't run with food in their stomachs, complaining of stitch, nausea or stomach discomfort. It is down to individual preference, but if your goal is improved performance, then it is possible to 'train' yourself to run with a small amount of food inside you. The potential benefits are more energy and greater endurance.

Try different high-carbohydrate options, such as a slice of toast, a banana, a small cereal or energy bar, a pot of yoghurt or a handful of dried fruit (such as raisins, apricots or sultanas). If you can't face solid food, try a liquid meal: diluted fruit juice or squash, a smoothie, flavoured milk or a sports drink. In any case, drink 150–250 ml water before setting out. This will help rehydrate you (especially important if you train first thing in the morning) and reduce the risk of dehydration during your workout. If you cannot eat anything before an early-morning workout, make sure that you eat well the day before, which will ensure muscle glycogen levels are replenished.

rise in insulin (good), and a smaller risk of hypoglycaemia (good). In other words, eating immediately before your session – provided you don't over-do it – won't harm your performance.

So, if you can't have a meal 2–4 hours before exercise, then eat a smaller meal or snack 5–60 minutes beforehand. The timing and the amount will depend on your schedule, but it should comprise mostly carbohydrate along with some protein and fat – you should feel satisfied but not too full. Again, it doesn't matter whether you choose high- or low-GI carbohydrate (Stannard, 2000).

On the other hand, if you have eaten a meal 2–4 hours before your session, then there's little to be gained from having more food in the hour before exercise – unless you are feeling hungry again. It is a good idea to experiment with different amounts and types of foods and vary the timing around exercise. For example, if hunger strikes 2 hours after eating a meal, then add more fat or protein to your meal (these nutrients promote satiety) or have a further snack just before the start of your session. Exercising with a growling stomach isn't conducive to good performance and may cause you to stop early.

Should I train low and compete high?

Training with low glycogen stores may be worth trying as part of a periodised training plan. It is used by some elite endurance athletes to improve their performance in competitions. The idea is to consume a low-carbohydrate diet during training, then a high-carbohydrate diet a few days before an event to fill your glycogen stores – a concept that's been termed 'train low, compete high'. By training with low levels of glycogen, your muscles adapt by burning fat instead of glycogen. So they make more mitochondria (that burn fat) and more fat-burning enzymes, which (theoretically) prolongs your endurance (Hawley and Burke, 2010; Burke *et al.*, 2011). So when you switch to a high-carbohydrate diet before your competition, you'll not only have the ability to burn more fat but you'll also have a full tank of glycogen to draw on. The downside is that exercising with low glycogen stores feels much harder so you may have to drop your pace. The research is in its early stages and while scientists have measured higher concentrations of fat-burning enzymes in athletes, they haven't yet proved that this translates into better performance during competition (Hawley *et al.*, 2011; Maughan and Shireffs, 2012).

Pre-exercise meals

The following meals have a low or moderate GI and are best consumed 2–4 hours before exercise:

Q&A

Will sugar before training give me a quick energy fix?

Sugary foods and drinks have a high GI and can raise blood glucose levels rapidly. When these levels are raised just before exercise there is the potential for a rebound drop in blood glucose levels (hypo-glycaemia) during exercise. Typical symptoms include lightheadedness, nausea, and early fatigue during exercise.

If you haven't eaten a meal for 4 hours or longer and you're planning to exercise for an hour or more, then sugar could help maintain blood glucose levels – but so would other more nutritious options! Provided you have only a small amount (less than 25 g) 30 minutes before exercising, a sugary snack or drink is unlikely to harm your performance. But make sure it is only a small amount as too much sugar may send your blood glucose levels and insulin soaring. Rather than making you feel more energetic, sugar could sap your energy. If you need a pre-training energy boost, it's safer to choose foods such as bananas or dried fruit and nuts that are less likely to cause rapid increases in blood sugar and insulin levels.

- Stew made with chicken, fish or beans, vegetables and potatoes.
- Jacket potato with beans, cheese, meat, fish or poultry, plus salad.
- Pasta with pesto sauce, vegetables and cheese.
- Chicken, fish or beans with rice and vegetables.
- Porridge made with oats and milk, plus fruit.
- Fish pie (fish in sauce with mashed potatoes) and vegetables.
- Stir-fried poultry, prawns or tofu with vegetables and noodles.

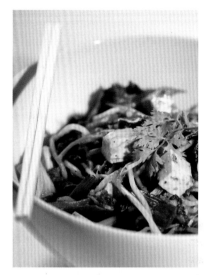

Pre-exercise snacks

The following snacks have a moderate to high GI and are best consumed 30–60 minutes before exercise:

- A pot (125 g) of yoghurt plus 150 g fresh fruit.
- 1–2 bananas.
- 25 g dried fruit and 25 g nuts.
- Sandwich with chicken, fish, cheese, egg or houmous and salad.
- A flapjack (50 g).
- A granola or oat-based cereal bar.
- 1–2 slices of toast with peanut butter.

Eating during training

Feeling nauseous if you drink during a hard session

If you struggle to drink anything when you're exercising hard, try having a sip of squash or cordial, and swishing it around in your mouth. Just the sensation of sugar in the mouth – without actually swallowing it – is enough to give you a performance boost. Scientists have found that the sweet taste of carbohydrate is enough to alleviate fatigue and help you exercise harder/longer during sessions lasting around 45–60 minutes. The exact reason isn't known, but the sugars in the drink act on sensors in the mouth, which transmit messages to the brain. These then act on the brain's reward centres, inducing pleasure and masking fatigue. Studies have shown that this simple trick improves performance during endurance exercise even though no or minimal carbohydrate are actually consumed (Rollo and Williams, 2011)! It's also a good way of avoiding extra carbohydrate/calories during exercise if you're trying to lose weight. But it doesn't mean not drinking anything – you still need to drink water and prevent dehydration (see page 59).

Q&A

What should I eat before a competition?

You should take your own supplies for the journey as well for race day as suitable foods may not be available. Keep to the guidelines for training outlined above, but bear in mind that competition nerves may reduce your appetite or affect your digestion. In general, stick to familiar foods and don't try anything new. Be certain that what you're eating and drinking is uncontaminated and safe. Drink plenty of water and avoid fast foods, salty or very sugary foods. Eat little and often (see Chapters 7–11 for more detailed advice).

Eating during training

How much carbohydrate should I consume during exercise?

If you're training longer than 1 hour

Extra carbohydrate from a drink or food may improve your performance if training longer than an hour. Studies have shown that consuming carbohydrate, whether in liquid or solid form, during exercise lasting over 60 minutes can help you keep going longer (Burke *et al*, 2011). These additional carbohydrate will top up blood glucose levels, fuel your muscles and spare muscle glycogen, particularly in the latter stages of your session when glycogen reserves are likely to be low.

If you're training 1–3 hours

To give your muscles a decent carbohydrate boost during exercise, particularly in the final glycogen-depleted stages, you need to take in at least 30 g of carbohydrate/hour during your session. Researchers at the University of Texas in Austin recommend 30–60 g/hour, depending on your body weight (heavier exercisers need more) and exercise intensity (more for harder workouts) (Coggan and Coyle, 1991; Rodrigues *et al*, 2009). That's equivalent to about 120–240 calories of carbohydrate/hour.

If you're training for longer than 3 hours

If you're exercising hard for longer than 3 hours, then consuming higher amounts (60–90 g) of carbohydrate/hour in the form of a sports drink containing glucose and fructose (or maltodextrin and fructose) in a 2 to 1 ratio may help improve your performance, helping you keep going longer at a higher intensity (IOC, 2011). One study suggests that 68–78 g carbohydrate/hour is the optimal dose for events lasting 3 hours (Smith *et al.*, 2013). Adding fructose to the mix overcomes the problem of glucose saturation, which happens when you drink an isotonic drink containing only glucose or only sucrose. The glucose transporters can only transport, or absorb, 60 g/hour. If you drink a more concentrated drink (hypertonic) then the extra glucose simply stays in the gut longer, which can make you feel nauseous or 'bloated'. However, fructose is absorbed by a different transporter so by consuming both glucose and fructose at the same time you can make use of both transporters and increase the overall absorption rate of carbohydrate.

This is clearly advantageous during long-distance high-intensity exercise, e.g. marathon running, ultra-distance running, long-distance cycling and triathlon events when you're urning a high percentage of carbohydrate/glycogen for three hours or more. One study found that performance in a cycling time trial improved by 8 per cent when drinking a glucose/fructose drink compared with a glucose-only drink (Jeukendrup, 2008). So, for these events it may be worth switching to a sports drink, bar or gel that contains a 2 to 1 ratio of glucose to fructose. Alternatively, experiment with different foods, such as honey, raisins and bananas, containing a mixture of glucose and fructose. This may be an equally effective and less expensive alternative.

What exactly should I consume during exercise?

During exercise lasting between 1 and 3 hours, choose drinks and foods with a high or moderate GI, as you need to get the carbohydrate into your bloodstream rapidly. The following fuel options meet this criteria. If you opt for drinks you'll be getting both carbohydrate and fluid, but if you opt for food then you should drink water with it rather than a sugar-containing drink otherwise you could be getting too much carbohydrate. Experiment with different drinks and foods, and try mixing and matching drinks and foods. It is important to devise your individual fuelling strategy during training so you'll know what suits you in competition. For example, you may prefer a carbohydrate-containing drink for the first hour, then food plus water for the rest of the session. Alternatively, you may prefer to alternate carbohydrate-containing drinks with food and water throughout your session. In general, moderate- and low-GI options would be more suitable for longer sessions lasting 2 hours or more:

- Diluted squash and cordial – contain sucrose, which provides both glucose and fructose in a 1 to 1 ratio. They have a GI of 58–66 ('moderate' GI).

- Fruit juices diluted 1 to 1 with water – contain a 1 to 1 ratio of glucose to fructose and have a slightly lower GI (40–55) than most squashes and cordials, which is classed as 'low'.

- Isotonic sports drinks – contain mostly glucose, maltodextrin (a short chain of glucose molecules) and sucrose, and have a GI of 65–100 ('high' GI), depending on the brand.

- Energy gels and energy bars – contain glucose, maltodextrin and sucrose and have a GI of 74–83 ('high' GI).

- Bananas – contain a 1 to 1 ratio of glucose and fructose and have a GI of 52 ('low to moderate' GI).

- Dried apricots – contain a 2 to 1 mixture of glucose to fructose and have a GI of 31 ('low'), ideal for fuelling longer sessions lasting more than 3 hours.

- Raisins and most other dried fruit – contain a 1 to 1 ratio of glucose and fructose and have a GI of 64, which is classed as 'moderate'.

Q&A

Do I need extra carbohydrate during exercise?

If you're exercising for less than an hour

There's no need to consume anything other than water. Extra carbohydrate from a drink or food are unlikely to benefit your performance – unless you haven't eaten beforehand. In this case, if you began exercise with low glycogen stores, then consuming extra carbohydrate during exercise will help maintain blood glucose levels, fuel your muscles, and allow you to keep going longer. It takes between 20 and 40 minutes for the carbohydrate to reach the muscles, so start consuming it early in your session.

- Granola and cereal (oat) bars – contain starch and sucrose and have a GI around 60 ('moderate').
- Rice cakes – these are made from puffed rice, basically starch, which breaks down rapidly to glucose, so have a 'high' GI of 78–82.

Which carbohydrate is best: liquid or solid?

Whether you choose solid or liquid carbohydrate makes no difference to your performance, provided you get enough fluid. For most actitivities, drinks are the most convenient option. They provide fluid, quench your thirst and deliver a fixed concentration of carbohydrate so you know how much you are getting.

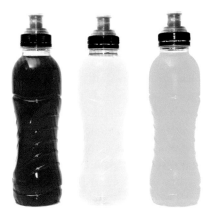

But carrying a sports drink with you on a long run, for example, is not always easy. It is heavy and can slow you down in a race. Solid carbohydrate has the advantage of being considerably lighter – just make sure you can get water somewhere en route. Do not skimp on your usual drink volume otherwise you will end up with excess carbohydrate sitting in your stomach.

If you decide to take food it needs to be portable, palatable, non-perishable and very easy to eat. (*See* below for suggestions.)

How often should you consume carbohydrate?

Start consuming carbohydrate early in your workout, ideally in the first 30 minutes. It takes around 20 to 40 minutes (depending on the source) for the carbohydrate to reach your muscles and for the energy boost to kick in, so don't wait until you feel tired.

Your goal is to maintain a steady supply of carbohydrate entering your bloodstream. If you are exercising for 1–3 hours, aim to consume 15–30 g every 15–30 minutes. Experiment to find the best amounts of drink or food for you.

The following table shows the equivalent of 15 g portion of carbohydrate.

TABLE 2.1 CARBOHYDRATE IN DRINK AND FOOD

Drinks	Foods
200 ml cordial (dilute 1 to 8)	17 g jelly beans
200 ml squash (dilute 1 to 6)	18 g dried mango
250 ml isotonic sports drink (e.g. Lucozade sport)	22 g (a small handful) raisins
400 ml hypotonic sports drink (e.g. Powerade ION)	25 g flapjack
270 ml apple juice (diluted 1 to 1)	25 g granola or cereal-type bar
170 ml 2 to 1 glucose/fructose sports drink (e.g. Lucozade sport elite)	65 g (half a large) banana
	3 rice cakes

Won't the extra carbohydrate stop me from losing weight?

If you're exercising to lose weight, opt for plain water instead of sports drinks. Carbohydrate-rich drinks, gels and bars all add extra calories and may even supply as many – or more – calories as you are burning off! If you are training hard for longer than 60 minutes and you're finding that your energy levels dip, choose a drink containing around 2–4 g carbohydrate/100 ml. This will provide extra carbohydrate to maintain blood glucose, but not too many to negate your weight loss goal.

Should I consume protein before or during exercise?

If you're doing a long hard gym session or strength workout lasting 2 hours, then consuming protein as well as carbohydrate immediately before and also during your session may help maximise the muscle-building benefits of your training. One study found that when athletes consumed a drink containing roughly equal amounts of carbohydrate and protein immediately before and then during a 2-hour weights workout they increased the amount of muscle they gained (Beelen *et al.*, 2008). This is because your body digests pre-exercise protein into amino acids during exercise and begins repairing damaged muscles.

The study used a specially formulated drink but you could get the same advantage by consuming 300 ml milk or a pre-workout sports drink containing both protein and carbohydrate. However, there's no benefit to be gained by consuming protein during endurance exercise as muscle repair is the same whether you consume a carbohydrate-only drink or protein plus carbohydrate (Beelen *et al.*, 2011).

Recovery nutrition

Why is recovery nutrition important?

What you eat and drink in the hours following your session is critical when it comes to improving your fitness and body composition. It is during this post-exercise period that your body gets stronger and fitter. A hard workout or event depletes your stores of glycogen and breaks down muscle tissue to a greater or lesser degree. Your aim is to rebuild these fuel stores and repair damaged muscle fibres before your next session. Failure to replenish fluids and fuel after training can quickly result in sore muscles, fatigue and under-performance at your next training session. Recovery includes the following:

- **Replace fluids** – your muscles cannot fully recover until your cells are properly hydrated (*see* pages 64–65).

- **Refuel** – you need to replace the fuel (carbohydrate) that you've used otherwise your muscles will feel sore and tired during your next session.
- **Rebuild** – you need to repair muscle cells that have been broken down during exercise.

How soon after exercise should I eat?

If you have a full day to recover before your next training session, or if you have done an easy (non-depleting) workout, you need not worry about refuelling immediately afterwards. Happily take your time after training and worry about your post-exercise meal when you feel hungry for it. As long as you eat well over the day, your muscles will be recovered for the next day's training session.

But if you plan to work out or compete within 24 hours, then speedy recovery is crucial. If you wait too long before eating or drinking, then you'll feel sluggish during your next session; if you get it right, then you'll recover faster. As a rule of thumb, the sooner you can begin refuelling after exercise, the quicker your body will recover.

There is what scientists call a 'recovery window', a period immediately after exercise when the speed of glycogen replenishment and muscle manufacture is greater than normal. Your muscle cells are more sensitive to insulin and the enzymes that are responsible for making glycogen are most active immediately after your workout, leaving you a 2-hour window to reload your muscle glycogen. Carbohydrate is converted into glycogen one and a half times faster than normal during this post-exercise period.

If you wait more than 2 hours, then your body's ability to convert what you eat or drink to glycogen drops by 66 per cent. The longer you wait, the longer it will take to start the recovery process. So have a carbohydrate- and protein-rich drink or snack (*see* page 70) as soon as possible after your workout – ideally within 30 minutes and no later than 2 hours.

What do I need for recovery?

For optimal recovery, the major nutrients you need in order of priority are:

1. **Carbohydrate** – these are particularly important for aiding recovery for endurance athletes. You'll need 1–1.5 g for each 1 kg of your weight, so the heavier you are, the more carbohydrate you'll need to refill glycogen stores.
2. **Protein** – regardless of your weight, you need approximately 20 g of protein for muscle repair.
3. **Antioxidants** – these will improve muscle recovery and reduce muscle inflammation/soreness.

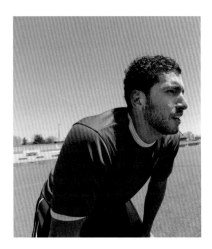

How much carbohydrate should I consume after exercise?

The amount of carbohydrate you need to consume depends on how much fuel you used during your session. The harder and longer you trained, the more carbohydrate you need to replace. As a guide, high-intensity endurance training (e.g. fast running, cycling or swimming) will deplete glycogen more than low-intensity activities (e.g. walking, jogging or yoga) or intermittent activities that include rest periods (e.g. weight training or recreational tennis). As a guide, studies recommend 1–1.5 g of carbohydrate/kg of body weight in the immediate post-exercise period (Rodrigues *et al.*, 2009) but you should adjust this depending on your activity. For instance, a person weighing 70 kg would need to consume 70–105 g of carbohydrate. This is especially important if you have less than 8 hours between sessions.

High- or low-GI carbohydrate after exercise?

It doesn't matter what type of carbohydrate you consume, although it's probably beneficial to opt for a moderate- or high-GI source. The combination of carbohydrate with protein during the 2-hour post-exercise period spikes insulin to a greater degree than carbohydrate alone. This, in turn, leads to a rapid uptake of glucose and amino acids from the bloodstream by the muscle cells. You can include a little fat in this post-exercise snack (e.g. peanut butter on toast) as it will not affect insulin release or muscle protein uptake. (See 'Refuelling snacks' on pages 53–55 for further suggestions.)

However, choose low-GI meals thereafter. Researchers at Loughborough University have found that eating low-GI meals during the 24 hours following exercise improves endurance during your next workout. What's more, it also encourages the body to burn more fat and less carbohydrate, which helps shed unwanted pounds as well as improve performance.

What should I eat after exercise?

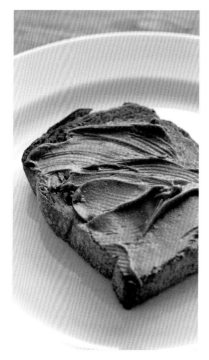

For speediest recovery, you should include both carbohydrate and protein in your post-exercise snack or meal. The combination of these two nutrients stimulates greater insulin release, which prompts the muscle cells to take up glucose and amino acids from the bloodstream. It also minimises protein breakdown and encourages muscle rebuilding. Studies have found that a ratio of about 3 parts carbohydrate to 1 part protein boosts glycogen storage (Zawadski *et al.*, 1992; Phillips *et al.*, 2007). It also promotes faster muscle repair and growth after a weights workout or strength training (Van Loon, 2007; Bloomer *et al.*, 2000), as well as after endurance exercise lasting longer than 1 hour. US researchers have also shown that protein with carbohydrate reduces post-exercise muscle soreness (Luden *et al.*, 2007).

How much protein should I consume after exercise?

Whether you've done endurance or strength exercise, you need protein afterwards to promote muscle recovery. Your post-workout meal or snack should, ideally, comprise about 20 g protein, although anywhere between 15–25 g would be beneficial. This will help promote faster muscle repair and greater muscle growth (Moore *et al.*, 2009; IOC, 2010; Rodrigues *et al.*, 2009; Phillips and Van Loon, 2011).

However, muscle recovery doesn't stop after 2 hours – it continues for several hours, perhaps up to 24 hours. Your muscle cells are able to take up amino acids more readily during this time, which means muscle manufacture will be faster than normal. So you should continue consuming protein at regular intervals throughout the day. Aim to have around 15–25 g protein at each meal and also include protein in your snacks.

In a one study, Canadian and Australian researchers found that protein evenly spaced through the day was optimal for muscle building (Moore *et al.*, 2012). Athletes who consumed 4 meals containing 20 g of whey protein every 3 hours gained more muscle protein than those who consumed either 8 x 10 g or 2 x 40 g whey protein over the same time period.

If you want to maximise muscle mass gain, it is also a good idea to consume some protein shortly before bedtime. One study found that athletes who consumed a protein drink before sleep had greater muscle protein uptake than those who had a placebo (Res *et al.*, 2012).

What type of protein is best after exercise?

All types of protein are useful for muscle repair, but if you're looking to maximise muscle growth after exercise, opt for high-quality proteins that contain all essential amino acids (Churchward-Venne *et al.*, 2012). Milk, whey, casein (the latter two are derived from milk), egg and meat have produced best results in studies.

These foods are also rich in the amino acid leucine (*see* page 105), which is an important 'signalling amino acid'. When it reaches the muscle cells, it triggers protein manufacture, which in turn leads to increased muscle strength. Whey is particularly high in leucine but you can also get it from milk.

Q&A

If I don't feel hungry after training, should I force myself to eat?

Ironically, hard endurance training, particularly in warm conditions, can sometimes suppress your post-workout appetite. This is because more of the blood flow is concerned with exercising muscles, so the hunger signals your brain receives from your gut sensors become weakened. If the thought of eating straight after a workout makes you feel queasy, try liquid meals such as milk, yoghurt drinks, flavoured milk, milkshakes or meal replacement (carbohydrate/protein) drinks. (*See* 'Refuelling snacks' on pages 53–55.)

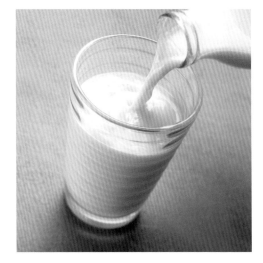

The following quantities of foods supply 20 g of protein:

- 3 eggs
- 600 ml milk (or flavoured milk)
- 27 g whey protein powder
- 85 g Cheddar cheese
- 85 g meat or poultry
- 450 g plain yoghurt
- 250 g strained Greek yoghurt
- 100 g fish, e.g. salmon, plaice

Milk, the best recovery food?

Milk is one of the best recovery foods. It is less expensive than commercial recovery sports drinks and it's been proven to aid muscle growth, promote muscle repair, reduce muscle soreness and rehydrate the body – after both resistance and endurance exercise, in men as well as women. Compared with traditional sports drinks, 500 ml milk consumed after training produces greater gains in muscle mass and strength as well as a greater aerobic capacity, and reduced body fat levels (Cockburn *et al.*, 2012; Ferguson-Stegall *et al.*, 2011; Josse, 2010; Elliot, 2006; Hartman *et al.*, 2007; Wilkinson, 2007; Karp *et al.*, 2006). It also rehydrates you as well as, if not better than, isotonic sports drinks (Shirreffs *et al.*, 2007).

In short, milk helps you recover faster and perform better in your next workout. A 2008 study by researchers at Northumbria University found that athletes who drank 500 ml of semi-skimmed milk or chocolate milk immediately after training had less muscle soreness and more rapid muscle recovery compared with commercial sports drinks or water (Cockburn *et al.*, 2008).

What's more, a 2009 study from James Madison University in the USA found that football players who drank chocolate-flavoured milk after training had less muscle damage and faster muscle recovery compared with those who consumed a sports drink (Gilson *et al.*, 2009).

Just how milk works isn't clear, but it is thought that the dairy peptides formed during digestion alter protein metabolism in the muscle and promote training adaptations.

Will antioxidants improve my recovery?

Muscle soreness is due to several factors, but one of the factors responsible is the build-up of free radicals (molecules that have one or more unpaired electrons in their orbit) generated during exercise. In the short term, free radicals can damage cell membranes and make the muscles sore. While regular exercise increases the body's natural defences against free radicals, you can boost them further by consuming plenty of foods rich in antioxidant nutrients (*see* page 32). High concentrations of antioxidants are found in fruits, vegetables, nuts, seeds, whole grains, lentils and beans. These foods may help protect the body from free

Q&A

Is it true that the calories I eat after a workout won't be stored as fat?

Not exactly: while carbohydrate calories after exercise will be converted preferentially into glycogen, they can also be converted into fat if you consume too much. The enzymes that turn carbohydrate into glycogen in your muscles can only comfortably handle 50–70 g carbohydrate every 2 hours. Eat too much in a short period and the resulting 'overspill' will be converted into fat. Try to keep a check on portion sizes and opt for snacks and meals with a low glycaemic load (GL; *see* page 13) such as yoghurt, a jacket potato with tuna, or a cheese sandwich. Avoid meals or snacks with a high GL and large portions of low-GI foods; for example, big bowls of pasta, jam sandwiches or even large volumes of energy drinks may give you more carbohydrate than you need.

radicals and reduce inflammation and muscle soreness. One study found that cherry juice (a natural source of phytochemicals and anthocyanins) before and after a marathon improved recovery (Howatson *et al.*, 2010). Another found that it improves muscle strength recovery after weight training (Bowtell *et al.*, 2011). However, there's little evidence that taking extra antioxidants in the form of supplements has any benefit.

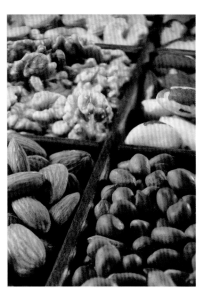

Nutrition, exercise and immunity

Many athletes find that intense training can leave them susceptible to colds and infections. It is ironic that moderate training boosts your immune system but hard training can lower your defences against germs and viruses – especially when combined with poor eating habits. The reason? Heavy prolonged training results in increased levels of stress hormones (e.g. adrenaline and cortisol), which inhibits your immune system. For a few hours after an intense session, your immune cells are depressed, making you more susceptible to infection during this period. Here are some ways to reduce your chances of infection during hard-training periods:

- Ensure you eat enough calories to match your needs – more on the days you exercise.
- Avoid hard training in a carbohydrate-depleted state. Low glycogen stores are associated with increases in cortisol levels and suppression of immune cells.
- If you're dieting and eating less carbohydrate, increase your protein intake.
- Try taking supplements of echinacea for up to 4 weeks during a period of hard training. Studies with athletes and non-athletes have shown that echinacea boosts the body's own production of immune cells and results in greater protection against minor illnesses.
- During long tough workouts, consume 30–60 g of carbohydrate/hour to stave off the rise in stress hormones and the associated drop in immunity (Halsen *et al.*, 2004).
- Ensure you are consuming plenty of foods rich in immunity-boosting nutrients – vitamins A, C, D, E, and B6, zinc, iron and magnesium. Best sources are fresh fruit, vegetables, whole grains, beans, lentils, nuts and seeds.
- Vitamin D plays a key role in immunity so make sure you're getting plenty from dietary sources (oily fish, eggs) or sunlight, otherwise take a daily supplement of around 10 μg of Vitamin D (*see* page 131).
- A modest antioxidant-rich supplement, such as cherry juice or elderberry extract, may help to boost your defences and reduce the risk of upper-respiratory infections. Avoid mega-doses.

■ Drink plenty of fluid. This increases your saliva production, which contains anti-bacterial proteins that can fight off air-borne germs.

■ Try taking probiotics either in the form of yoghurt or yoghurt drinks, or as a supplement. This can increase the number of beneficial bacteria in the gut and increase immunity.

Real foods or supplements?

Real foods are better than processed/formulated foods or supplements when it comes to getting the nutrients you need after exercise. This goes for carbo-hydrate and protein, as well as vitamins, minerals, antioxidants and fats. You can read food labels, and check on websites such as http://www.food-database.co.uk, for the amounts of carbohydrate and proteins in various foods, but below are some easy options containing 20 g protein (plus carbohydrate).

Refuelling snacks

After strength and power training

The following options provide around 20 g of high-quality protein to promote muscle building:

■ 600 ml milk. Any type of milk will provide the protein needed to maximise muscle adaptation after strength and power training. It also contains the optimal amount of the branched chain amino acid leucine to promote muscle building after exercise.

■ 500 ml yoghurt and fruit milkshake. Use 500 ml of milk plus yoghurt and fresh fruit (in general, bananas, strawberries, pears, mango and pineapple give the best results) for an excellent mixture of protein, carbohydrate and those all-important antioxidants.

■ 450 ml yoghurt. Choose plain yoghurt after a strength workout, or fruit yoghurt after an endurance session lasting an hour or more. Both contain high-quality proteins that will accelerate muscle repair; fruit yoghurt has added sugar containing the ideal 3 to 1 carbohydrate to protein ratio for speedy glycogen refuelling.

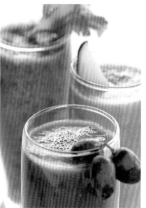

■ 330–500 ml whey protein shake. Shakes made up with milk or water are an easy and convenient mini-meal in a glass.

Q&A

Why do I find it hard to recover after a workout?

Are you overtraining? Rest is an essen-tial part of a training programme – your muscles need time to refuel and repair. Take at least one, if not two, days off from exercise per week (*see* 'The signs of overtraining' on page 54).

Are you eating enough carbo-hydrate? If you've increased your training intensity or volume, you may need to step up your carbohydrate intake to 7–10 g/kg of body weight. One study found that runners con-suming 5 g/kg of body weight/day during an intense training period experienced greater fatigue and muscle soreness plus a drop in performance and mood. These symptoms were reversed when the runners increased their carbo-hydrate intake to 8 g/kg/day (Achten *et al.*, 2004).

Are you anaemic? If your iron stores are depleted, you'll feel exces-sively tired during exercise. Anaemia is common, so ask your GP for a blood test that measures your serum ferritin (stored iron). If your regular diet tends to be a bit low in iron, consider a daily multivitamin containing at least 15 mg of iron. Also, try to include more iron-rich foods in your diet: red meat, fish, eggs, green leafy vegetables, nuts, beans and lentils.

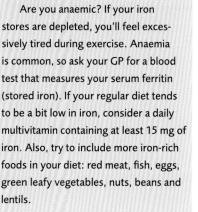

Opt for one containing 20 g protein. Powders and ready-to-drink versions generally contain a balanced mixture of carbohydrate (usually as maltodextrin and sugar), protein (usually whey), vitamins and minerals.

- 50 g of almonds or cashews plus 250 ml yoghurt – nuts not only provide 10 g of protein but also B vitamins, vitamin E, iron, zinc, phytonutrients and fibre. Yoghurt supplies another 10 g of protein. The fat in the nuts may reduce insulin a little, but will not affect muscle building

- 250 ml strained Greek yoghurt. This is also perfect after a strength workout, because strained Greek yogurt is more concentrated, containing about twice the protein of ordinary yoghurt.

- 500 ml ready-to-drink milkshake – opt for a shake that contains around 20 g protein for convenient refuelling after exercise. Alternatively, make your own speedy version by mixing 3 tsp of milkshake powder with 500 ml of milk.

- 2 x 100 ml yoghurt drinks plus 300 ml milk-based drink. Probiotic yoghurt drinks are useful for boosting immunity, thanks to their probiotic bacteria, as well as supplying protein (3 g), carbohydrate (12 g) and calcium.

- 80 g 'protein' bar. Bars containing a mixture of carbohydrate and whey protein are a convenient option after workouts. Opt for one containing around 20 g protein.

After endurance training

The following options provide the ideal 3 to 1 ratio of carbohydrate plus protein to promote muscle repair as well as glycogen refueling:

- 600 ml flavoured milk. This has been hailed as the perfect sports drink for after endurance exercise, following a study published in the *International Journal of Sport Nutrition and Exercise Metabolism* (Karp *et al.*, 2006). The study showed that chocolate-flavoured milk improved endurance more than conventional carbohydrate-only sports drinks because it contains the ideal ratio of carbohydrate to protein to help refuel tired muscles.

- 500 ml milk with a banana. Any type of milk will provide the protein needed to maximise muscle adaptation after exercise. After long intense sessions, the extra carbohydrate from the banana will further refuel energy stores ready for the next session.

- 500 ml hot chocolate. This warming option, made by mixing 3 tsp of hot chocolate (or 1 tsp cocoa powder plus 3 tsp of sugar) with 500 ml hot milk, is ideal during cold weather for refuelling glycogen and protein.

THE SIGNS OF OVER-TRAINING

- An increase in resting heart rate of around 10 per cent, or about 5 beats per minute above your normal rate.
- Reaching training heart rate zone much sooner into a training session than usual.
- Increased time for heart rate to recover between intervals.
- Inability to make progress in fitness goals.
- Extreme fatigue.
- Depression or lack of enthusiasm for training.
- Regular injuries (such as sprains and strains), colds or upper respiratory tract infections.

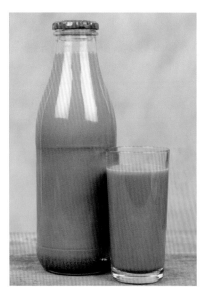

- A 'high-protein' sandwich. Make your own with 85 g meat, chicken, turkey, fish or cheese and a couple of slices of wholegrain bread, then add some salad to make a great refuelling snack.

- A bowl of porridge – made with 500 ml milk and 65 g oats, porridge is an ideal recovery food as it provides the ideal ratio of carbohydrate and protein, along with B vitamins, iron and fibre. It has a moderate to low GI, so is ideal if you're not training the same muscles within 24 hours.

- 500 ml milk or milkshake plus a flapjack. This snack gives you the optimal amount of milk protein for muscle repair plus low GI carbohydrate from the flapjack to promote glycogen refuelling over the next few hours.

- 300 ml milk or milkshake plus 125 g yoghurt plus 1 slice of wholegrain toast and honey. Ideal if you want rapid recovery; you'll get all the muscle-re-building benefits from dairy proteins as well as high-GI carbohydrate from wholegrain toast.

- Chocolate banana shake: blend 200 ml milk, 1 banana, 250 ml yoghurt, 1 tablespoon chopped walnuts, 1 scoop chocolate milkshake or whey powder, and 6 to 8 ice cubes. The walnuts provide omega-3 fats, vitamin E and iron.

Timing of day-to-day nutrition

While the amount and timing of carbohydrate before, during and after exercise is important for performance, you also need to consider the timing of your day-to-day diet. Total intake of calories, carbohydrate, protein, fat, etc. over the course of days, weeks and months must be adequate or else training and performance will be negatively affected. First and foremost, the body must meet its daily energy needs. Insufficient overall calories will limit the storage of carbohydrate as muscle or liver glycogen. You should make it a priority to eat regularly throughout the day. Athletes with a consistent fuelling pattern tend to be leaner and have more energy. Eat a balanced breakfast that combines carbohydrate (whole grains) and protein for sustainable energy. Here are some ideas:

- Eggs on wholegrain toast; milk and fruit
- Porridge with milk and banana
- Yoghurt with fruit, nuts and honey

Q&A

I work out in the evening and often don't return home until 9 or 10 o'clock. Should I eat anything at this late hour?

Always eat and drink after a hard workout no matter how late it is. Your body needs carbohydrate, protein and other nutrients to replenish fuel stores and recover after training. Skipping that post-workout meal will delay recovery and leave you feeling sluggish the next day. Provided you don't over-eat, these calories will not be turned into fat.

To ensure you are properly fuelled before your evening workout, aim to consume the majority of your calories and nutrients during the early part of the day – have a good amount for breakfast and lunch, with two or three balanced snacks in between meals. After working out, have a milk-based drink (milk, milkshake, flavoured milk or hot chocolate) to get your protein and carbohydrate. If you've done high-intensity endurance exercise that's depleted muscle stores of glycogen, add a further snack or light meal as soon as possible. Suitable options include a flapjack with fresh fruit, cheese on toast, jacket potato with tuna, pasta with chicken, or a banana with yoghurt. Avoid weight gain by counting this meal towards your daily intake instead of additional to your usual daily meals. Plan ahead to ensure you have all the right foods and ingredients to hand. That way, you'll avoid the temptation of fast foods, sugary snacks or ready meals after your workout.

Opt for meals that provide a good balance of carbohydrate, protein and fat. Here are some ideas for balanced meals that provide a good ratio of carbohydrate, protein and fat.

■ Chicken and vegetable stir-fry with rice

■ Pasta with olives, tomato sauce, grilled fish and salad

■ Grilled meat with vegetables and potatoes

■ Chicken or bean casserole with vegetables

■ Pan-fried fish with vegetables and rice

■ Beef or lentil chilli with rice and vegetables

Plan to have healthy snacks available to consume between meals, approximately every 3–4 hours, according to your schedule and hunger. These will provide enough fuel to sustain intense training. Here are some ideas:

■ Fruit, e.g. bananas, apples, clementines, strawberries

■ Nuts, e.g. cashews, almonds, peanuts

■ Strained Greek yoghurt (contains more protein than ordinary yoghurt)

■ Milk, hot chocolate, latte, milkshakes

■ Wholegrain toast

■ Flapjacks and oat-based bars

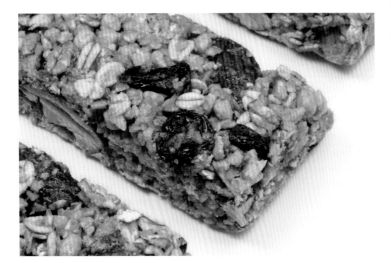

Q&A

I feel ravenous after a workout – how can I avoid binge eating?

An increased appetite is the body's way of telling you to eat. After a hard workout, you need to replace the fuel you have just used – but no more than that! It may be tempting to reward your workout efforts with an indulgent snack, but unless you keep a check on the calorie content, you may end up eating more than you've just burned off.

To prevent weight gain while satisfying your body's requirement for protein and carbohydrate after your session, focus on high-protein foods (such as strained Greek yoghurt, meat, poultry or fish) that promote satiety and aid muscle repair. Add some vegetables, salad and fresh fruits, which contain filling fibre as well as important nutrients.

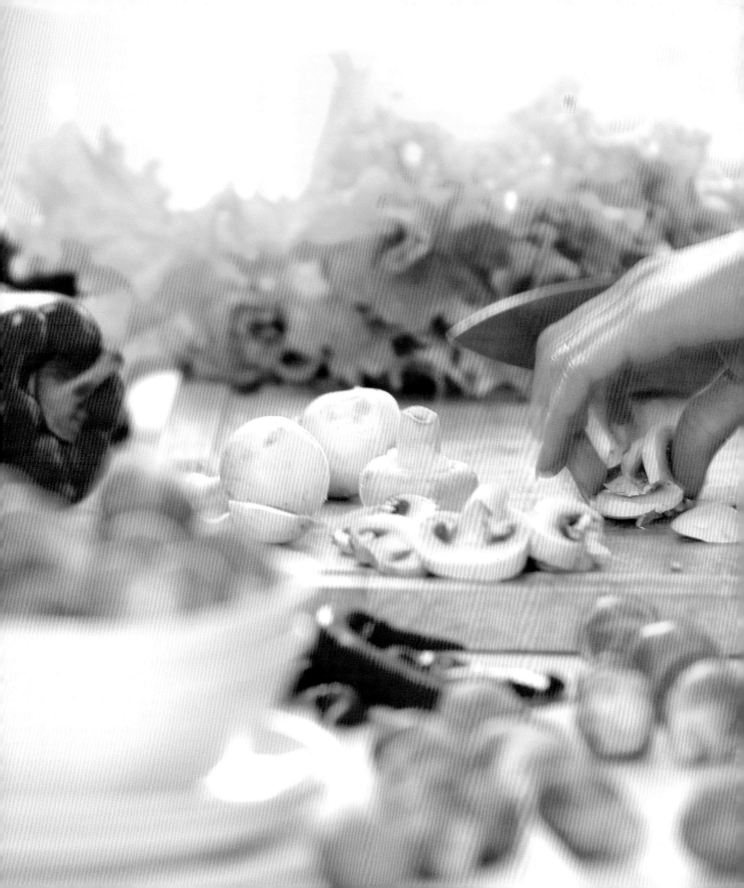

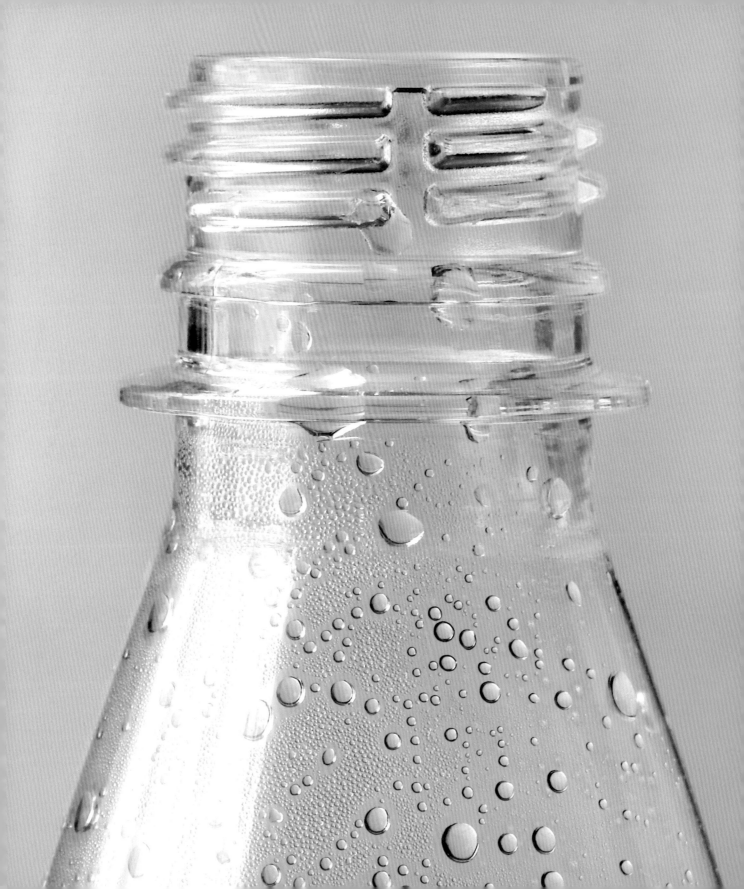

3 HYDRATION AND PERFORMANCE

Every day you lose fluid by sweating, breathing and urinating. But it's the sweating that you need to pay attention to because as soon as you start exercising you start to dehydrate.

Sweating is a vital function. It rids your body of excess heat produced during exercise, maintaining your core body temperature within safe limits – around 37–38°C. Without sweating you would quickly over-heat and die. Fluid loss can be high – up to 500 ml in 30 minutes – depending on how hard and long you are training as well as the surrounding temperature and humidity. Also, heavier people sweat more and some people simply sweat more than others.

If you're exercising for less than an hour, the risk of dehydration is usually small and is unlikely to affect your performance. But if you're exercising for longer, especially in hot humid conditions, then loss of fluid will be greater and this may harm your performance. In these situations, maintaining hydration is crucial if you want to avoid heat-related illness and perform at your best. At the same time, you need to ensure that you don't overhydrate as this can also result in adverse symptoms. This chapter explains how to develop your perfect hydration plan.

How can dehydration affect my performance?

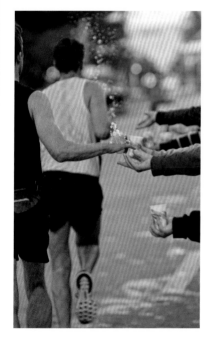

Your body can lose a certain amount of sweat without your performance being affected, but at some point that loss of fluid starts to take a toll. This usually occurs once you have lost around 2–3 per cent in body weight – for example, after about an hour of intense exercise in hot humid conditions – and this can lead to fatigue and a drop in performance during high-intensity endurance activities (Goulet, 2012; Sawka et al., 2007; Shirreffs and Sawka, 2011; Cheuvront et al., 2003; Sawka, 1992).

In one study, running speeds over 5 km and 10 km dropped by 6–7 per cent in runners who were dehydrated (2 per cent body weight loss) compared to full hydration (Armstrong et al., 1985). This translated into a drop in performance of 2.62 minutes over 10 km. In another study, mild dehydration (2 per cent body weight loss) resulted in a higher heart rate, core temperature and perceived exertion (i.e. the exercise felt harder) during a 2-hour cycle trial (Logan-Sprenger *et al.*, 2013).

However, the majority of dehydration studies have been carried out in the lab instead of real-life situations (i.e. races) where loss of fluid has less impact on performance. Researchers have found that dehydration up to 4 per cent does not reduce performance in real-life situations, but dehydration greater than 2 per cent will reduce performance in lab exercise studies (Goulet, 2013).

Once dehydration has reached a certain threshold, though, your body is unable to cool itself efficiently, which puts extra stress on the heart and lungs and means your heart must work harder to pump blood around the body. If you don't consume enough fluid, your blood will become more viscous (or 'thicker') and your heart will need to beat faster to pump the blood around your body (Cheuvront *et al.*, 2005). If dehydration continues, it can have more serious health consequences. A 5 per cent drop in body weight can result in headache, light-headedness, disorientation and shortness of breath.

Dehydration can affect strength and power training. One study found that dehydration resulted in a loss of strength – the amount of weight male lifters could bench press was lower by about 6 kg when they were dehydrated compared to when they were rehydrated (Schoffstall *et al.*, 2001). Dehydration may also increase levels of the catabolic hormone cortisol, and reduce levels of the anabolic hormone testosterone, thus potentially compromising the muscles' adaptation to training.

Is it possible to drink too much?

Overhydration can also have a negative impact on your health and on your workout. Too much fluid causes the sodium in the body to become too diluted, a condition called hyponatraemia, or low blood sodium concentration (*see* page 64). Ironically, the symptoms are similar to those of dehydration: a drop in athletic performance, nausea, lethargy, dizziness and disorientation. Continued hyponatraemia can lead to serious health consequences, such as blackouts and fits.

How can I get the balance right?

The key to avoiding dehydration and overhydration is to stay in your hydration zone. This is the level of hydration that allows you to perform optimally. You can get a good idea as to whether you are within your zone by weighing yourself before and after exercise. You should never consume so much fluid that you actually end up gaining weight. Equally, you should try to avoid losing more than

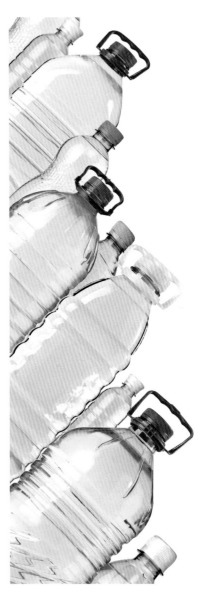

2 or 3 per cent of your body weight. For example, if you weigh 68 kg (150 lb), 2 per cent of your body weight is 1.4 kg (3 lb). So your hydration zone would be between 66.6 kg and 68 kg.

What is the most important hydration advice?

All researchers agree on one thing: you need to start a workout or competition hydrated to minimise the risk of dehydration during exercise. This way you'll have the best chance of putting in your best performance. If you begin dehydrated, this can adversely affect your performance, reducing your power output and your endurance and causing early fatigue (Gigou *et al.*, 2010).

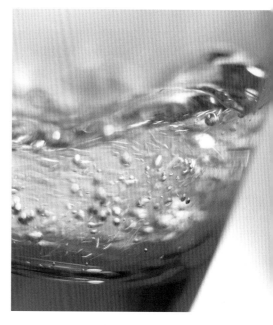

The best strategy is to keep hydrated throughout the day rather than load up with fluid just before your workout. Try to make a habit of drinking water regularly. Have a glass of water first thing in the morning and then schedule drinks during your day. If you train in the evening, ensure you drink plenty of water during the day. If you train early in the morning, make sure to have a drink as soon as you wake up.

The European Food Safety Authority recommends an intake of 2.5 litres of water for men and 2 litres of water for women per day (Jequier and Constant, 2010) – that's approximately 8 glasses.

It's better to drink little and often rather than drinking large amounts in one go, which promotes urination and a greater loss of fluid. Carry a bottle of water with you everywhere: to the gym, office and in the car, as a constant reminder to drink.

How much should I drink before exercise?

The American College of Sports Medicine recommends drinking 5–7 ml of fluid per kg of body weight 4 hours before exercising (Sawka *et al.*, 2007). This is approximately 350–490 ml for a person weighing 70 kg, roughly equivalent to a small bottle of water. The idea is that you should have enough time for your body to excrete what it doesn't need before you set off. It also ensures your body makes up for any previously incurred fluid deficit. Again, don't drink it all in one go – divide into several smaller amounts and sip at regular intervals.

How can I tell if I'm dehydrated?

You can monitor your hydration status by checking the colour of your urine (the 'pee test'). University of Connecticut researchers found that urine colour correlates accurately with hydration status. A pale straw colour indicates good hydration. If it's darker and has a strong odour, then that's a sign that you need to drink more fluid before you start exercising.

What should I drink before exercise?

When it comes to choosing the best pre-exercise drink, water is one of the best ways of hydrating the body. Opt for a drink with sugar (e.g. squash or diluted fruit juice) only if you haven't eaten anything – in which case the sugars in the drink will help maintain blood sugar levels and fuel the muscles. Otherwise, water is a perfect pre-exercise choice, together with a pre-exercise meal or snack.

Is drinking to thirst optimum?

The ACSM currently advise everyone to drink to thirst (Sawka *et al.*, 2009). Feeling thirsty is your body's way of telling you that you need to drink more. Previously, experts advised drinking before you feel thirsty, but this was withdrawn in the light of the number of cases of overhydration (hyponatraemia) during marathons and ultra-distance events.

A study of Boston marathon runners in 2005 found that 13 per cent had hyponatraemia (Almond *et al.*, 2005). As a result, the governing body for marathon physicians (International Marathon Medical Directors Association) made a recommendation that athletes should 'drink to thirst' to avoid hyponatraemia during these events.

Some scientists, such as Professor Tim Noakes at the University of Cape Town, believe that official advice on hydration has been influenced by the marketing claims of the sports drink industry, who have brainwashed athletes to overhydrate. Noakes contends that quite large fluid losses don't lead to dehydration or heat-related illness, and that elite endurance athletes can tolerate significant sweat loss (over 3 per cent) without any negative effect on their performance (Noakes, 2012). He believes that the associated weight loss via sweating may even enhance performance in elite athletes as this improves their power to weight ratio. For example, if a 70 kg athlete loses 2 per cent of body weight (1.4 kg), then he or she will have 1.4 kg less to carry around, so less power will be needed at any given speed.

However, while the ACSM recommendation to drink to thirst may be appropriate for some athletes (e.g. marathon runners who run relatively slowly and take several hours to complete the course), it may not apply to everyone. For example, if you're a faster runner, competing in a shorter event, doing strength training, high-intensity endurance training, intermittent activities or swimming, it's harder to know when you're thirsty and how much to drink. In practice, it can be easy to miss, ignore or override thirst and this may prevent you from performing to your full potential. One

Q&A

Can caffeinated drinks such as coffee and tea dehydrate you?

Coffee and tea contain caffeine, which is a mild diuretic, but they do not dehydrate the body, as was once thought. According to several US studies, drinking caffeine-containing drinks immediately before a workout won't cause dehydration nor have any detrimental effect on your performance (indeed, it may even enhance your endurance, *see* page 125). But, at rest, caffeine drinks may 'make you go' more frequently.

A daily intake of 3 cups of coffee (less than 300 mg of caffeine) results in no larger urine output than water, according to University of Connecticut researchers (Armstrong, 2002; Armstrong *et al.*, 2005). At this level, caffeine is considered safe and unlikely to affect your performance or health.

Drinking coffee and tea regularly builds up your caffeine tolerance, so you experience smaller diuretic effects.

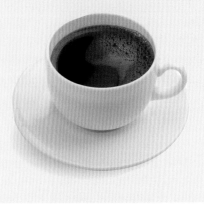

study of runners seeking medical attention after the Boston marathon from 2001 to 2008 found dehydration is almost six times more common than overhydration (Siegel *et al.*, 2009). So a balance needs to be found between preventing both hyponatraemia (overhydration), as well as dehydration, heat stress and poor performance (underhydration).

How much should I drink during exercise?

There are no strict rules on how much you should drink during exercise. It depends on how heavily you are sweating, which in turn depends on your size, your exercise intensity and the temperature and humidity of your surroundings. Generally, bigger people sweat more because they have a smaller skin surface area to weight ratio so it takes more fluid to dissipate the heat. Also exercising at higher intensities and in hot humid conditions increases your sweat rate. It's a myth that sweating heavily means you're unfit. The truth is, sweating is the body's way of regulating temperature so if you sweat readily and profusely it simply means you are getting rid of heat. It does not necessarily indicate your level of fitness.

You may prefer to drink to thirst or follow a schedule that replaces fluid according to your sweat losses (as learned during training by weighing yourself pre- and post-exercise). For most workouts and climates, 400–800 ml/hour will prevent dehydration as well as overhydration. Aim to consume fluids at a rate that keeps pace with your sweat rate. You'll sweat more in hot and humid conditions and when working out harder/faster. It's better to drink little and often – say 100–150 ml every 15 minutes – as this results in greater retention and less urination. You should start drinking early during your workout as it takes about 30 minutes for the fluid to be absorbed into your bloodstream.

Working out how much to drink

Experts advise drinking to thirst, but here's a rough guide to calculating your fluid losses and working out how much to drink:

1. **Know your baseline hydrated weight.**
   Make sure your urine is a light straw colour and then weigh yourself. This will give you your baseline fully hydrated weight.

2. **Estimate your average sweat rate.**
   This will vary according to your exercise intensity and surrounding temperature, but the easiest way to work out how much fluid you lose in sweat is to weigh yourself before and immediately after your

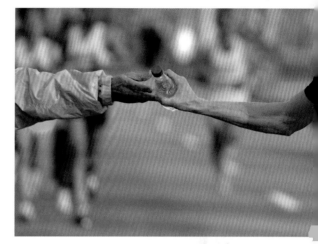

DEHYDRATION SYMPTOMS

The initial signs and symptoms of mild dehydration appear when the body has lost about 2 per cent of its total fluid. These mild dehydration symptoms include:

- Feeling thirsty
- Unusually lacking in energy
- Fatiguing early during exercise
- Feeling too hot
- Skin appears flushed and feels cool and clammy
- Passing only small volumes of dark-coloured urine
- Nausea
- Poor concentration and reduced alertness

Advanced symptoms may include:

- A bad headache
- Becoming dizzy or lightheaded
- Appearing disorientated
- Shortness of breath

exercise session. Your starting weight should be your baseline hydrated weight. Remember not to drink anything for this test.

3. **Work out your hydration requirement.**
   Calculate the difference between your pre- and post-workout weight You can assume that almost all of your weight loss is sweat (although that's not strictly accurate as a small amount will come from the breakdown of carbohydrate and fat). So a weight loss of 0.5 kg represents a fluid loss of about 500 ml. For each 1 kg lost, you should consume 1.5 litres of fluid after exercise, so if you lose ½ kg, you need to make sure that you drink ¾ litre of fluid per hour to fully restore fluid levels.

What should I drink during exercise?

If you're exercising for less than 30 minutes, then fluid losses through sweating are unlikely to be great enough to harm your performance. If you're exercising for longer than 30 minutes you will certainly benefit from drinking something during exercise. But with the growing array of sports drinks it's a confusing choice for most people.

If you're exercising less than 1 hour

For most activities, water is all you need. It is absorbed relatively quickly into your bloodstream and keeps your body hydrated. It's cheap, plentiful and readily available. Extra carbohydrate won't benefit your performance so it's not necessary to consume anything else.

If you're not keen on the taste of water, though, and cannot force enough down, flavour it with a little 'sugar-free' squash or cordial. This helps improve palatability but won't harm or improve your performance. If you prefer to drink ordinary squash, cordial or diluted fruit juice, this will introduce extra sugar (carbohydrate), but provided it's diluted to less than 8 g sugar/100 ml it won't harm your performance. Concentrated drinks containing more than 8 g sugar/100 ml take longer to absorb so may reduce your performance.

Alternatively, just swilling a carbohydrate-containing drink (e.g. squash, cordial or a sports drink) in your mouth could give you a performance boost. Carbohydrate sensors in your mouth send signals to the brain that act on its reward and pleasure centres, so you feel more motivated to keep exercising hard (*see* page 43). However, it's still better to consume the drink if you can.

WHAT IS HYPONATRAEMIA?

Hyponatraemia is defined as having a low blood salt (sodium) concentration (<135mmol/L). This can happen during events lasting several hours – such as cycling, marathon running and hiking – when you drink water excessively. It can also occur when you lose a lot of sodium in sweat and drink water all the time. Excessive sweating combined with drinking only water dilutes the concentration of salts in the body to a dangerously low level. Both scenarios can result in symptoms of hyponatraemia: nausea, lethargy, dizziness and mental confusion. If left untreated, it can lead to seizure, coma and death.

Those most at risk of hyponatraemia are the slowest runners who take a long time to get round the course, and therefore aren't losing that much fluid through sweating. Running at a slow pace also makes it easier to drink 'on the run' and drink more than you need. Best advice? If you plan to exercise for more than 4 hours in warm weather, drink no more than 800 ml per hour, be guided by thirst (don't force yourself to drink) and ensure that you don't drink so much that you weigh more after exercise than before.

If you're exercising for more than 1 hour

Drinks containing carbohydrate – squash, cordial, diluted fruit juice or commercial sports drinks – may be better than plain water when you are exercising hard for longer than 60 minutes. The sugars they contain not only provide fuel for your exercising muscles (thus sparing glycogen), but also speed up the absorption of water into your bloodstream.

Ideally, you should aim to consume 30–60 g of carbohydrate/hour, depending on how hard you are exercising. That's equivalent to 400–800 ml of a 6 per cent drink (6 g sugar/100 ml), such as cordial or squash diluted 1 to 6.

If you're exercising for more than 2 hours

For longer high-intensity sessions, particularly during hot humid conditions when fluid losses are particularly high, a drink containing both carbohydrate (sugars) and sodium may improve your endurance and performance. The sugars speed water absorption, maintain blood glucose levels and fuel your muscles, while the extra sodium helps water retention. The latter is important only when sweat rates are high and prolonged, not when sweat rates are low. If you lose large amounts of fluid and sodium through sweating then blood volume can drop, core temperature can rise and performance will suffer.

Should I always replace electrolytes during exercise?

If you're exercising for less than 2 hours, you won't need to take in extra electrolytes (sodium) in the form of a drink (e.g. sports drinks) or food (Shirreffs and Sawka, 2011). Sodium (and other electrolytes in sports drinks such as potassium, magnesium and chloride) doesn't speed fluid delivery nor have any benefit on your performance (Noakes, 2012; Sawka *et al.*, 2007). The only value of sodium (and other electrolytes) in sports drinks is to help your body retain water and stimulate thirst – and this isn't necessary during most activities that last for less than 2 hours. What's more, sodium in sports drinks will not prevent cramps or heat illness (Noakes, 2012).

In general, sports drinks containing sodium are really only beneficial if you're exercising at a high intensity for more than 2 hours (and therefore losing significant amounts of sodium in sweat), or in extremely hot humid conditions when your sweat losses are exceptionally high. However, one study at the University of Ottawa suggests that sodium may not be necessary if you're exercising in fairly cool conditions

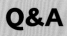

Q&A

Which are better for rehydrating you: cold or warm drinks?

Cold drinks not only quench your thirst better, but may also help improve your performance if you're exercising in hot and humid conditions. One study found that athletes who drank a cold drink (4°C) before and during exercise in the heat were able to cycle 23 per cent longer than those consuming a warm drink (37°C) (Lee *et al.*, 2008). The cold drink helped slow the rate of heat gain and reduced the athletes' heart rates, sweat rates and perceived exertion.

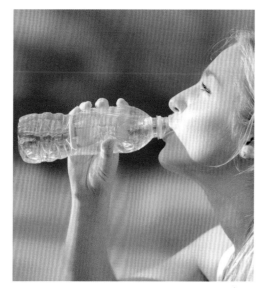

(Cosgrove and Black, 2013). Cyclists who consumed a salt tablet (plus water) did not perform better than those who just drank water during a 72-km time trial of 3 hours' duration in cool conditions.

Although sweat can taste 'salty', you don't lose very much sodium during most activities. Sweat is always more diluted than body fluids, which means that you're losing proportionally more water than sodium. So it's more important to replace water than to replace sodium during exercise. Your body regulates the amount of sodium lost in sweat (and urine) to equal the amount you consume through food and drink. So if you consume a lot of sodium then your sweat will contain more than those who consume less sodium. People in hot countries survive on a fraction of the amount of salt eaten by people in the UK.

Unless you're exercising for longer than 2 hours in hot humid conditions and sweating profusely, then it is not necessary to consume a sports drink containing electrolytes.

Sports drinks guide

Water is the best option if you're exercising for less than an hour or if you're exercising at a fairly low intensity that doesn't deplete your glycogen or make you sweat much (e.g. in cool conditions). Most people may not consider plain water a sports drink, but it is when it aids your performance.

But if you're exercising at a high intensity for longer than an hour or you're sweating heavily, then a homemade or commercial sports drink may improve your performance and hasten your recovery. They are essentially sugar (and salt) solutions, and can be divided into four main categories:

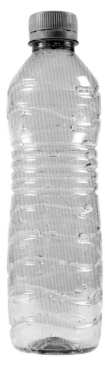

- Low-calorie, hydration, 'lite' or fitness drinks
- Isotonic drinks
- Dual source sports drinks
- Recovery drinks

The difference between the above is down to the concentration of sugars. As a rule the higher the sugar content the slower the water absorption rate, but the greater the fuel delivery – you have to decide whether you need mainly fluid or fuel.

Sports drinks include commercial drinks as well as homemade drinks. As the former are expensive and, for most sports and fitness activities, unnecessary, consider making your own from everyday ingredients, such as squash or cordial, for a fraction of the cost. The formulation you choose is essentially down to your performance goals, budget and convenience.

Low-calorie, hydration, 'lite' or 'fitness' drinks

Hydration drinks contain between 2 g and 4 g sugar/100 ml, which is about half that of most isotonic drinks, along with small amounts of sodium. They are hypotonic drinks as they contain a lower concentration of dissolved particles (sugars and electrolytes) than the body's fluids.

They will hydrate you but offer no real benefit over water. The main appeal is probably their taste – as they are sweetened and flavoured, they work to increase your desire to drink, so you're less likely to get dehydrated. The amount of sugar (and calories) is very low, which won't improve your endurance, but may appeal to you if you are exercising to lose or maintain weight, i.e. you don't want extra calories. The sodium in the drink won't speed water absorption or aid performance, but it may stimulate thirst and encourage water retention.

When they may be useful:

A specific sports drink isn't really necessary if you're exercising for less than an hour, but if you're losing significant fluid through sweating (e.g. in hot humid conditions) and don't like the taste of water, then hydration drinks would be a good option.

Make your own:

Add a dash of sugar-free or ordinary cordial or squash to your water bottle (salt is unnecessary during exercise lasting less than 2 hours).

Isotonic drinks

Isotonic sports drinks are essentially drinks containing 4 g to 8 g sugar/100 ml (usually glucose, sucrose, fructose and maltodextrin) and electrolytes (sodium, potassium, magnesium and chloride). Isotonic means they contain the same concentration of dissolved particles (sugar and electrolytes) as body fluids, which promotes quicker hydration compared with plain water. They also contain sweeteners, preservatives and colours and some may also provide selected vitamins. The additives in sports drinks – as with any food or drink – are considered safe but you may wish to avoid high intakes, as the long-term risks (particularly of additive combinations) are unknown.

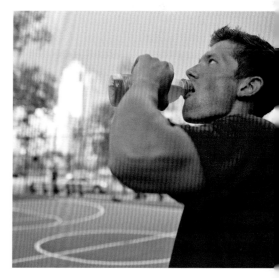

The main benefit of isotonic sports drinks is their sugar content. Sugar speeds the absorption of water, tops up blood sugar levels, and provides extra fuel for intense exercise lasting over an hour.

Their sodium content increases the urge to drink, aids water retention, and improves the drink's taste. It does not speed water absorption and is not necessary for most activities lasting less than 2 hours. Other electrolytes and vitamins in the drink have no immediate effect on your performance – they just make it a bit 'healthier'!

Research from the University of Texas found that drinking water during 1 hour of cycling improved performance by 6 per cent compared with no water, but drinking an isotonic sports drink resulted in a 12 per cent improvement in performance (Below *et al.*, 1995). Researchers at the University of Loughborough found that sports drinks improved running time by 3.9 minutes over 42 km compared with drinking water (Tsintzas *et al.*, 1995).

Try to avoid drinks containing more than 8 g of sugar (hypertonic) as these slow the rate at which fluid is absorbed, and can cause stomach discomfort.

Alternatively, you can fuel your workouts with real food. In one study at Appalachian State University, bananas were shown to be as effective as a 6 per cent carbohydrate sports drink in fuelling performance in a 75-km cycling time trial (Kennerly *et al.*, 2011).

When they may be useful:

If you're exercising at a high intensity for longer than 60 minutes, then isotonic sports drinks may help improve your endurance. By providing the working muscles with additional fuel you can delay fatigue. The optimal amount is 30–60 g/hour for activities between 1 and 3 hours, or 60–90 g for activities longer than 3 hours. One litre of an isotonic sports drink will provide around 60 g of carbohydrate.

Make your own:

To make an isotonic drink containing 50–60 g carbohydrate/litre, add any one (not all) of the following options to a 1-litre water bottle and top up with water:

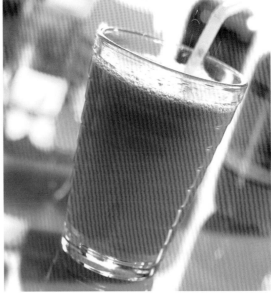

100 ml cordial
130 ml squash
500 ml apple or grape juice.

For exercise lasting more than 2 hours, add 0.5–0.7 g (one eighth of a teaspoon) salt.

Dual source sports drinks

These 'new generation' sports drinks contain two types of carbohydrate: glucose (or maltodextrin) and fructose in a ratio of 2 to 1. The idea is that combining fructose with glucose or maltodextrin (a short chain of glucose molecules made from corn starch) allows the body to absorb carbohydrate faster, and therefore deliver them to the muscles faster than regular isotonic drinks. This is clearly an advantage when you are exercising at high intensities for prolonged periods (3 hours or longer) and therefore burning carbohydrate at a high rate.

Why do they contain two carbohydrate sources? Normally, the body cannot absorb more than 1.1 g glucose/minute – any excess sits in the stomach longer and can result in discomfort – which is why scientists recommend consuming no more than 30–60 g carbohydrate/hour during prolonged endurance exercise. However, when you mix fructose and glucose (or maltodextrin), carbohydrate absorption can be increased to 1.5 g/minute (or 90 g/hour), which increases the speed of carbohydrate delivery to the muscles (Wallis *et al.*, 2005). However, a more recent study suggests that 78 g/hour may be the optimal dose (Smith *et al.*, 2013). Faster absorption is due to the fact that fructose is absorbed by a different mechanism from glucose. Each sugar has its own 'transporter' that takes it from the intestines to the bloodstream. So, by consuming two different types of carbohydrate (glucose/maltodextrin and fructose) you can utilise the two different transporters instead of one and overcome the problem of glucose saturation.

Dual source sports drinks may feasibly help improve your performance and endurance during exercise lasting more than 3 hours – for example, in marathons, triathlons, cycling events and ultra-distance events, where glycogen depletion would be a limiting factor. Do they work? Researchers at Birmingham University found that when cyclists consumed a 2 to 1 fructose drink during 3 hours of cycling, they completed a one-hour time trial 8 per cent faster compared with drinking either water or a glucose-only sports drink (Currell and Jeukendrup, 2008).

When they may be useful:

These drinks may be a good option if you're exercising at a high intensity for more than 3 hours. They supply a higher amount of carbohydrate than regular isotonic drinks, which will help spare your muscle glycogen stores and increase your endurance.

Make your own:

Mix 60 g of glucose (or a mixture of glucose and maltodextrin) and 30 g of fructose in 1 litre of water. If this tastes too sweet or you find that it is too concentrated for you (e.g. it sits in your stomach during training), experiment with different amounts and ratios to find what suits you best. Fructose is sweeter than

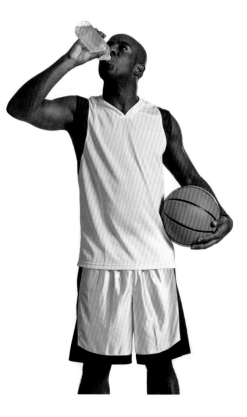

glucose and you may prefer to mix it with more maltodextrin than glucose to get the right balance of sweetness. Add a dash of sugar-free squash to boost flavour if you like.

Recovery drinks

These contain a mixture of carbohydrate and protein. The carbohydrate is usually a mixture of sugar and maltodextrin, and the protein may be whey or a mixture of whey, casein and soy. They are designed to be consumed immediately after exercise because consuming protein with carbohydrate stimulates muscle protein synthesis (i.e. muscle repair and growth) and therefore speeds recovery to a greater extent than carbohydrate alone.

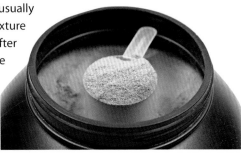

The amounts and ratio of carbohydrate to protein varies between brands, but research has shown that a 3 to 1 ratio of carbohydrate to protein promotes most rapid glycogen refuelling (Phillips *et al.*, 2007). You'll need 1–1.5 g of carbohydrate/kg of body weight (Rodrigues *et al.*, 2009), but you should adjust this depending on your activity. After long intense endurance sessions when you've depleted significant amounts of glycogen, you'll need more carbohydrate than after shorter sessions or strength training. The optimal amount of protein that promotes muscle building is 15–25 g (Moore *et al.*, 2009). You'll need more (i.e. a dose at the upper end of the range) after strength and power training, and less (i.e. a dose at the lower end of the range) after endurance activities.

Whey is a 'fast-acting' protein which is rapidly digested and absorbed. It also has all the essential amino acids and high levels of the branched chain amino acid, leucine, which has been shown to trigger muscle protein synthesis. Studies have shown that whey is superior to casein and soy in promoting muscle repair after resistance exercise (Tang, 2009; Churchward-Venne *et al.*, 2012). However, casein and soy are added to some brands because they are absorbed slower than whey and provide a 'timed release' of protein to the muscles. The whey delivers quickly while the casein and soy provide a more sustained rise in blood levels of amino acids, extending the window for muscle building.

When they may be useful:

Recovery drinks may be useful if you're planning to exercise again within 24 hours. The 2-hour period after exercise represents an ideal opportunity to maximise muscle recovery and glycogen refuelling because recovery takes place one and a half times faster than normal. However, if you're not intending to exercise for another 24 hours or if you've just done a light (non-depleting) training session, then it's less critical to refuel immediately afterwards. Provided you get your daily protein and carbohydrate (and other nutritional requirements) over the next 24 hours, then you'll recover just the same by your next session.

Make your own:

600 ml of whole, semi-skimmed or skimmed milk provides the all-important 20 g of high-quality protein along with 30 g of carbohydrate, electrolytes (sodium) and other nutrients (*see* page 51). Milk also helps rehydrate the body more effectively than sports drinks (Shirreffs *et al.*, 2007).

Alternatively, make your own recovery drink with 600 ml milk and 2 tablespoons (30 g) milkshake powder (add more or less according to the length, intensity and type of exercise). Or blend 500 ml milk, a banana, 100 ml yoghurt, and a scoop (25 g) of milkshake powder (after endurance exercise) or whey protein powder (after strength exercise).

Are fizzy drinks beneficial or detrimental during exercise?

Fizzy drinks such as cola are popular among endurance athletes, but this is probably due more to taste and perceived benefits rather than science!

Fizzy drinks are an unlikely option for a sports drink because their sugar content (10 g/100 ml) is higher than the optimal range for isotonic drinks (4–8 g/100 ml). They are hypertonic (contain a higher concentration of dissolved particles than body fluids), which means they empty from the stomach relatively slowly – making fluid absorption slower if compared to plain water. Nevertheless, cola is popular with many triathletes, cyclists and long-distance runners in the latter stages of races.

The main appeal of cola is due to its caffeine – a 330 ml can of Coke has between 32 mg (regular Coke) and 42 mg (Diet Coke) caffeine. This is about half that contained in a cup of coffee or a can of energy drink, and possibly less than many people imagine – you would need around 200 mg caffeine to get a performance-enhancing effect. It is possible, though, that the caffeine in cola enhances performance by reducing the perceived effort of exercise, improving concentration and increasing endurance, but you would need to drink around 1 litre.

According to studies, carbonation has no detrimental or beneficial effect on a drink's ability to rehydrate the body during exercise or deliver carbohydrate to exercising

SPORTS DRINKS DECODED

- **Glucose** – the basic sugar unit and the body's immediate source of cellular energy.
- **Sucrose** – ordinary white sugar, consisting of one molecule each of glucose and fructose.
- **Fructose** – tastes sweeter than sucrose and produces a smaller blood sugar rise.
- **Maltodextrin** (glucose polymer) – produced commercially from cornstarch; comprises between 4 and 20 glucose units. Is much less sweet than sucrose.
- **Taurine** – an amino acid; claims have been made that it helps combat muscle breakdown, although there is no sound research to back this up.
- **Beta-alanine and histidine** – amino acids that make carnitine, which helps buffer lactic acid produced during very high-intensity exercise.
- **Leucine and valine** – branched chain amino acids that may help reduce muscle damage and aid muscle recovery, although you can get them from foods such as milk, eggs and meat.
- **Vitamin E** – an antioxidant that may help reduce free radical damage, although you can get it from foods such as nuts and avocado.
- **Caffeine** – may increase mental acuity and performance, and decrease perceived effort.

muscles. Researchers at Washington University School of Medicine gave cyclists fizzy or flat drinks containing either 10 per cent carbohydrate or no carbohydrate on four separate occasions (Zachwieja *et al.*, 1992). Both the fizzy and flat drinks emptied from the stomach at the same speed, and raised blood sugar levels to a similar extent.

If you prefer drinking carbonated drinks on the move and find the bubbles don't upset your stomach, then go ahead – but they won't give you any advantage over flat drinks. If it's cola you crave, dilute it one or two parts to one part water to give you a better carbohydrate-concentration (4–8 per cent) for maximum absorption. Because it is a very acidic drink with the ability to dissolve tooth enamel you should swish water around your mouth after a drink.

Replacing lost fluids: how much should I drink after exercise?

The sooner you begin replacing the fluid you have lost through sweat, the sooner you will recover and cut the risk of post-workout dehydration. Fail to drink enough and you will feel listless with a risk of headache and nausea. As a rule of thumb, you need to drink 750 ml of water for every 0.5 kg of body weight lost during your workout (1 kg of lost weight is equal to 1 litre of sweat, which needs to be replaced with 1.5 litres of fluid). Try to drink around 500 ml over the first 30 minutes, little and often, then keep sipping until you are passing pale urine. Drinking slowly rather than guzzling the lot in one go will hydrate you better. If you pass only a small volume of dark yellow urine, or if you feel headachy and nauseous, then you need to keep on drinking.

What should I drink after exercise?

Cell recovery and muscle growth can only take place once cells are fully hydrated so it's important to replace fluids lost through sweating as soon as possible after exercise. The type of drink you choose depends on how much sweat you have lost and how rapidly you want to recover.

If you have exercised for *less than an hour* and/or lost little fluid through sweating, then opt for water or diluted cordial or squash. These drinks will do a perfectly good job of replacing lost fluid (and glycogen) and therefore restore normal fluid balance in your cells. There's no need to consume a specially formulated sports drink or recovery drink as your sodium losses will have been relatively small. These can be easily replaced in your diet.

But after longer sessions lasting *an hour or more*, or after intense exercise in hot humid conditions when sweat losses have been high, opt for a drink

MYTH: DEHYDRATION CAUSES CRAMPS

There is no evidence that people who get cramps are more dehydrated and it's also a myth that cramps are due to lack of salt. One study of 209 Ironman athletes found no significant difference in the levels of dehydration or electrolyte loss between those who developed cramp and those who didn't, which challenges the prevailing electrolyte-depletion hypothesis of cramps (Schwellnus *et al.*, 2011).

A more plausible explanation is the 'altered neuromuscular control hypothesis', which suggests that an altered neuromuscular control occurs during fatigue (Minetto *et al.*, 2013). This makes sense because cramping often occurs at the end of tough workouts or at the beginning of unaccustomed workouts when neuromuscular alterations occur. People who get cramp tend to be those who do high-intensity exercise. Researchers also believe that there is an element of genetic susceptibility and that some people are simply more prone to cramp than others. If you get cramp during exercise, slow down, stretch, and try to relax the affected muscle(s). Correcting any muscle imbalances and developing a more efficient technique for your sport may also help avoid cramp.

containing *sodium* (alternatively you can consume water plus food with sodium). The sodium will help enhance fluid retention and the restoration of normal fluid balance. Sodium will also make you feel thirstier, encouraging you to drink more.

Water (or drinks without sodium) isn't the best option because it can increase urine production and make you excrete more fluid than you drink. Large volumes of water dilute the sodium in the bloodstream, reducing its 'osmolality', signalling an increase in urine production. Also, water can quench your thirst before you're fully hydrated so you may not drink enough to restore normal fluid balance in your cells. So, if you want rapid recovery and/or plan to exercise again within a few hours, adding sodium either in the form of a drink or in the form of food will reduce urine production and promote water retention.

Ideally your recovery drink should contain a mixture of *protein* and *carbohydrate* as well as *sodium*. Studies have shown that this unique combination of nutrients promotes better rehydration after exercise compared with a normal carbohydrate-sodium sports drink (James *et al.*, 2013). You can opt for a commercial recovery drink or make your own (*see* pages 70–71 – above).

Milk (any type) is a good option for a recovery drink because it provides both water and sodium along with protein and carbohydrate (*see* page 51). Studies have shown that it is more effective than isotonic sports drinks for promoting rehydration after exercise (Shirreffs *et al.*, 2007). What's more, milk and other milk-based drinks (such as milkshakes, hot chocolate or lattes) offer additional nutrients, such as calcium and B vitamins.

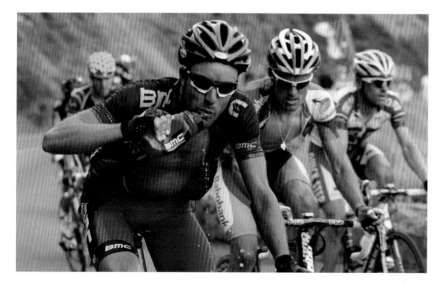

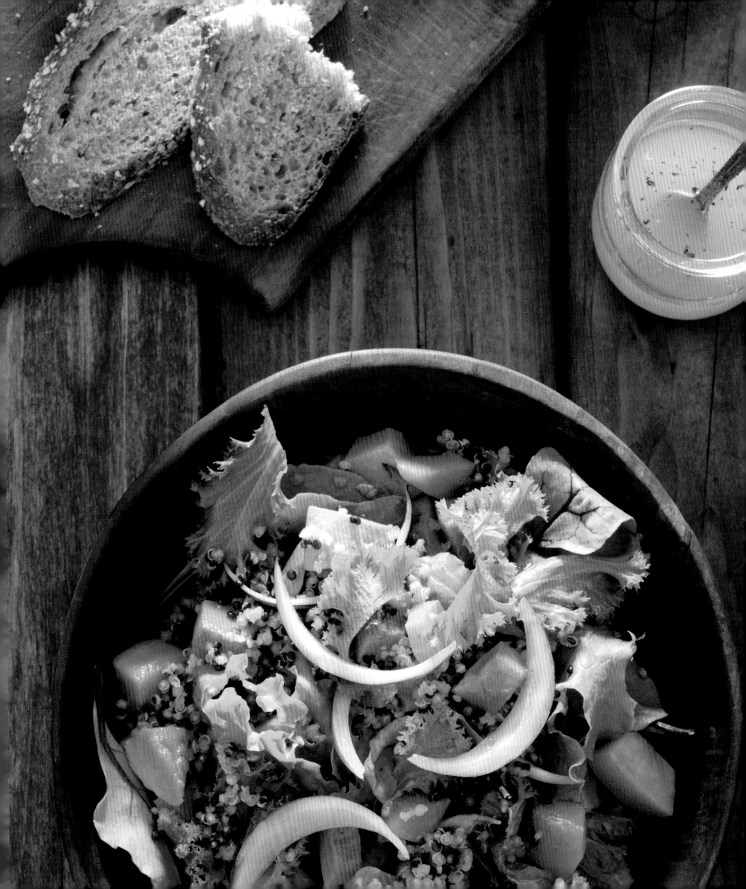

4 EATING FOR FAT LOSS

Whether you wish to lose a few pounds or have a bigger weight loss goal, exercise provides a healthy way to burn off extra calories. The problem is that even if you work out daily, it is hard to lose weight through exercise alone. Increasing your activity will speed your fat loss, but you also need to make some changes to the way you eat.

Many popular diets are based on gimmicks or unproven science and often involve cutting out certain food categories or limiting certain nutrients. Neither strategy will help you sustain weight loss.

The secret to successful long-term fat loss is to reduce total calories without compromising your intake of essential nutrients. In practise, this means adjusting your carbohydrate intake and making dietary changes that are sustainable.

Instead, focus on the foods your body was designed to eat, not processed foods, and adjust your carbohydrate intake to suit your exercise programme. It's a matter of listening to your body, responding to your natural appetite cues, and eating the amount of food you need.

There isn't one diet that is right for everyone. What you should eat depends on a lot of things including: age, gender, current health, activity levels, goals, environment, financial status and personal preferences, etc.

This chapter provides you with a set of scientifically proven guidelines to help you lose fat, maintain muscle, and achieve your optimal weight.

First, a quick lesson about body fat …

Body fat is not a redundant depot of unwanted calories. Although it does serve as a fuel store, it has a number of other important functions in the body. First, you need a certain amount of body fat ('essential fat') to stay alive and for your body to function normally. Fat is essential for the functioning of the brain, nerves and bone marrow, and it cushions the internal organs and keeps them warm. It is also important for healthy skin, hair and nails. Women need a certain amount of body fat to maintain normal hormonal balance and menstrual function. All this accounts for about 3 per cent of body weight in men and 9–12 per cent of body weight in women. If you go below these levels, then you risk health problems. Women can develop menstrual irregularities and bone loss.

The remainder is stored under the skin and around the abdominal organs. Here it serves a number of other critical roles in your body. Fat cells are involved with hormone production (they produce the appetite-regulating hormone leptin, and also modify oestrogen) and they also regulate the immune system. People with very low body fat levels are more prone to infection and illness.

What body fat percentage should I aim for?

Scientists recommend body fat levels of 18–25 per cent for women and 13–18 per cent for men. These ranges are associated with the lowest health risk in population studies. However, lower body fat levels are advantageous to performance in many sports: body fat levels in the region of 10–18 per cent in women and 5–10 per cent in men are common among elite athletes.

But make sure your goal is realistic and that you don't try to attain a body fat level that is too low. Having a very low body fat percentage does not necessarily result in improved performance. Going below a certain threshold depresses the immune system, upsets hormonal balance and, for women, increases the risk of developing amenorrhoea (cessation of periods), infertility, osteopenia (bone mineral loss), stress fractures and osteoporosis. It's not possible to prescribe a body fat that's perfect for everyone – the optimum level of fat that produces peak performance is different for each sport and each individual. It's best to think of an optimal body fat range that maximises your performance and minimises health risks. Use the above figures as a guide and then a combination of trial and error (as well as your good judgement) to find a weight and body fat that is right for you.

For competitive athletes, there's a weight and body fat at which you perform at your best. However, you cannot maintain your competitive weight year-round – it's fine to gain a little weight (fat) between competitions. Try to keep within 8 per cent of your competitive weight. For example, if you compete at a weight of 65 kg, aim to stay within 5 kg of that weight – i.e. below 70 kg – between competitions.

To count calories or not?

Calories are the most important factor when it comes to weight loss. Ultimately you need to consume fewer calories than you expend to achieve your fat loss goal, but you do not necessarily need to count them. Simply focusing on the source, or quality, of your calories is often sufficient to create a calorie deficit.

Counting calories, checking labels and portion sizes can be time-consuming and there's usually a big margin of error involved. But on the plus side, it can make you more aware of your dietary habits and give you a better idea of what you're eating. By being more conscious of what you eat, you will be able to eat more healthily. Of course, counting calories isn't essential, but it is a tool that can help get you started in the right direction.

If you don't like the idea of calorie counting, focus instead on avoiding sugar and processed foods and eating nutrient-dense unprocessed foods.

WHAT ARE CALORIES?

In simple terms, a calorie is a unit of energy. Specifically, it's the amount of energy required to heat 1 g of water by 1°C. As this is a very small amount of energy, food labels use larger units called kilocalories (kcal), which is 1,000 calories. When people mention calories in the everyday sense, they are really talking about kilocalories.

Now, set yourself a goal...

To help you succeed at losing weight, set a realistic goal and reward your positive behaviour. A goal has to be personal, specific, realistic and measurable:

- *Personal* – you have to believe in your goal and truly want to achieve it. For example, 'I know that losing 5 lb will allow me to run faster and make the top 10 in my next half-marathon.'

- *Specific* – you need to clearly define what you want to achieve. For example, 'I want to reduce my waist size by 6 cm in six weeks.'

- *Realistic* – your goal has to be realistic and attainable for your body shape and lifestyle.

- *Measurable* – you need to track your progress and state how you will know when you've reached your goal. Keeping a food diary and training log will help you monitor your progress and allow you to see whether you met the goal.

Your goal should also be:

- *Agreed* – agree your goal with someone else (e.g. your coach or a friend) and write it down. This signals a commitment to change and makes it more likely that you will be successful.

- *Time-scaled* – once you have decided on your goal, you should prioritise steps, organise plans, and establish a timescale for reaching your goal.

- *Reward yourself* – rewarding yourself when you have reached a goal helps you stay motivated and focused. Rewards can be something simple like going to watch a film for reaching a weekly target or a new pair of training shoes for reaching a six-month goal.

Four weight loss myths debunked

There are many myths when it comes to fat loss that could be preventing you from reaching your health and performance goals. Here's the truth about four of the most common weight loss myths:

Myth 1: *Exercising on an empty stomach makes you lose weight faster*

Exercising on an empty stomach – such as first thing in the morning – may force your body to burn more fat than carbohydrate for fuel, but it won't necessarily help you lose weight faster. Researchers at Northumbria University asked 12 male volunteers to do a moderate-intensity treadmill workout at 10 a.m. either after an overnight fast or after eating breakfast (Gonzalez *et al.*, 2013). They found that those who exercised on an empty stomach burned up to 20 per cent more fat compared with those who ate a meal before training.

A study by Belgian researchers found that the muscles could be 'trained' to burn a higher percentage of fat by exercising in a fasted state (Proeyen *et al.*, 2011). Athletes completed a workout, either after they had fasted or after consuming carbohydrate. After six weeks, those who trained after fasting burned a higher percentage of calories from fat and increased the number of fat-burning enzymes in their muscles.

However, all this doesn't mean you'll lose more fat. A study at Loughborough University found that those who exercised before breakfast ate the same number of calories over the course of the day as those who exercised after breakfast (Deighton *et al.*, 2012).

The bottom line is that if you're exercising to lose fat, then exercising on an empty stomach may in theory burn more fat, but it won't necessarily help you shed the pounds faster. What matters is your overall daily calorie intake relative to your output.

Myth 2: All calories are equal

In principle, all calories are equal in terms of the energy they deliver. However, the amount of energy you get from a food depends on where those calories come from (i.e. protein, carbohydrate or fat). In other words, 100 calories worth of chicken or broccoli is not the same as 100 calories worth of sugar.

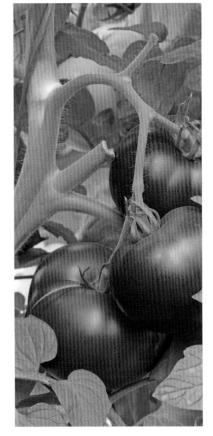

Different foods have different effects on your body, even if they contain the same number of calories. Once ingested, proteins, carbohydrate and fats are digested, absorbed and metabolised by the body. The energy required for these processes differs between the various macronutrients. Some of the calories you consume are used up digesting the food and turning it into fuel available to the body. This is called the thermic effect of food, or thermogenesis. For example, the body uses more calories to digest and metabolise protein than it does carbohydrate or fat. When you consume protein, approximately 25–30 per cent is 'wasted' or lost as heat. In contrast, 6–8 per cent of the calories consumed in the form of carbohydrate and 2–3 per cent of the calories in fat are used up in digesting it (Jequier *et al.*, 2002). In other words, carbohydrate and fat are relatively easy for the body to turn into energy. Protein needs to be broken down into amino acids, which is a far more complex process. So if you eat 100 calories of protein, only about 70–75 will be absorbed – the rest is lost as heat.

You also need to consider the effects the different macronutrients have on satiety (how full up they make you feel). Protein has the highest satiating effect, with refined carbohydrate having the lowest satiating effect. So 100 calories of steak will make you feel more satiated than 100 calories of crisps.

Some types of calories can increase your appetite and cause you to eat more. For example, sugar promotes overconsumption because it increases the palatability of foods and drinks (*see* page 9). Protein, fat and low-GI (non-sweetened) carbohydrate, on the other hand, are less likely to make you want to eat more after consuming them.

In summary, when looking purely from a measurement perspective, all calories are equal, but in terms of weight management and health, they are not. That's why you need to focus on the quality of the calories you're eating and not simply count calories.

Myth 3: You need to cut or burn 3,500 calories to lose a pound

The 3,500-calories-equals-a-pound rule is regarded as dogma when it comes to dieting but is not very accurate. This bit of arithmetic comes from a small starvation study done in the 1950s. It has no scientific basis and doesn't take account of your body composition, your current weight or metabolism.

Cutting 3,500 calories to lose a pound may 'work' for the first 10 to 12 days of a diet as you lose water weight, but when the body weight drops you carry less mass and start to burn fewer calories for the same activities. After a period of time, you stop losing weight even if you continue to cut back by the same amount. This is called 'adaptive thermogenesis' and refers to the lowering of your metabolic rate as your body weight goes down and you eat fewer calories (Rosenbaum and Leibel, 2010). Essentially it's your body's way of conserving energy when energy is in short supply (Tremblay *et al.*, 2013). One study found that when people were put on a restricted-calorie diet, they had a lower metabolic rate than could be explained by their weight loss (Heilbronn *et al.*, 2006).

What's more, when you create a calorie deficit by eating less, you don't just lose fat but you burn off protein too. So any weight loss comes from a loss of both fat and muscle mass.

Myth 4: Fat makes you fat

This myth is based on the premise that at 9 calories/g, fat is more fattening than other nutrients. The truth is that fat is no more likely to make you fat than any other nutrient – possibly less so. Fat plays an important structural role in the body, helping to form cell membranes and make hormones.

Fat may be high in calories, but it is also satiating so it gives the body the feeling of being full – providing you eat fat in as natural a form as possible (e.g. milk, cheese, nuts, fish) and not in a highly processed form (e.g. biscuits, cakes and

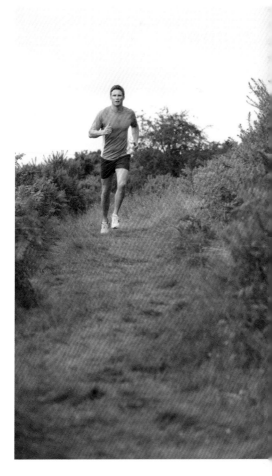

pies). Contrary to popular belief, fats can actually help you lose weight because they help appetite control. Refined carbohydrate and sugar, on the other hand, don't promote satiety and can make you want to eat more.

Rather than avoiding fat to lose fat, add natural unprocessed fats, such as butter, olive oil, nuts, seeds, oily fish and avocados, to your diet, while cutting down on sugar and refined carbohydrate.

Ten steps to fat loss

Everyone loses (and gains) weight differently and there's no one diet that will work the same for everyone. In fact there is no 'right' diet, nor is there any evidence that one particular diet works better with an individual's specific metabolism (Pagoto and Appelhans, 2013). The truth is that ALL diets will work if you follow them. Some people are predisposed to gain weight easily and must work harder than the average person to burn it off. But one thing is certain: that losing fat requires a sustained daily effort. Here we look at ten ways that will help you lose fat without sacrificing hard-earned muscle.

1. Eat real food

Losing fat is far easier if you focus on 'real' foods, for example, minimally processed foods such as meat, poultry, fish, eggs, beans, lentils, nuts, seeds, fruit, vegetables, whole grains, tubers, milk, cheese, yoghurt, butter, olive oil and butter.

Real food is filling, satiating and delicious. When you focus on eating these foods you will feel less hungry, and have less desire to eat 'junk' food. Eating real food limits the amount you eat without needing much restraint. It helps reduce the total number of calories you eat. For example, it takes fewer calories to fill up with vegetables than with crisps. Try eating vegetables or salad first at every meal before everything else. You'll find that you'll eat fewer calories as these foods have a high satiety rating. Put simply, you'll burn more calories, feel more satiated, and lose more weight if you get most of your calories from 'real' food rather than from processed food even if the calories are the same.

Avoid high-sugar foods and drinks, and any processed foods labelled 'low fat', 'reduced fat' or 'fat-free'. These fat-reduced foods are often higher in sugar, starch or salt than the full-fat versions to make up for the flavour and texture that's lost when food manufacturers take out the fat.

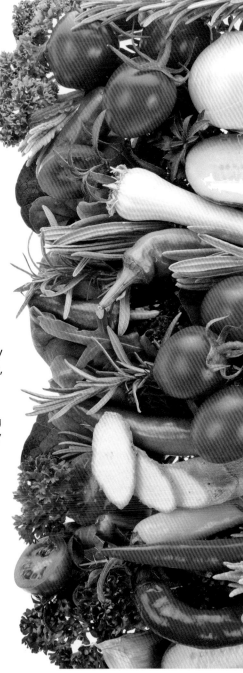

In fact, reduced- and low-fat foods may actually make you gain weight as their high sugar content triggers insulin release, which drives sugar from the bloodstream into cells to be converted into fat (once glycogen stores are full). They fail to satisfy your appetite and reduce levels of dopamine (a feel-good hormone) in the brain and can cause overeating. Because these foods claim to be 'low in fat', we automatically assume they are healthy and tend to eat bigger portions (i.e. more calories) as shown in a study by Cornell University in the USA where people who were given products labelled 'light' or 'reduced fat' ate up to 50 per cent more than they did with the standard product.

2. Adjust carbohydrate

The key to fat loss is to adjust your carbohydrate intake. This doesn't mean cutting carbohydrate completely or forgoing pasta and potatoes, but reducing carbohydrate to a level that gives you just enough fuel for your training, but not too little to cause fatigue or illness. Training at high intensities with low glycogen levels may result in fatigue, lethargy and poor performance. Over time, eating too little carbohydrate may lead to overtraining, where your performance drops and your health suffers.

If you do high-intensity endurance training, then you'll certainly need carbohydrate immediately before and after training as you can't fuel intense exercise (more than 70 per cent of maximal aerobic capacity) from fat alone. On the other hand, if you do mostly lower-intensity training (less than 70 per cent of maximal aerobic capacity), then cutting carbohydrate and training with lower muscle glycogen levels should not adversely affect your performance.

Reducing carbohydrate not only lowers your calorie intake, but it also lowers your insulin levels, which puts your body in fat-burning mode rather than fat-storage mode. The job of insulin is to transport glucose and fatty acids from the blood into cells. When insulin levels are high (e.g. after eating a high-carbohydrate meal), the body stops burning fat and burns carbohydrate instead. It also makes the body store excess carbohydrate (as glycogen or fat) and fat. By reducing your carbohydrate intake, you will lower blood glucose levels and insulin production, which means less fat storage and more fat burning. In other words, the body will turn to fat (not carbohydrate) for fuel.

By cutting carbohydrate from high-sugar foods and drinks you'll also find it much easier to control your appetite. High intakes of sugar (fructose) can alter the balance of brain chemicals as it acts on the same hormonal pathways that reward behaviour. Rather than satisfying your appetite it may increase it (*see* page 8).

So, how much carbohydrate should you eat? There are no hard and fast rules – it's essentially a matter of minimising sugars and processed starches, and replacing them with foods rich in protein and healthy fats. These foods reduce appetite, promote satiety, and cause an automatic restriction in calories (making calorie counting unnecessary in many cases). Protein also spares muscle, so you should be able to maintain your hard-earned muscle while losing fat.

You'll need to eat less than your 'maintenance' level and you'll need to eat more on training days when your energy needs are higher. For most people, this is likely to average 3–5 g carbohydrate/kg of body weight/day (Phillips and van Loon, 2011).

Table 4.1 gives you a suggested amount of carbohydrate based on your activity level. For example, if you're in the 'moderate-intensity training' category (exercising for an hour a day), you should eat 3–5 g carbohydrate/kg of body weight/day. Try to get most of your carbohydrate in the 2–4-hour time period before exercise and the 2–4-hour time period after exercise so that your performance won't suffer and you will have enough energy to train hard.

High-carbohydrate foods should be the mainstay of your meals before and after intense training sessions. Aim for around 50–200 g of carbohydrate 2–4 hours before exercise, depending on how close your meal is to your workout, and also how long and hard you plan to train. If you have very little time between eating and exercising, or if you plan to exercise for less than an hour, then eat less. On the other hand, if you have longer to digest your food or if you plan to do a hard session lasting more than an hour, then eat more carbohydrate.

Consuming adequate carbohydrate is particularly important in the period immediately following intense exercise as this can speed recovery and help prevent overtraining. Your muscles are more sensitive to insulin in the 2-hour period following exercise, and glycogen manufacture is one and a half times faster than normal. Aim for about 1 g/kg of body weight, or 60 g for a 60 kg person, but adjust this according to the duration and intensity of your workout. If you have exercised longer than 2 hours, you may need more as your glycogen stores will be depleted. If you have exercised for less than an hour (or at a low intensity), then you will need less. Adding 15–25 g protein to your post-exercise recovery drinks and meals will promote optimal recovery after hard training (*see* page 50).

By eating less carbohydrate and storing less glycogen, you can literally 'train' your muscles to use more fat and less carbohydrate for fuel. If there is less blood glucose or muscle glycogen available, the muscles will turn to fat for fuel. So limiting carbohydrate and eating fat causes the muscles to adapt to fat for endurance activities. However, this only applies to endurance activities performed at a low to moderate intensity, such as walking, cycling and running, and not high-intensity endurance (e.g. running fast) or anaerobic activities (e.g.

Q&A

Are low-carbohydrate diets healthy?

An analysis of 23 randomised controlled trials concluded that low-carbohydrate diets are effective for producing weight loss as well as lowering important risk factors for heart disease, including abdominal fat, blood pressure and blood fats (Santos *et al.*, 2012). Another study found that people following a low-carbohydrate high-fat diet lost more body fat than those following a high-carbohydrate low-fat diet, and reduced their risk of metabolic syndrome (Volek *et al.*, 2009).

weight lifting). You need carbohydrate to fuel high-intensity activities. Without it, you will fatigue quickly and your performance will drop. In summary, if you lower your carbohydrate, you may need to reduce the intensity of your training or devise a way of consuming carbohydrate in the time period before, during and after training.

Burning fat rather than carbohydrate may in fact improve some types of endurance training – at least in theory. By training your muscles to use fat for fuel you will preserve your limited and more 'valuable' glycogen stores. This makes sense on paper because the body has vastly greater fat storage compared with glycogen storage.

However, there's no evidence yet from studies that this results in better performance during competitions! At the end of the day, carbohydrate intake is very individual – if a lower-carbohydrate diet works for you and you're feeling full of energy, then carry on. If you're getting great results on a high-carbohydrate diet and you are not overweight, then there's no reason to cut your carbohydrate.

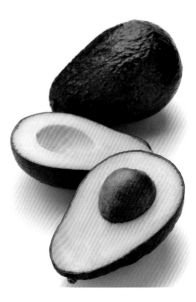

TABLE 4.1 HOW MUCH CARBOHYDRATE SHOULD I EAT FOR FAT LOSS?

Activity level	Recommended carbo-hydrate intake g/kg of body weight/day	Carbohydrate/day for a 50 kg person	Carbohydrate/day for a 60 kg person	Carbohydrate/day for a 70 kg person
Very light training (low-intensity or skill-based exercise)	1–3 g/kg	50–150 g	60–180 g	70–210 g
Moderate-intensity training (approx 1 hour/day)	3–5 g	150–250 g	180–300 g	210–350 g
Moderate- to high-intensity training (1–3 hours/day)	5–7 g	250–350 g	300–420 g	350–490 g
Very high-intensity training (> 4 hours/day)	7–10 g	350–500 g	420–600 g	490–700 g

3. Don't be afraid of fat

Fat may be high in calories but it is also satiating, so it gives the body the feeling of being full, again the emphasis is on consuming calories in as natural a form as possible (e.g. milk, cheese, nuts, fish) and not in processed foods (e.g. pies, cakes and biscuits).

The key to weight control is satiety, the feeling of fullness and satisfaction that you should have at the end of a meal. The reason most diets fail is that they are too restrictive (and often limit fat, which promotes satiety!) and don't satisfy hunger. Low-fat diets are not satiating. The bottom line? To lose weight and stay lean, stick with full-fat versions of real foods and listen to your appetite. That way, you'll eat fewer calories overall.

Feeling full and satisfied while eating nutritious foods you like makes it much easier to lose unwanted pounds. Without fat in the mix, you are left hungry soon after eating, seek out another low-fat 'fix', thus setting up a vicious cycle of over-eating.

The biggest mistake is reducing fat while cutting carbohydrate – you'll end up starving! Eating foods that satisfy your hunger will mean that you consume fewer calories – it's that simple.

Higher-fat diets may be more successful in promoting weight loss than low-fat diets. In one study, people who ate a higher-fat Mediterranean-style diet (35 per cent of calories from fat) lost more weight than those following a low-fat diet for two years (Shai *et al.*, 2008).

4. Up your protein intake

Make sure you include adequate amounts of protein. Not eating enough protein may induce hunger and muscle loss when you're dieting.

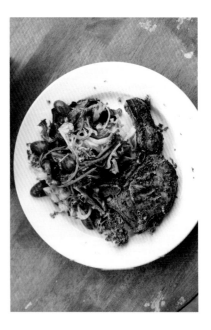

Protein has also been shown to reduce appetite and induce satiety ('fullness') more than carbohydrate, which is why it is particularly useful when you're trying to lose (or maintain) weight (Westerterp-Plantenga *et al.*, 2012). Protein slows the time it takes for food to move from your stomach to your intestines, helping you feel full longer. It also reduces levels of hunger hormones, such as ghrelin, and increases levels of satiety hormones such as glucagon and cholecystokinin, which tell the brain that you're full. One study found that the more protein and less carbohydrate people ate, the less hungry they felt (Belza *et al.*, 2013). Those who ate the most protein had the highest levels of satiety hormones and the lowest levels of hunger hormones.

Carbohydrate simply doesn't provide the same satiated feeling that protein does. Therefore if you increase your protein intake without making any conscious attempt to eat less, you'll naturally eat less anyway due to reduced appetite. This is another important sense in which protein, carbohydrate and fat calories are not equal (*see* page 78).

One study found that protein not only helped people feel less hungry, but it also resulted in significant weight loss (Weigle *et al.*, 2005). When dieters increased their protein intake from 15 per cent to 30 per cent of total calories, they felt much fuller even though they ate the same number of calories. When they were then allowed to eat as much as they wanted, they voluntarily reduced their daily intake by 441 calories per day and lost almost 11 pounds in 12 weeks.

Increasing your protein intake will also help maintain your muscle mass while losing body fat. A study found that when athletes ate 1.6 g protein/kg of body weight (twice the RDA) or 2.4 g/protein/kg of body weight (three times the RDA), they lost more fat and less muscle compared with those who just ate the RDA for protein – 0.8 g/kg of body weight (Pasiakos *et al.*, 2013). All three groups lost the same amount of weight, but those eating extra protein had a more favourable body composition at the end of the dieting period. Increasing protein from two to three times the RDA made no difference, so the optimal amount of protein is likely to be between 1.6 g and 2.4/kg/body weight (Phillips and Van Loon, 2011). That's 112–168 g for a 70 kg person.

Include a portion of high-quality protein (meat, poultry, fish, dairy foods, eggs) with each meal. The exact amount will depend on your fitness programme or sport, but aim for 1.6–2.0 g of protein/kg of body weight. For speedy recovery, you should also include around 15–25 g protein in your post-exercise snack (*see* page 50).

5. Eat when hungry

It may sound obvious, but if you eat only when you're hungry and listen to your body's appetite cues then your weight will automatically find its set-point (provided you also follow the rest of the advice in this chapter). If you're not hungry you probably don't need to eat yet. There's no need to eat if your body doesn't need the fuel.

6. Choose naturally fibre-rich foods

If you eat mostly unprocessed food you'll automatically reap the benefits of fibre. Foods such as fruit, vegetables, beans, fish and whole grains do a better job of satisfying your hunger than foods rich in sugar and refined starch. Low-satiety foods, such as cakes, biscuits and chocolate, are easy to over-eat, empty from your stomach quickly, and leave you hungry again in a relatively short time.

By taking up more space in your stomach, fibre-rich foods help to fill you up and reduce your appetite. Fibre expands in the gut,

HOW TO CUT DOWN ON SUGAR

1. Avoid:
   - Soft drinks – these contain very high levels (typically 35 g sugar/330 ml can) and the sugar is rapidly absorbed by the body.
   - Fruit juices – surprisingly contain the same amount of sugar as soft drinks.
   - Sweets – they provide sugar and no other nutrients.
   - Biscuits and cakes – these are high in sugar and refined carbohydrate.
   - Low-fat or reduced-fat foods – biscuits, desserts, etc. that have the fat removed are often very high in sugar.
2. Drink water instead of soft drinks and fruit juice.
3. Try substituting some of the sugar in recipes with natural sweet ingredients such as cinnamon, nutmeg, vanilla, almond extract, ginger or lemon.
4. Simply avoid processed foods and satisfy your sweet tooth with fresh fruit instead.

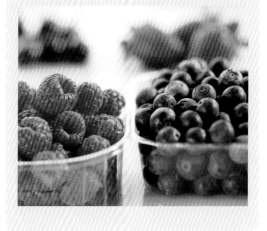

thereby making you feel fuller. It slows the rate that foods pass through your digestive system and stabilises blood sugar levels. One study has shown that people who increased their fibre intake for 4 months ate fewer calories and lost an average of 5 lb. For each 1 g increase in total fibre consumed, their weight decreased by 0.25 kg and fat decreased by 0.25 percentage point (Tucker and Thomas, 2009).

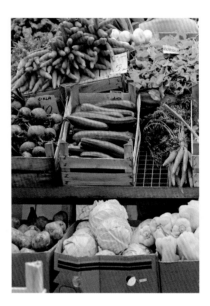

Also, fibre-rich foods require more chewing, which helps slow down your eating and stops you over-eating. Eating slowly gives your brain the chance to recognise that you're full.

Whole fruits are more filling than dried or pureed versions and vastly more filling than juice. You can eat an awful lot of apples, for example, without taking in a lot of calories. They make your stomach feel full because they take up so much space. But a glass of apple juice doesn't satisfy your appetite in the same way, even though it has the same number of calories.

7. Track your progress

You can track your progress by measuring your waist circumference and weighing yourself once a week. Focusing only on your weight and weighing yourself every day can be misleading and reduce your motivation. There is little point in measuring yourself more often than weekly as your weight can fluctuate day to day depending on hydration levels.

When you stand on the scales you are measuring muscles, bone and internal organs as well as fat. You may gain muscle weight but lose fat, but this won't register on the scales. Using either your waist circumference or your body fat percentage will help you track your fat loss and give you a more accurate idea of your progress.

Waist circumference

Your waist circumference is a good reflection of your abdominal fat and your total body fat percentage, and studies show it is more accurate than BMI in predicting your risk of heart disease and type 2 diabetes (Janssen *et al.*, 2002). Ideally your waist should be less than 80 cm (for women) and less than 94 cm (for men)

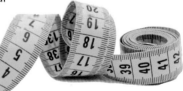

A loss of 1 cm around your waist equates to fat loss of approximately 1 kg. Put the measuring tape around your middle, slightly above your navel – at the midpoint between your hip bone and the bottom of your ribs. Exhale and relax – don't suck in your stomach.

Body fat percentage

Percentage body fat can be measured using skin-fold callipers or bioelectrical impedance. These techniques will tell you how much of you is muscle and how much is fat:

- Skin-fold measurements using callipers should be carried out by a trained person who would measure the thickness of the layer of fat beneath the skin at various sites of the body. It works on the theory that 50 per cent of total body fat is stored under the skin. Most assessments involve measurements at four sites: the triceps, biceps, below the shoulder blades, and mid-way between the hip and navel. The accuracy depends on the level of skill of the person taking the measurements. It is less accurate for very lean and obese individuals.

- Bioelectrical impedance measures the resistance to a small electrical current passed through two points of the body. The more fat present, the greater the resistance. A person's hydration status (and, for women, stage of the menstrual cycle) can affect the reading. It is also less accurate for very lean and very overweight individuals.

8. Don't skip breakfast

Occasionally skipping breakfast may help reduce your daily calorie intake (Clayton and James, 2015) but is not a good weight loss strategy if you want to train hard later in the day. Researchers from Loughborough University, UK, found that those who omitted breakfast experienced a 4.5% drop in their performance in a cycling time trial (after lunch but before dinner) (Clayton *et al.*, 2015).

Skipping breakfast may also make you burn fewer calories by reducing your spontaneous physical activity. A study from the University of Bath, UK, found that people who eat breakfast burn more calories – about 442 calories – by being active, mainly in the morning after eating than those who skip breakfast (Betts *et al.*, 2014). However, contrary to popular belief, eating breakfast does not increase your metabolic rate.

It makes sense to eat more food when your energy needs are greatest and less when your needs are lower. For most people, this means eating early in the day. Breakfast therefore provides your body with fuel when you need it most. The calories you eat at this time will be used to fuel your daily activities and workouts, instead of being stored as body fat (as they are if eaten in the evening). What you eat for breakfast is important too. Researchers have found that eating high-protein foods for breakfast significantly improves appetite control and stops food cravings later in the day (Leidy *et al.*, 2013). Those who ate foods such as eggs, meat or fish for breakfast felt more satisfied and went on to eat fewer calories in the day than those who ate a bowl of cereal. Protein and fat both cut hunger, and increased satiety, compared with foods rich in carbohydrate.

Here are some high-protein breakfasts:

- 200 g of 2 per cent fat Greek yoghurt with 25 g nuts

- 2 scrambled eggs and 1 slice of toast

- Milkshake made with 300 ml semi-skimmed milk, 150 g pot of low-fat fruit yoghurt and 125 g berries

- 120 g smoked haddock fillet with spinach and 1 poached egg

- 50 g smoked salmon with 1 scrambled egg on ½ a bagel

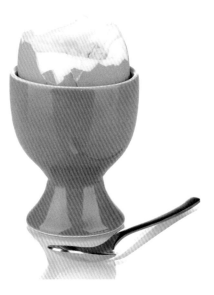

9. Get enough sleep

Getting enough sleep is also important when it comes to weight control. Studies have shown that the less you sleep, the more you are likely to eat during the day (St-Onge *et al.*, 2012). This is because lack of sleep boosts levels of the hormone ghrelin, which makes you feel hungry, while lowering levels of the hormone leptin, which makes you feel full (Spiegel *et al.*, 2004). This hormonal imbalance sends a signal to the brain that more food is needed when, in fact, enough has been eaten. Research at the University of Chicago shows that sleeping for 4 hours or less increases levels of the stress hormone cortisol, which makes you feel hungry (Leproult and Van Cauter, 2010).

In one 2009 US study, those who averaged 5.5 hours' sleep ate 221 more calories than those who slept about 8.5 hours (Nedeltcheva, 2009). Although they didn't eat bigger meals they did snack more in the evening than the well-rested group, and consumed more carbohydrate. Another study in the *American Journal of Epidemiology* found that women who got less than 5 hours' sleep were 33 per cent more likely to gain weight over 16 years than those that get 7–8 hours' sleep (Patel *et al.*, 2006). People who get 5 hours' sleep gained 1 kg during the 16-year study, although their calorie intake was no higher than those getting more sleep. Researchers speculate that a lack of sleep somehow depresses your metabolism so you burn fewer calories throughout the day.

Here are some ways to help you get a better night's sleep:

1. Get up at the same time, even at weekends. In the long term, this will help the body get into a regular sleep pattern.

2. Avoid daytime naps and go to bed only when you are sleepy.

3. Avoid caffeine after 2 p.m. – it takes time for caffeine to leave the body.

4. Limit your alcohol intake 3 hours before bedtime. While alcohol might make you feel relaxed, it disrupts your sleep and you are likely to wake up feeling less refreshed.

5. Limit exercise in the 4 hours before bedtime. Physical activity can make it difficult to get to sleep for several hours afterwards.

6. Spend as much time as possible in daylight (at least 15 minutes every day). This is good for your circadian rhythm (your 'body clock').

7. Make sure that your bed is comfortable, your bedroom is dark enough, and that it stays at a reasonable temperature.

8. Avoid television and laptops in bed.

9. Have a hot bath an hour before bedtime – the cooling down after a bath makes you sleepy.

10. Do the right type of exercise

Exercise is an important part of any fat loss programme. Not only does it burn calories but it also has a favourable effect on your body composition, helping maintain muscle while losing fat. Some people find they become hungrier and eat more when they begin a new exercise programme (the 'compensation effect'), but you can avoid this by upping your protein intake. Protein increases satiety more than carbohydrate or fat (*see* page 84). Also, by eating real food and avoiding processed foods, you'll find your appetite automatically adjusts.

For the best fat-burning results, make sure you include both resistance exercise and cardiovascular (endurance or aerobic) exercise in your weekly schedule. The American College of Sports Medicine recommends two weight training sessions a week in addition to five 20–40-minute sessions of aerobic activity.

Resistance training

The most effective strategy for building or toning muscles and burning fat simultaneously is resistance or weight training. This doesn't necessarily mean lifting heavy weights – conditioning exercises using light or moderate weights tone muscle and prevents the loss of lean body tissue when you're losing fat. The American College of Sports Medicine recommend 2–3 days a week for beginners, progressing to 4–5 times a week for the more advanced (Garber *et al.*, 2009). In general, train each muscle group for 2–4 sets of exercises with a weight you can lift only 8–12 times, taking 30 seconds' rest between sets. You won't necessarily burn more calories lifting weights than doing aerobic exercise, but the increased muscle mass you develop as a result will improve your body.

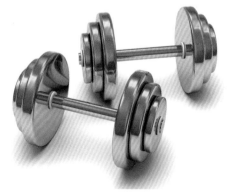

Cardiovascular exercise

Cardiovascular exercise burns calories and increases the body's ability to burn fat. It is any kind of activity that uses the large muscle groups of the body and can be kept up for 20–40 minutes, with your heart rate in your target training range (60–85 per cent of maximum heart rate). Try running, elliptical training machines, swimming, cycling, fast walking and group exercise classes. Vary your activities so you don't become bored. Remember, the higher the resistance, the more muscle you will build, so high-resistance activities such as rowing, stair-climbing, incline running and hard cycling are good for strengthening as well as defining muscles. The American College of Sports Medicine recommends 150 minutes per week to improve your health (Donnelly *et al.*, 2009) or 200–300 minutes to lose weight. That's equivalent to 5 sessions of 30 minutes (for health) or 5 sessions of 60 minutes (weight loss).

A sensible target would be 20–40 minutes per session, 3–5 times per week, but don't overdo it. Increase the intensity and duration of your sessions gradually, aiming for 60 minutes 5 times a week.

Ten more fat-loss tips

1. Plan ahead

Plan your meals for the week and work out exactly what you need. If you make a list before you go shopping, you're more likely to stick to it. Also, planning ahead means you won't get home from work tired and hungry only to discover there's nothing healthy in your fridge to eat.

2. Limit your food choices

Research carried out at Tufts University in Massachusetts found that when people are presented with a wider variety of foods, they eat considerably more (McCrory *et al.*, 1999). Also, when eating a single food, your eating rate slows down, you are satiated more quickly and, therefore, you will eat less. The pleasure of eating a food increases up to the third or fourth bite then drops off. If you have lots of different foods on your plate you prolong the sensory pleasure, which stops you feeling full. The message here is to simplify your diet: place fewer types of food on your plate.

3. Practise portion control

It may sound obvious, but larger portions make you eat more. Researchers have found that when people are given larger food portions they eat more than those given a small portion. In one study at the University of New South Wales,

Q&A

Which burns more calories: weights or cardiovascular training?

During resistance training you burn fewer calories than cardiovascular training – around 250 calories vs. 500 calories per hour (on average). Both exercise modes have a similar 'afterburn' – i.e. the number of calories in the period immediately after exercise. So if you have only a limited amount of time available to exercise, then cardiovascular exercise is probably best for weight loss. However, it is better to have a mix of both resistance and cardio-vascular exercise – this way you will burn fat and build muscle, which will keep you strong and healthy and prevent injury. One study found that people who did a combination of cardiovascular and resistance exercise lost more fat than those doing cardio-only exercise, but also gained more muscle (Willis *et al.*, 2012).

women who were served a large portion consumed 34 per cent more pasta than those served a small portion (Cavanagh *et al.*, 2013). This amounted to about 87 calories of extra calories. Another study at Cornell University in New York found that people ate 45 per cent more popcorn when given a large portion (Wansink *et al.*, 2005). Even when the popcorn was stale, they still ate 33 per cent more.

The size of your plate, the bowls you serve yourself from, and the size of the utensils you use can also make you eat more. Switching to eating from a smaller plate makes the amount you put on it look larger and means you will automatically eat less. So, try serving yourself from smaller bowls and using smaller serving spoons as a lesson in portion control.

4. Start with salad or soup

According to a 2004 study at Pennsylvania State University, eating a large portion of low-energy-density foods, such as salad or fruit, as a starter can cut the number of calories eaten during the main meal by 12 per cent (Rolls *et al.*, 2004). The fibre and water in the salad/fruit takes the edge off the appetite, causing you to eat less of the higher-calorie foods. Starting your meal with a bowl of chunky, fibre-rich soup can cut your calorie intake by 20 per cent, according to a study by the University of Pennsylvania (Flood and Rolls, 2007). The idea is that the fibre in soup fills you up meaning you'll eat less of the higher-calorie foods that follow.

5. Eat without distractions

Don't eat in front of the TV, or while you are working at the computer because you are less likely to notice what you are eating. Studies have shown that the distraction of TV postpones the point at which people stop eating, with TV watchers eating approximately 12–15 per cent more than those who do not eat in front of the TV. In addition, people who watch TV for more than 4 hours a day consume one-third more calories because they have more opportunity to nibble and less opportunity to exercise.

Making time for formal meals at a table rather than grabbing food while on the run or in front of a screen could help you to cut down on unhealthy snacking. Another study found that when women ate five biscuits while playing a computer game they felt less full and wanted more. Those given the same amount of food without any distraction felt sated (Brunstrom and Mitchell, 2006).

6. Eat mindfully

You'll eat fewer calories if you sit down and take time to eat your meal rather than eating on the go. Eating too fast almost certainly leads to over-eating. It means

---

MYTH: BUILDING MUSCLE SPEEDS YOUR METABOLISM

Contrary to popular belief, building muscle doesn't increase your metabolism or add significantly to your daily calorie burn. The oft-quoted statistic that a pound of muscle burns 30–50 calories/day has no scientific basis. In fact, muscle burns just 6 calories/lb (13 calories/kg).

Your basal metabolic rate (the number of calories burned at rest) is largely determined by genetics and total body weight, and is not significantly altered by diet or exercise. That makes sense when you consider that your muscles account for only 28 per cent of the calories you burn at rest – compared to your heart, kidneys, liver and brain which combine to make up as much as 70–80 per cent of your BMR.

However, that's not to say you need not bother adding muscle. Resistance training has many other advantages – it improves athletic performance, makes you look better, helps stop the natural loss of muscle with ageing, makes the chores of everyday life easier, and can reduce the risk of injury. Additionally an hour of resistance training burns 250–400 calories (depending how much rest you take between sets), plus you burn a few more calories post-exercise ('afterburn').

that your hypothalamus – the part of the brain that senses when you are full – doesn't receive the right signals, which explains why you may feel hungrier sooner if you rush a meal. Mindful eating – eating slowly and genuinely relishing each bite – has its origins in Buddhist teachings, where eating food is considered a form of meditation. It will curb your desire to eat more than you need. It's about experiencing food more intensely, taking time to eat food carefully and paying attention to the colours, smells, textures, flavours, temperatures, and even the sounds of your food. When you eat, just eat. Turn off the electronica and focus on the food. Take a (small) bite of food and then put your knife and fork down. Chew patiently and contemplate the flavour and texture of your food, aiming for 25 to 30 chews for each mouthful.

7. Cut down on alcohol

Alcohol calories count too: if you consume several alcoholic drinks in an evening, they can sabotage your fat-loss plan. Alcohol calories can't be stored and have to be used as they are consumed – this means that calories excess to requirements from other foods get stored as fat instead. Alcoholic drinks are often high in calories, for example one small glass of wine contains 120 calories and a bottle of lager contains 130 calories.

8. Recognise thirst

Many people confuse thirst with hunger. It's hard to know sometimes whether it's really food or water your body needs. Both thirst and hunger signals are controlled in the same area of the brain, so it sends the same signal whether you are hungry or thirsty (Mattes, 2010). If you don't recognise the sensation of thirst, you may assume that you are hungry and eat instead of drinking water. Next time you're feeling peckish, drink a glass of water and wait 10 minutes to see if you are still hungry.

9. Avoid liquid calories

Liquid foods move through the body quickly and don't provide the same sense of satisfaction as solid foods. That's why 100 calories of liquid don't satisfy you as 100 calories of solid food would, even though they contain the same number of calories.

MYTH: EATING FREQUENTLY BOOSTS YOUR METABOLISM

Eating several small meals through the day ('grazing') instead of two or three does not increase your metabolism or help you lose fat faster. In one study, there was no difference in weight loss between overweight people who consumed 3 meals a day and those who consumed the same calories as 6 meals a day (Cameron *et al.*, 2010). Other studies have found no correlation between metabolic rate and eating frequency – people who ate 6 times a day did not have a higher metabolic rate than those who ate 2 times a day (Taylor and Garrow, 2001). Although eating temporarily increases the metabolism (the 'thermic effect of food'), this will not greatly increase your total daily calorie burn. A review of 179 studies concluded that eating frequency has no effect on weight loss (Palmer *et al.*, 2009).

However, eating several small meals a day does have other benefits. It lowers blood cholesterol levels, improves appetite control and curbs your hunger. In one study, people who ate several meals had less hunger than those who ate the same amount of food in just 2 meals (Stote *et al.*, 2007). This could help prevent over-eating. When athletes were given 250-calorie snacks, they ate fewer calories at mealtimes, gained lean mass and lost fat (Bernardot *et al.*, 2005). This may be explained by energy partitioning. When small frequent meals are eaten, the calories you consume are more likely to fuel your body's immediate energy need or convert to glycogen than get stored as fat. So if you're a regular exerciser, eating several small meals while dieting may help preserve your muscle mass.

The average person gets around 20 per cent of their daily calories from drinks. So cutting sugar-sweetened drinks is a simple way to save calories. Swap soft drinks for water and limit your alcohol intake to one drink per day. Sweetened drinks ('diet' drinks) are not recommended because they maintain your sweet tooth and may increase your appetite (*see* page 94).

10. Don't shop for food when you're hungry

If you go shopping when you're hungry you will be tempted to fill up your trolley with high-calorie foods like crisps and cakes. One study at Cornell University found that hungry people chose a greater number of high-calorie foods when they shopped either in a supermarket or online (Tal and Wansink, 2013). Those who shopped after eating a meal chose fewer high-calorie foods. Make a shopping list before you go to the supermarket or shop online, that way you'll avoid unplanned supermarket splurges in unhealthy foods and be less likely to make impulsive food choices.

Core menu plans for fat loss

The following core menu plans show the amounts of foods needed to meet your calorie and macronutrient requirements for fat loss. There are two plans providing approximately 2,000 and 1,800 calories suitable for individuals weighing more than 75 kg and less than 75 kg respectively, and exercising at moderate intensity for approximately one hour a day. If you exercise longer than an hour a day or at a very high intensity, then you should increase the portion sizes to take account of your greater calorie expenditure. Similarly, if you exercise for less than an hour or at a low intensity, then you should reduce the portion sizes. There is also a 1,500-calorie menu plan suitable for rest days when you don't do any training.

You should use the core menu plan as a template for developing your individual daily eating plan. Where the menu plan gives a choice of food type (e.g. 'carbohydrate'), simply pick your preferred option (e.g. pasta or potatoes) or substitute an equivalent (high-carbohydrate) food (e.g. quinoa or noodles). Try to vary your choice of fresh fruit and vegetables as much as possible according to what's in season as this will give you a greater range of micronutrients, antioxidants and phytonutrients. Many of the lower-carbohydrate recipes in Part 3 can be

Q&A

Which is best for fat loss: high- or low-intensity exercise?

High-intensity cardiovascular exercise, such as running, burns more body fat than low-intensity activities, such as walking, because it burns more calories. It also conditions the heart and lungs better and encourages the body to burn more fat – and less carbohydrate – 24 hours a day.

However, high-intensity interval training (HIIT) is even more effective for fat burning as well as cardiovascular fitness. The basic concept of HIIT is to train at different speeds for a number of intervals. Researchers at Laval University in Quebec found that 9 times more fat was lost in the group that used HIIT, compared to the group that used traditional steady-intensity cardio (Tremblay *et al.*, 1994). It also increases your metabolic rate for the following 24 hours. In other words, your body's fat-burning process continues long after your workout, even when you are at rest.

HIIT can be performed with a variety of activities or machines – running, swimming, treadmills, bikes, elliptical trainers or skipping-ropes. Pick your equipment of choice, and make sure to warm up properly to prevent injury. Be aware of your own limits, and work out accordingly. After a 10-minute warm-up, try 30–45 seconds of high-intensity exercise, alternating with 1 minute of recovery. Repeat the interval 4 or 5 more times and then cool down for 10 minutes.

incorporated into your plan; simply use the amount of carbohydrate, protein and fat in the core menu plan as a guide.

As a start, measure and weigh your portions carefully to get an idea of what different amounts of foods look like. You will then find it quicker and easier to judge how much to eat.

You should also track your progress – if it's too slow and you're not losing fat, then you may need to cut your portion sizes. Similarly, if it's too rapid and you're losing muscle as well as fat, then you may need to increase your portion sizes.

The menu plans do not give quantities for water or other drinks as the amount you need is quite individual and will vary from day to day according to the climate and your sweat rate. Check your hydration status with the 'pee test' (*see* page 61) and ensure you drink sufficient fluids to maintain proper hydration.

Also note that the menu plans provide guidance on 'real' foods but do not give recommendations for sports supplements or products. You should read the information in Chapter 6 before deciding to incorporate any product into your daily eating plan.

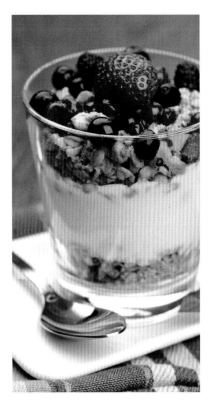

Q&A

Should I replace sugar with sweeteners?

Switching from ordinary soft drinks to diet drinks may sound like a good way to save calories and lose weight but, in fact, the opposite is true. Several studies have found that using sweeteners either make no difference to weight loss or cause people to gain weight. In fact, sweeteners may stimulate the appetite and cause greater weight gain than sugar. In the San Antonio Heart Study, people who drank sweetened drinks gained more weight over an 8-year period compared with those who did not consume them (Fowler *et al*., 2008). The most likely explanation is that when you taste sweet food or drink, your body expects to get calories, so it releases insulin that prepares the body for the energy intake. When this doesn't happen you're left feeling hungry and unsatisfied and end up snacking more and putting on weight. Another reason to avoid sweeteners is that they maintain a desire for sweet food.

MENU

Core menu plan for fat loss for a >75 kg person (training day)

Breakfast	Water 2 eggs; 2 x wholegrain toast 100 g fresh fruit
Snack	25 g nuts 125 g whole-milk yoghurt Water
Lunch	Water Protein: 100 g chicken, meat, fish or 2 eggs or 50 g cheese Vegetables or salad Carbohydrate: 2 slices wholegrain bread or 50 g wholegrain pasta or rice or 200 g potato Fat: 15 g olive oil or butter 100 g fresh fruit and 125 g whole-milk yoghurt
Training (<1h)	Water
Post-training	600 ml whole milk
Dinner	Water Protein: 150 g chicken or fish or 3 eggs or 75 g cheese Vegetables or salad Carbohydrate: 100 g potato or 50 g (uncooked weight) wholegrain pasta or rice Fat: 15 g olive oil or butter 125 g whole-milk yoghurt

Nutritional analysis:

2,047 calories

153 g protein (30 per cent calories)

88 g fat (38 per cent calories)

174 g carbohydrate (32 per cent calories)

MENU

Core menu plan for fat loss for a <75 kg person (training day)

Breakfast	Water 2 eggs; 1 x wholegrain toast 100 g fresh fruit
Snack	25 g nuts 125 g low-fat Greek yoghurt Water
Lunch	Water Protein: 100 g chicken, meat, fish or 2 eggs or 50 g cheese Vegetables or salad Carbohydrate: 2 slices wholegrain bread or 50 g wholegrain pasta or rice or 200 g potato Fat: 1 tbsp olive oil or butter 100 g fresh fruit and 125 g low-fat Greek yoghurt
Training (<1h)	Water
Post-training	600 ml skimmed milk
Dinner	Water Protein: 150 g chicken or fish or 3 eggs or 75 g cheese Carbs: 2 slices of wholegrain bread/50 g wholegrain pasta or rice/200 g potato Vegetables or salad Fat: 1 tbsp olive oil or butter 125 g low-fat Greek yoghurt

Nutritional analysis:

1,725 calories

156 g protein (36 per cent calories)

52 g fat (27 per cent calories)

148 g carbohydrate (34 per cent calories)

MENU

Core menu plan for fat loss (rest day)

Breakfast	Water 2 eggs; 1 x wholegrain toast 100 g fresh fruit
Snack	25 g nuts Water
Lunch	Water Protein: 100 g chicken, meat, fish or 2 eggs or 50 g cheese Vegetables or salad Carbohydrate: 1 slice bread or 25 g wholegrain pasta or rice Fat: 15 g olive/coconut oil or butter 100 g fresh fruit and 125 g whole-milk yoghurt
Snack	400 ml milk 100 g fresh fruit
Dinner	Water Protein: 150 g chicken or fish or 2 eggs or 50 g cheese Vegetables or salad Fat: 15 g olive/coconut oil or butter

Nutritional analysis:

1,543 calories

123 g protein (32 per cent calories)

76 g fat (44 per cent calories)

100 g carbohydrate (24 per cent calories)

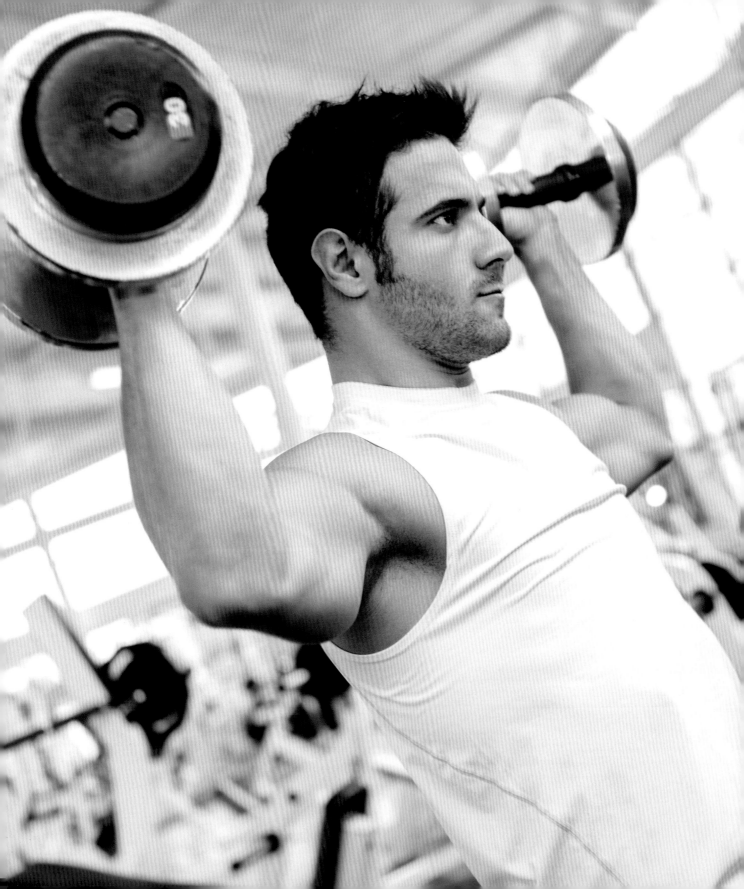

5 EATING FOR MUSCLE GAIN

Perhaps you are naturally very lean and struggle endlessly to add more weight. Or maybe you find it difficult to build muscle without gaining fat and need to achieve better muscle definition. Either way, the answer lies in devising an eating plan that allows you to put on muscle without unwanted fat.

To gain muscle and strength, it's necessary to combine a healthy food intake with a consistent resistance training programme. Without both, you will not gain muscle. Resistance training is the first part of the process: it breaks down muscle tissue, providing a stimulus for muscle growth and creating a demand for additional protein (as well as other nutrients). The second part of the process is recovery; this is when muscle growth takes place and when your diet becomes paramount.

Getting the right amount of calories, protein, carbohydrate and fat as well as vitamins and minerals is the key to optimal muscle growth, recovery and performance. This chapter gives you information on what, when and how much to eat before and after training, and helps you devise a daily eating plan that supports your muscle-building programme.

Why do some people gain muscle more easily than others?

The amount of muscle weight you can expect to gain depends on several genetic factors, including your body type, muscle fibre mix, the arrangement of your motor units and your hormonal balance, as well as your training programme and diet.

An ectomorph (naturally slim build with long lean limbs, narrow shoulders and hips) will find it harder to gain muscle than a mesomorph (muscular, athletic build with wide shoulders and narrow hips). An endomorph (stocky, rounded build with wide shoulders and hips and an even distribution of fat) gains both fat and muscle readily.

THE SCIENCE OF MUSCLE PROTEIN SYNTHESIS

To build muscle you need to combine a resistance training programme with a healthy intake of nutrients. The idea is to stress the muscles just hard enough during your workout to break down muscle proteins and cause very small (micro) tears in the fibres. This 'damage' triggers muscle protein synthesis (MPS), or muscle growth (Rennie and Kipton, 2000). After your workout, the muscle releases cytokines (hormone-like molecules) that signal muscle repair for up to 48 hours. These activate various pathways such as MTOR and AKT that begin the process of MPS. MTOR, which is short for the Mammalian Target of Rapamyacin, is the functioning unit that senses nutrient and oxygen levels in cells. AKT signals cell division and growth. These pathways enable amino acids to pass from the bloodstream into the muscle cell and then get transported within the cell to where they will be assembled into new muscle proteins. Thus, these new proteins are added to the muscle fibres, making the muscle stronger and denser.

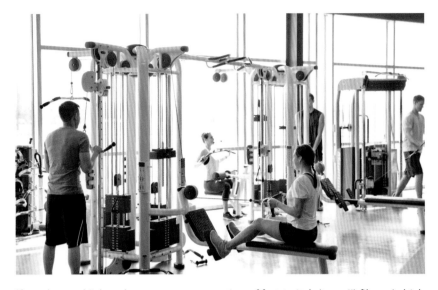

If you have a higher-than-average proportion of fast-twitch (type II) fibres (which generate power and increase in size more readily than the slow-twitch (type I or endurance) fibres), you will probably respond faster to a strength-training programme.

People who tend to gain strength and size very rapidly may have an above-average number of muscle fibres in each motor unit. For the same effort, they generate a higher force output than the average person. This creates a bigger stimulus for muscle growth.

On the other hand, people with a higher natural level of the male (anabolic) sex hormones, such as testosterone, will also gain muscle faster. That is why women cannot achieve the muscle mass or size of men unless they take anabolic steroids.

How fast can I expect to gain weight?

When it comes to muscle gain there is no quick fix that will allow you to pack on more muscle quickly. It's physiologically impossible to gain more than ½ kg (1 lb) of muscle per week although, for most people, ½–1 kg per month would be a more realistic goal if you use an effective training programme supported by the right diet (ACSM, 2009; Houston, 1999). Mass gains of 20 per cent of your starting body weight are common after the first year of training, but the rate of weight gain will gradually drop off over the years as you approach your genetic potential.

Remember that gaining muscle is a long-term goal and not something that can be achieved in a few weeks. If you're dedicated and consistent in your efforts, you'll make progress. Obviously, your age, genetics, body type, training experience and work ethic will affect your gains. Women usually experience about 50–75 per cent of the gains of men – i.e. ¼–¾ kg/month – partly due to their smaller initial body weight and smaller muscle mass, and partly due to lower levels of anabolic hormones. It's better to keep focused and realistic by training hard, eating healthily and ensuring you recover properly; this will result in you achieving a more muscular physique.

How many calories?

In order to build muscle you need to consume more calories in a day than your body burns, because building new muscle requires extra energy (calories). This cannot be over-emphasised! One study found that athletes following a resistance-training programme gained the same amount of body weight and muscle mass whether they got extra calories from protein or carbohydrate (Rozenek *et al.*, 2002). However, it is better these additional calories come from a balanced ratio of carbohydrate, protein and fat, and not 'junk food calories'.

To gain lean weight at the optimal rate you should begin by increasing your usual daily calorie intake by 20 per cent. Of course, this assumes that you know what your maintenance calories actually are. If you do, just add 20 per cent. If not, estimate your calories using the formula on page 4. Or use this quick estimate:

To gain weight: 42–48 calories/kg of body weight for weight gain
To maintain weight: 35–40 calories/kg of body weight

For example, if you normally consume 2,700 kcal daily without gaining weight, to gain muscle mass you will need to eat 2,700 x 1.2 = 3,240 kcal.

However, you may need to adjust your calories depending on your individual metabolism. Bear in mind that not all of the extra calories will be turned into muscle. Some of them will be 'wasted' as heat as your metabolic rate increases when you over-consume calories (around 7 per cent). This is called adaptive thermogenesis and may partly explain why some people (ectomorphs) struggle to gain weight despite eating large quantities of food! Similarly, when you cut calories to lose weight, your metabolic rate drops to conserve energy.

Another reason why some people find it difficult to gain weight ('hard gainers') is non-exercise activity thermogenesis ('NEAT'), which are the calories you burn doing activities that aren't exercise, for example, fidgeting, moving around. Hard gainers usually have a high NEAT energy expenditure – they burn lots of calories through excess activity.

Is it possible to build muscle without gaining fat?

To build muscle you need to consume a calorie surplus. The problem is some of these excess calories will go towards the repair and growth of new muscle, and some of the calories may spill over and be stored as fat. It's possible to minimise fat gain while gaining muscle, but don't expect to reduce it – you cannot build muscle and lose fat at the same time. Instead, you should prioritise your goal, i.e. build muscle or lose fat and focus on one at a time. The trick is to keep your calorie surplus high enough for muscle growth, but not so high that it results in fat storage. Follow these simple rules:

- Get your calories from real foods – it's far harder to gain fat if you focus on 'real' foods, i.e. minimally processed foods such as meat, poultry, fish, eggs, beans, lentils, nuts, seeds, fruit, vegetables, whole grains, milk, cheese, yoghurt, butter, olive oil and butter. These foods increase satiety and reduce hunger (for more on this see Chapter 4).

- Don't go overboard with your calorie surplus – most people only need a surplus of 300–500 calories a day. Going any higher than this is likely to start a spill over and your body may store these extra calories as fat.

- Track your calories – use a calorie counter app such as myfitnesspal or a simple pad and pen to keep a food diary. You don't have to be very accurate, but you do need to have a good idea of your daily calorie intake.

- Train for muscle gain – an intense, effective workout routine is essential to stimulate growth and put your calorie surplus to use. If you don't follow a consistent training programme, then the extra calories you consume will turn into fat.

- Include some cardiovascular exercise – incorporating a few short (10–20 minutes), high-intensity interval cardiovascular sessions a week is a good way to keep those unwanted fat gains under control. This kind of exercise supports muscle growth while eliminating excess fat storage.

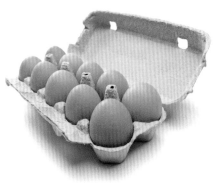

How much carbohydrate should I consume?

You need to consume enough carbohydrate to achieve high muscle glycogen levels, the main fuel for resistance training. Eating too little carbohydrate means training with low levels of muscle glycogen, which risks excessive protein (muscle) breakdown.

A good guide as to whether you are eating enough carbohydrate is your performance. If you get easily fatigued and struggle to complete your workout, or you find you're not able to progress your workouts by lifting heavier weights, performing more reps or more sets, then you are probably training with low glycogen levels. Try increasing your carbohydrate intake by an extra 50–100 g daily to restore glycogen levels.

On the other hand, eating too much carbohydrate won't give you extra energy, nor help you train harder. Ironically, you may feel more tired and lethargic, particularly if you eat too much sugar and refined carbohydrate ('white' bread, pasta, rice and cereals) before your workout. These foods can spike your insulin levels, which results in lower blood glucose levels. This rebound effect can make you feel tired, weak and lightheaded. Instead, eat a low-GI meal that includes protein and fat as well as carbohydrate 2–4 hours before exercise. If you need an energy boost before training and you haven't eaten for more than 4 hours, then have a smaller meal or snack.

Once your glycogen stores are filled, excess carbohydrate are converted into fat, meaning that you might put on weight. Try to listen to your body and you'll soon find the balance between too little and too much carbohydrate.

Table 1.1 on page 4 gives the carbohydrate intake for different training schedules. In general, carbohydrate requirements increase with increasing training duration and intensity (Rodriguez *et al.*, 2009; IOC, 2011). So, the longer and more intense your training sessions, the more carbohydrate you will need to fuel your workout. However, you should factor in rest periods between sets – while they are essential for recuperation, they don't strictly count towards your daily activity tally. For example, in a 2-hour gym session, you may be spending only 45 minutes training, and 75 minutes resting. Your daily carbohydrate requirement would be 5–7 g/kg of body weight/day. This equates to (5 x 70) to (7 x 70) = 350–490 g for a person weighing 70 kg. Even if you're lifting heavy weights, this amount of carbohydrate will be more than enough to fuel a typical workout. However, this is only a guideline and you should adjust this according to your specific training goals, how active you are during the rest of the day, and how you feel during and after training.

Protein is key

Protein is the next most important part of your weight-training diet. The building blocks of protein, amino acids, are used for repairing and rebuilding the muscle fibres that you have damaged during your workout.

Resistance training breaks down muscle tissue and thereby creates a demand for additional protein. Since protein helps muscles recover faster, athletes who consume the right amount will optimise their muscle gains and are less likely to get injured, according to the International Society of Sports Nutrition (Campbell

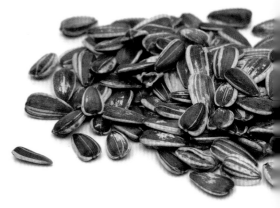

et al., 2007). Conversely, if you don't get sufficient amounts of protein you are limiting the results you get from your training. What's more, a high-protein intake has been shown to help maintain a strong immune system.

How much protein?

It is widely accepted that athletes have higher protein requirements than the general population (Rodriquez *et al.*, 2009; Phillips *et al.*, 2007; Campbell *et al.*, 2007). The exact amount of protein necessary for muscle building has been hotly debated for many years, but the scientific consensus from the IOC Conference on Nutrition in Sport 2010 is an intake of 1.3 g–1.8 g protein/kg of body weight per day for athletes generally; with intakes at the higher end of this range (1.6–1.8 g) for strength and power athletes (Phillips and van Loon, 2011). This translates to 112–126 g daily for a 70 kg person, considerably more than the Guideline Daily Amount (GDA) for the general population (45 g for women and 55 g for men). This extra protein is needed to compensate for the increased breakdown of protein during exercise and to facilitate muscle repair and recovery after intense training.

A longer-term effect of continued resistance training is that it increases protein retention. In other words, resistance training reduces the relative amount of protein consumed that is lost in urine. So, experienced strength athletes actually need less protein weight for weight than novices.

Most people eat more protein than they actually need, so deficiencies are rare and protein supplements are not necessary – you can still get these levels of protein from a balanced diet. You can get more than enough protein from 3–4 daily portions of chicken, fish, dairy products, eggs and pulses. Even vegetarians can meet their protein needs by eating dairy products, eggs, and non-animal proteins such as beans, lentils, nuts and soya.

Eating too little protein occasionally isn't a problem as the body can adapt to low intakes in the short term by recycling amino acids (rather than excreting them). But, in the long term, low protein intakes can cause fatigue and slow recovery after workouts. It can result in a loss of muscle tissue and strength.

THE FUNCTIONS OF PROTEIN

Protein consists of chains of amino acids that combine in various ways to form part of the structure of every cell in your body, including muscles, tendons, skin and hair. It also serves other functions including enzyme, hormone and antibody production.

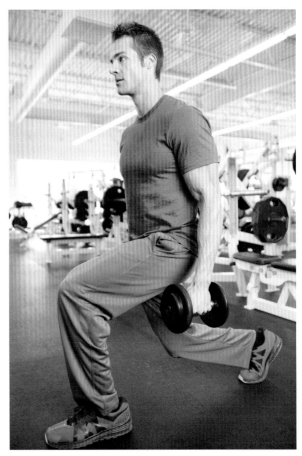

Are higher intakes of protein beneficial or harmful?

Some strength athletes and bodybuilders prefer to consume more than the recommended 1.8 g/kg of body weight in the belief that high levels of protein will produce greater muscle gains. However, extra protein won't give you any performance benefits. Studies have demonstrated that eating more than you need for daily repair does not result in additional muscle growth, strength, stamina or speed (Lemon *et al.*, 1992).

A high-protein diet is unlikely to pose any health risk provided the amount of protein consumed isn't excessive. Any protein that isn't needed for tissue repair and growth is partly excreted (in the form of urea) and partly used as a fuel source. It's a myth that high-protein diets cause kidney damage – there's no evidence to support this belief (Tipton and Wolfe, 2007). It stems from studies that found people with pre-existing kidney problems experienced stress on their kidneys when processing protein in their diet. But, for healthy people, excess protein does not harm the kidneys.

It's also a myth that excess protein makes you fat – but eating excess calories will. It's harder for the body to convert excess protein calories to fat than to convert excess calories from carbohydrate or fat. When you consume protein, 25–30 per cent of the calories are lost as heat in the process of digestion. Also, protein induces greater satiety than carbohydrate or fat, as it raises levels of satiety hormones such as glucagon, so it's actually quite difficult to eat too many calories on a high-protein diet (Halton and Hu, 2004).

Why is leucine important for muscle building?

Scientists have discovered that one of the essential amino acids, leucine, can help speed recovery and stimulate muscle growth after exercise and is particularly important for those wanting to build muscle mass. It acts as a signal to the muscle cells to make new muscle proteins; in other words, it kick-starts the process of regenerating and building muscles (Norton and Layman, 2006) Leucine activates a compound called mTOR (mammalian target of rapamycin), a molecular switch that turns on the machinery that manufactures muscle proteins.

Low leucine concentrations signal to mTOR that there is not enough dietary protein present to synthesise new muscle protein, so mTOR deactivates. High leucine levels signal to mTOR that there is sufficient dietary protein to synthesise new muscle protein, so mTOR 'turns on'. So, leucine is critical for muscle growth because without it, protein synthesis cannot take place.

FOODS SUPPLYING 2 G LEUCINE AND 20 G PROTEIN

600 ml milk
85 g Cheddar cheese
450 g plain yoghurt
3 eggs
85 g meat or chicken
100 g fish
17 g whey powder

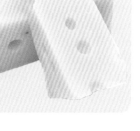

In a study at the University of Maastricht, athletes who consumed a leucine/carbohydrate/protein supplement after resistance training had less muscle protein breakdown and greater muscle protein synthesis than those who consumed a supplement without leucine (Koopman *et al.*, 2005).

However, it isn't necessary to take in leucine in the form of supplements. It is found widely in foods, the best sources being animal (high-quality) proteins: eggs, dairy products, meat, fish and poultry. It is also found in high concentrations in whey protein. You'll need around 2 g leucine to get maximum muscle-building benefits; that's the amount found in approximately 20 g of an animal-protein source. The box on the previous page shows the amounts of various foods that you would need to consume to get 2 g leucine and 20 g protein.

When is the best time to consume protein?

The timing of your protein intake around exercise sessions is important. Many studies have shown that athletes gain more muscle when they eat some of their protein before and also after training than when they consume the same amount of protein each day but consume none before and after their workouts (Willoughby *et al.*, 2007; Tipton *et al.*, 2003).

After intense exercise, the rate of protein manufacture is low and protein breakdown high. However, you can shift this balance and kick-start muscle protein recovery by supplying your muscles with approximately 20–25 g protein (as well as carbohydrate) during the 2-hour post-exercise period. Studies suggest that this amount of protein ensures that enough amino acid building blocks are present to repair muscle tissue (Moore *et al.*, 2009).

A review of studies on protein needs by researchers at McMaster University, Canada, concluded that protein should be consumed with carbohydrate in a 3 to 1 ratio after exercise (Tipton *et al.*, 1999). They found that this particular protein and carbohydrate combination was more effective in promoting muscle repair and glycogen storage than protein or carbohydrate alone.

Consuming protein with carbohydrate promotes a greater release of insulin, which stimulates the transport of glucose and amino acids into muscle cells. The more insulin is present in the bloodstream, the more glucose and amino acids can be carried into the muscles for glycogen and protein manufacture. When protein is consumed with carbohydrate, the insulin response can nearly double that invoked by carbohydrate alone. Insulin also blunts the rise in cortisol that would

MYTH: YOU CANNOT ABSORB MORE THAN 25 G PROTEIN IN ONE MEAL

Although only 20–25 g protein is needed for muscle repair and growth (Phillips and van Loon, 2011), it doesn't mean that you cannot digest and absorb more than this in one sitting. You will digest and absorb all of the protein you eat, whether it's 25 g or 50 g. It's just that not all of it will be used for *muscle building*. Anything surplus to this will be used for other functions in the body or be used as a fuel source. What's most important is that you meet your total daily protein requirement, and that you consume 20–25 g immediately after training when your muscles are most receptive to amino acids.

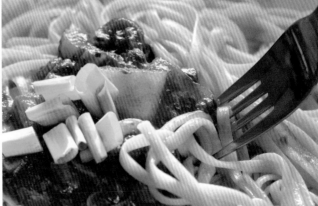

otherwise follow exercise. Cortisol suppresses protein synthesis and stimulates protein breakdown.

How much protein should I consume after training?

Canadian researchers found that 20–25 g is the optimal level for muscle growth immediately after a weights workout (Moore *et al*., 2009). When athletes consumed less than 20 g they gained less muscle; when they consumed more than this amount they experienced no further muscle gains. However, it's best to think of 20–25 g as a ballpark figure. If you weigh more than 85 kg (the weight of the athletes in the study) then you will need more, if you weigh less than 85 kg you may need less.

What types of protein are best for muscle growth?

Milk, whey, casein (the latter two are derived from milk), egg, meat, poultry and fish provide all the essential amino acids at levels that closely match the body's needs. Studies have shown that these types of protein stimulate muscle growth more than other types of protein.

These foods are also rich in the amino acid leucine, which is an important 'signalling amino acid' (see page 105). This amino acid has been shown to be a critical element in regulating protein manufacture in the body as well as playing a key role in muscle recovery after exercise. It triggers protein manufacture, which in turn leads to increased muscle strength.

However, non-animal protein sources, such as beans, lentils, nuts, soya and (to a smaller degree) grains also contribute amino acids to your diet and will count towards your total daily protein intake (see Table 1.5 on page 19 for the protein content of various foods).

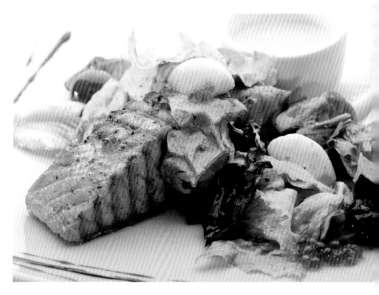

Is fat important for building muscle?

Fat isn't merely a fuel for training; it also plays a vital role in the manufacture of the muscle-building hormone testosterone. High testosterone levels stimulate muscle growth and increase strength. Studies have shown that higher-fat diets (40 per cent calories from fat) can boost testosterone levels (Dorgan *et al*., 1996). On the other hand, low-fat diets (less than 20 per cent calories from fat) reduce the body's production of testosterone (Hämäläinen *et al*., 1983).

A higher-fat diet may also help to increase levels of insulin-like growth factor (IGF-1), a key hormone that stimulates muscle growth and increases strength.

Studies show a correlation between a higher intake of dietary fat and IGF-1 levels. And low-fat diets are shown to lower IGF-1 levels. In fact, one study found that when people ate a low-fat diet for 11 days, IGF-1 levels dropped by 20 per cent (Ngo *et al.*, 2002). After two years on a low-fat diet, their IGF-1 levels fell by 55 per cent.

For optimal muscle building, you should aim to eat about 1.5–2 g fat/kg of body weight, or about 105–140 g for a 70 kg athlete. That typically equates to about 30–40 per cent of the total daily calories. This is a moderate amount of fat and is the amount that has been found to keep testosterone levels highest in athletes.

What should I eat post-workout?

Milk and milk-based drinks are near-perfect recovery drinks and good alternatives to many of the commercial protein/carbohydrate recovery drinks. Studies shows that consuming 500 ml of milk after exercise helps to maintain muscle performance during the recovery period (Cockburn *et al.*, 2012). Approximately 20 g of protein is needed to maximise muscle protein synthesis after exercise, therefore you should consume approximately 600 ml of milk to hit this target. This volume of milk also provides 30 g of carbohydrate, which is necessary to help replenish muscle glycogen stores and build muscle.

Milk also supplies minerals (such as calcium and magnesium) and vitamins, such as riboflavin. Opt for whole- or semi-skimmed milk or ready-to-drink milk drinks, or make your own recovery drink from milkshake powder or whey powder. Hot chocolate, latte and other coffee drinks made with milk are also suitable recovery options. Several studies have shown that consuming milk immediately after resistance exercise increases muscle growth and repair, reduces post-exercise muscle soreness, improves body composition and rehydrates the body better than commercial sports drinks (Elliot *et al.*, 2006; Hartman *et al.*, 2007; Wilkinson, 2007; Karp *et al.*, 2006).

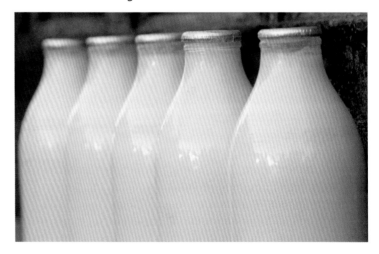

Recovery continues well past the immediate post-exercise period so you need to continue paying attention to your diet and fluid intake. Protein manufacture increases over the following 24–48 hours, generally peaking after about 24 hours. If you don't supply your body with adequate nutrients you risk incomplete recovery and sub-par adaptation to training. Eat regularly spaced nutritious meals that deliver protein and carbohydrate along with fibre, vitamins, minerals and fats.

Post-workout snacks

The following muscle-building options provide approximately 20 g of high-quality protein:

- 600 ml milk
- 600 ml flavoured milk
- 500 ml home-made milkshake – blend 350 ml milk, 150 ml yoghurt and around 100–200 g fresh fruit (any combination of bananas, strawberries, raspberries, blueberries or pineapple work well)
- 500 ml ready-made or home-made milkshake (made with 3 tsp of milkshake powder and 500 ml milk)
- 350–500 ml whey protein shake (made up with milk or water)
- 450 ml yoghurt
- 250 ml strained Greek yoghurt
- 50 g of almonds or cashews plus 250 ml yoghurt
- 80 g 'protein' bar

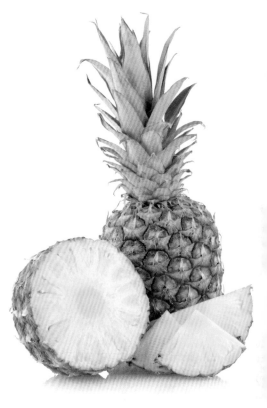

Will supplements help?

There are countless supplements claiming to enhance muscle growth but you should be cautious of extravagant claims that sound too good to be true. The chances are they don't work. Many nutritional supplements are lacking safety data and scientific proof and some have even been found to contain illegal substances!

The simple fact is that your diet and your training will determine at least 90–95 per cent of your success in building muscle (or for any sport). There's no short cut! Before considering taking any supplement, you need to look carefully at what you are eating and make sure that your meals are healthy and balanced. Only once you are confident that your diet and training programme are well balanced, should you think about supplements. Here are three supplements that may be worth considering (see Chapter 6 for more information on supplements).

Creatine

Numerous studies have shown that creatine supplements can improve performance in activities involving repeated bouts of high-intensity exercise with brief recovery periods (such as resistance training), as well as increase muscle strength and lean body weight (Gualana *et al.*, 2012; Buford *et al.*, 2007).

You can either use a 'loading protocol' of 0.3 g/kg of body weight for 5–7 days – equivalent to approximately 4 x 5 g = 20 g a day for a 70 kg person – or use a smaller daily dose of 2–3 g over 3–4 weeks. Both methods will achieve optimal levels in your muscles. Once you have saturated the muscles with creatine you can maintain these levels with 0.03 g/kg/day, or about 2 g per day.

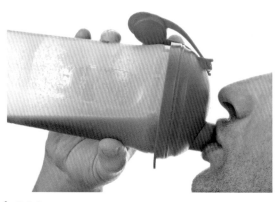

The best time to take creatine is immediately after your workout when the muscles are most receptive to the insulin-mediated uptake of creatine. Take creatine with carbohydrate (e.g. a banana, fruit juice or dried fruit) to maximise absorption.

It appears to be a safe supplement; the only side effect may be an upset stomach if you take too much without proper hydration. Anecdotally, some people are known to be 'non-responders'. This may be due to a diet high in meat in which the body is already saturated with dietary creatine prior to supplementation.

All-in-one supplements

All-in-one supplements contain high-quality protein (whey or a blend of whey and casein) and carbohydrate. Some contain vitamins, minerals, creatine and L-Glutamine. These types of shakes will not necessarily improve your performance, but are a convenient way to get your micronutrients and macronutrients for recovery. They're also a good option if you don't have the time to eat a post-exercise meal – although you should not regard them as substitutes for proper meals. Although expensive, think of them as a convenient supplement to your diet but not a replacement for real food.

Protein supplements

Protein supplements contain high levels of whey or casein, which are derived from milk. They are available in the form of powders, ready-to-drink products and bars. They are generally more expensive than real food (such as milk), but may be a convenient way of getting some of your daily protein immediately after training.

Whey protein is the most popular protein supplement and is available as isolate or concentrate. Concentrate contains about 80 per cent protein (as well as lactose and fat); isolate contains higher levels, around 90 per cent. However, consuming protein supplements does not inherently increase muscle protein synthesis. In studies where athletes were already consuming adequate amounts of protein in their diets, taking additional protein in the form of supplements before and after their workouts made no difference to muscle synthesis or strength (Weisgarber *et al.*, 2012). In general, if you are getting enough protein from food, there's probably little point in taking supplements.

The timing of your protein is important and this is perhaps where protein supplements may be useful. If you consume protein immediately after resistance training, you can speed muscle recovery. Clearly, any type of high-quality protein would be beneficial, but supplements would be a convenient way of getting your protein when you're out and about.

You may prefer to drink milk (which contains whey and casein naturally) as studies have shown that it is just as effective as supplements in promoting muscle synthesis after resistance training. Athletes who consumed milk gained more muscle than those consuming soy protein drinks during a 12-week resistance training programme (Hartman *et al.*, 2007).

Weight-gain tips

A sure-fire way to gain weight would be to eat more sugar and 'junk' food – they supply lots of calories, won't fill you up, and will encourage you to eat more – but you'll end up gaining fat not muscle. Instead, increase your calories by focusing on real food, and getting a balanced intake of fats, protein and 'quality' carbohydrate that won't put your body into fat-storage mode. Here are nine top tips:

1. Put more total eating time into your daily routine. This may mean rescheduling other activities. Plan your meal and snack times in advance and never skip or rush them, no matter how busy you are.

2. Increase your meal frequency. Try to eat at least three meals and three (or more) snacks each day.

3. Eat regularly – every 2–3 hours – and avoid gaps longer than three hours.

4. Plan nutritious high-calorie snacks – e.g. yoghurt, nuts, dried fruit, flapjacks, and oat-based bars.

5. Eat larger meals and increase portion sizes.

6. If you are finding it hard to fit in enough food, try nutrient-dense drinks such as whole milk, flavoured milk, milkshakes, and yoghurt and fruit smoothies to help increase your calorie and protein intake. Add ground nuts or seeds to shakes to further boost calories.

7. Eat full-fat milk and dairy products, use a little more (olive or coconut) oil for cooking, drizzle olive or walnut oil on salads and vegetables.

CHECK YOUR BODY COMPOSITION

Measuring your body fat percentage using skin-fold callipers or bioelectrical impedance will tell you how much of you is muscle and how much of you is fat (*see* page 87). In gaining weight, expect some of that to be fat. If you put on 3 kg of muscle and 1 kg of fat, you're making great progress. If you gained 2 kg of muscle and 2 kg of fat over the same period, you know your overall calorie and carbohydrate intake is too high, pushing up body fat levels.

If you're not gaining weight:
Eat one and a half times the amount of carbohydrate and protein at two of your meals a day. Use extra fats (butter, olive oil or coconut oil) and follow the rules to the left.

If you're gaining weight, but it's as much fat as it is muscle:
Halve the carbohydrate in your meals (excluding your post-workout meal).

If you gained muscle at first, but now your body fat has increased:
Halve your carbohydrate in your last two meals. If your body fat falls in two weeks, increase your carbohydrate.

8. Scatter extra grated cheese on dishes; add extra butter on toast, in sandwiches and in sauces.

9. Add extra nuts, dried fruit and honey to porridge; stir nuts and honey (or maple syrup) into Greek or whole-milk yoghurt.

Core menu plans for muscle gain

Here are three core menu plans, providing different amounts of energy, designed to help you gain muscle. They give you the amounts of foods needed to meet your calorie and macronutrient requirements. They provide approximately 3,000, 3,500 and 4,000 calories and are suitable for individuals weighing less than 65 kg, less than 75 kg and more 75 kg respectively, and doing approximately 1–2 hours moderate-intensity training a day. If you exercise for longer than an hour a day or at a very high intensity, then you should increase the portion sizes to take account of your greater calorie expenditure.

You should use the core menu plans as a template for developing your individual daily eating plan. Where the menu plan gives a choice of food type (e.g. 'carbohydrate'), simply pick your preferred option (e.g. pasta or potatoes) or substitute an equivalent (high-carbohydrate) food (e.g. quinoa or noodles). Try to vary your choice of fresh fruit and vegetables as much as possible according to what's in season as this will give you a greater range of micronutrients, antioxidants and phytonutrients. Many of the lower-carbohydrate recipes in Part 3 can be incorporated into your plan; simply use the amount of carbohydrate, protein and fat in the core menu plan as a guide.

Measure and weigh your portions carefully to start with to get an idea of what different amounts of foods look like. Thereafter, you should find it quicker and easier to judge how much to eat. You should also track your progress – if you're not gaining muscle, then you may need to increase your portion sizes overall; if you're gaining fat as well as muscle, then you may need to reduce the carbohydrate in your meals.

The menu plans do not give quantities for water or other drinks as the amount you need is quite individual and will vary day to day according to the climate and your sweat rate. Check your hydration status with the 'pee test' (see page 61) and ensure you drink sufficient fluids to maintain proper hydration.

The menu plans provide guidance on 'real' foods, but do not give recommendations for sports supplements or products. You should read the information in Chapter 6 before deciding to incorporate any product into your daily eating plan.

MYTH: TRAINING WITH LIGHT WEIGHTS PRODUCES MUSCLE DEFINITION

It's a myth that doing high repetitions of light weights produces definition – it improves muscle endurance, but isn't the best way to burn fat. To improve muscle definition, you need to reduce your body fat by cutting calories and doing fat-burning exercise (*see* Chapter 4 for more information on fat loss).

MENU

Core menu plan for muscle gain for a <65 kg person

Breakfast	Water 2 eggs plus 2 slices wholegrain toast 300 ml milk (or hot chocolate/coffee/milkshake) 100 g fresh fruit
Snack	25 g nuts 100 g fresh fruit Water
Lunch	Protein: 150 g chicken, meat, fish or 3 eggs or 75 g cheese Vegetables or salad Carbohydrate: 3 slices wholegrain bread or 75 g (uncooked weight) wholegrain pasta or rice or 300 g potato Fat: 15 g olive/coconut oil or butter 100 g fresh fruit and 125 g whole-milk yoghurt Water
Pre-training	2 bananas 125 g whole-milk yoghurt Water
Training (<2h)	100 ml cordial or squash (diluted 1 to 8)
Post-training	600 ml milk/milkshake/protein shake 125 g whole-milk yoghurt
Dinner	Water Protein: 150 g meat, chicken or fish or 3 eggs or 75 g cheese Vegetables or salad Carbohydrate: 75 g (uncooked weight) wholegrain pasta or rice or 300 g potato Fat: 15 g olive/coconut oil or butter 100 g fresh fruit and 125 g whole-milk yoghurt

Nutritional analysis:

Calories 3,006

198 g protein (26 per cent calories)

101 g fat (30 per cent calories)

351 g carbohydrate (44 per cent calories)

MENU

Core menu plan for muscle gain for a <75 kg person

Breakfast	Water Porridge (75 g oatmeal plus 500 ml milk) Banana 2 eggs plus 1 x wholegrain toast
Snack	2 x bananas 125 g whole-milk yoghurt Water
Lunch	Water Protein: 150 g chicken, meat, fish or 3 eggs or 75 g cheese Vegetables or salad Carbohydrate: 3 slices wholegrain bread or 75 g (uncooked weight) wholegrain pasta or rice or 300 g potato Fat: 15 g olive/coconut oil or butter 100 g fresh fruit and 125 g whole-milk yoghurt
Snack	2 bananas 125 g whole-milk yoghurt Water
Training (<2h)	100 ml cordial or squash (diluted 1 to 8)
Snack	600 ml milk/protein shake 125 g whole-milk yoghurt
Dinner	Water Protein: 150 g chicken, meat or fish or 3 eggs or 75 g cheese Vegetables or salad Carbohydrate: 75 g (uncooked weight) wholegrain pasta or rice or 300 g potato Fat: 15 g olive/coconut oil or butter 100 g fresh fruit and 125 g whole-milk yoghurt

Nutritional analysis:

3,425 calories

212 g protein (25 per cent calories)

111 g fat (29 per cent calories)

425 g carbohydrate (47 per cent calories)

MENU

Core menu plan for muscle gain for a >75 kg person

Breakfast
Water
Porridge (75 g oatmeal plus 500 ml milk)
Banana
2 eggs plus 2 x wholegrain toast

Snack
50 g nuts
100 g fresh fruit
Water

Lunch
Water
Protein: 150 g chicken, meat, fish or 3 eggs or 75 g cheese
Vegetables or salad
Carbohydrate: 4 slices bread or 100 g wholegrain pasta or rice or 400 g potato
Fat: 25 g olive/coconut oil or butter
100 g fresh fruit and 125 g whole-milk yoghurt

Snack
2 x bananas
125 g whole-milk yoghurt
Water

Training (<2h)
100 ml cordial or squash (diluted 1 to 8)

Snack
600 ml milk/protein shake
125 g whole-milk yoghurt

Dinner
Water
Protein: 150 g chicken, meat or fish or 3 eggs or 75 g cheese
Vegetables or salad
Carbohydrate: 75 g (uncooked weight) wholegrain pasta or rice or 300 g potato
Fat: 25 g olive/coconut oil or butter
100 g fresh fruit and 125 g whole-milk yoghurt

Nutritional analysis:
4,010 calories
227 g protein (23 per cent calories)
147 g fat (33 per cent calories)
480 g carbohydrate (45 per cent calories)

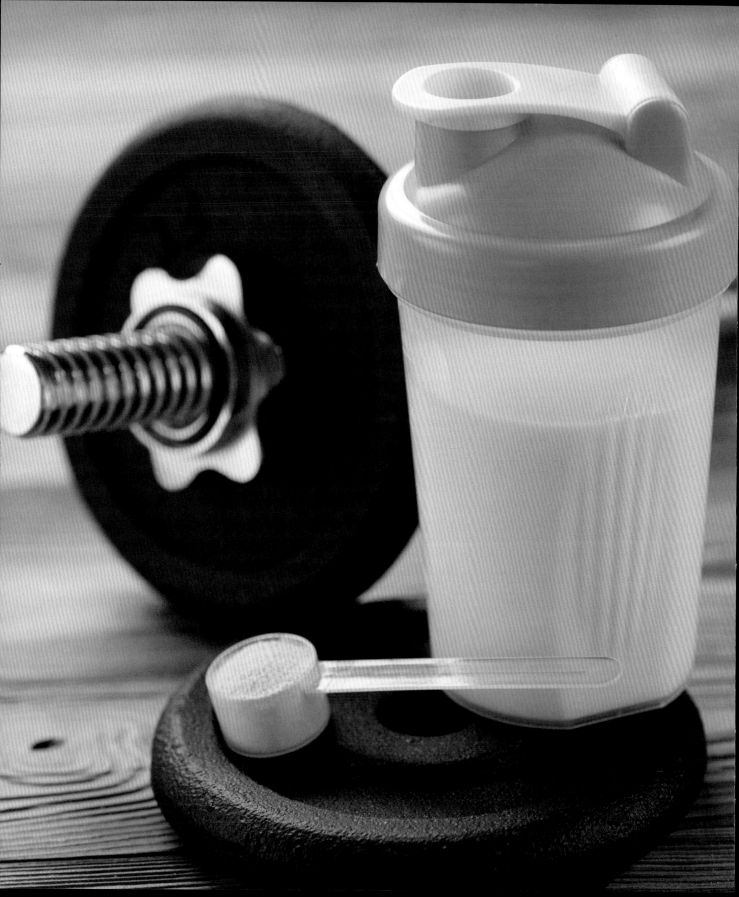

6 SPORTS SUPPLEMENTS

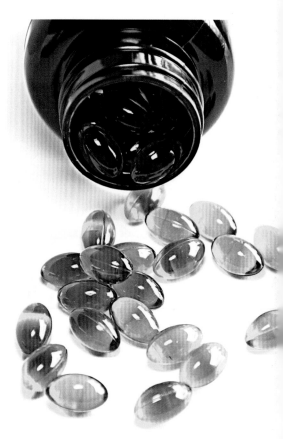

With the multitude of products on the market, it's hard to know if what you're taking is safe, effective and legal. Unlike medicines, there's no systematic regulation of supplements or herbal remedies, so there's no guarantee that a supplement lives up to its claims.

Many are advertised in fitness publications alongside impressive testimonials or sports celebrity endorsements, which can make the product's claims appear very convincing. But, despite the hype, many supplements have little, if any, scientific backing.

Some types of supplements such as energy bars, gels and drinks represent relatively little risk in terms of safety and legality, but another category of supplements poses more serious issues: ergogenic aids. Ergogenic aids are defined as *any external influence created to enhance sport performance.*

Are supplements safe?

The problem with dietary supplements is that they are classified as foods so they don't have to undergo safety tests. While some companies do follow good manufacturing practices, others do not.

Supplement manufacturers are not regulated in the same way as medicine manufacturers, meaning contents listed on the label may not be a true reflection of what they actually contain. There is the risk that such supplements could be contaminated with banned substances. This is known to be the case as many athletes have been tested positive through the use of such supplements. A 2012 investigation by the Medicines and Healthcare Products Regulatory Agency (MHRA) found that 84 illegal products such as energy and muscle-gain products are being sold that contain dangerous ingredients such as steroids, stimulants and hormones (MHRA, 2012).

In a study conducted by the International Olympic Committee of 634 supplements tested from 13 different countries, 94 supplements (15 per cent) contained prohibited substances (Geyer *et al.*, 2004). Another 10 per cent showed the possible presence of steroids. That means that 1 out of every 4 supplements contained prohibited substances. Products that tested positive were from all over the world. Of the 37 samples tested from the UK, 19 per cent tested positive.

A study in 2008 by HFL Sport Science found that 10 per cent of supplements and weight loss products purchased and tested in the UK were contaminated with steroids and/or stimulants at levels that could have resulted in positive testing for athletes.

How do you assure the quality of supplements?

You can never be 100 per cent sure that any supplement is free from banned substance. All sporting associations hold the athlete responsible for what goes into his or her body, so if you're an elite athlete bound by WADA and choose to take supplements, only use products that have been batch-tested and speak to a qualified medical practitioner if you have any concerns about any supplements.

Look for voluntary certifications by Informed Choice on the label, indicating that the product has been tested. Informed Sport is an organisation administered by HFL Laboratories that provides a supplement testing and a certification programme for sports nutrition products (http://informed-sport.com/). To date, only a small number of supplement manufacturers have registered their products with this programme, due to the high costs involved – you'll find all registered products listed on the Informed Sport website. However, realise that even when using certified products, you are still risking a positive drug test. Any product can be contaminated since there is nothing in place to prevent this.

Alternatively, choosing pharmaceutical-grade products may reduce (though not eliminate) the risk of inadvertently taking a contaminated or poorly labelled product. Choose reputable manufacturers who can justify their claims with scientific evidence, and have their products screened to minimise the risk of testing positive for a substance on the World Anti-Doping Agency's Prohibited List (WADA, 2013). Contact the supplement company to investigate what they do to screen for contamination.

How to evaluate supplements

- Don't be taken in by supplements that promise dramatic results. If the manufacturer's claims sound too good to be true, then they probably are.

- Be sceptical of adverts that contain lots of technical jargon or unnecessary graphs. If the information isn't clear and factual, leave the supplement well alone.

- Be wary of glossy adverts that rely on astonishing 'before' and 'after' photos rather than scientifically sound evidence for the supplement.

SUPPLEMENTS POSITION STATEMENT

'UK athletes are advised to be extremely cautious about the use of any supplements. No guarantees can be given that any particular supplement, including vitamins and minerals, ergogenic aids, and herbal remedies, is free from prohibited substances as these products are not licensed and are not subject to the same strict manufacturing and labelling requirements as licensed medicines. Antidoping rules are based on the principle of strict liability and therefore supplements are taken at an athlete's risk and personal responsibility.'

Issued in 2003 by UK sport, the British Olympic Association (BOA), the British Paralympic Association (BPA), National Sports Medicine Institute (NSMI), and the Home County Sports Councils (HCSC).

- Ask the manufacturer for evidence and studies that support the supplement's claims. If the information isn't available, don't touch that supplement.

- Check that any evidence is unbiased. Ideally, studies should have been carried out at a university (not funded solely by the manufacturer), and published in a reputable scientific journal.

- Don't take a supplement that has been recommended only by word of mouth. Check out exactly what is in it and whether it works before you buy it. Ask an expert if you have any questions.

- Be wary of supplements that contain similar endings to a banned substance. For example, supplements ending in 'one' are likely to have a similar chemical structure to testosterone.

This chapter looks at three categories of sports supplements: sport food supplements; ergogenic aids that have a solid evidence base for their use, and ergogenic aids that you should avoid at all costs.

Category 1: Sport food supplements
Sports drinks
These are typically not altogether necessary unless you are training for longer than one hour (see page 66 for more detailed information on sports drinks). There are three types of sports drinks:

1. Low-calorie ('lite') sports drinks
What's in them?
These drinks contain sugar, electrolytes (sodium, potassium, magnesium, chloride), flavouring, preservatives, colouring and sweeteners. They are hypotonic, which means they are less concentrated than body fluids, containing between 2 g and 4 g sugar/100 ml. They are absorbed faster than plain water, but slower than isotonic drinks.

Do you need them?
They provide hydration and some fuel (sugar), but not enough to increase your stamina or performance appreciably compared with water or flavoured water. The sodium makes them more palatable, drives your thirst, and helps the body hold on to fluid – but this will not improve performance or recovery if you're exercising for less than 2 hours. Choose them for their taste and convenience if you're exercising at a low intensity for less than an hour.

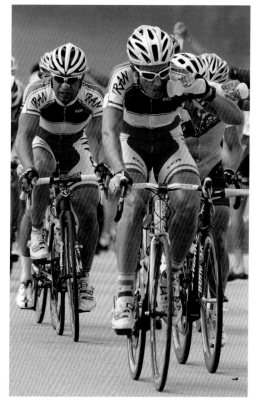

Make your own: Add a dash of sugar-free or ordinary cordial or squash to your water bottle (salt is unnecessary during exercise lasting less than 3 hours).

2. Isotonic drinks

What's in them?

These contain sugar, electrolytes (sodium, potassium, magnesium, chloride), flavouring, preservatives, colouring and sweeteners. They contain between 4–8 g sugar/100 ml (glucose, sucrose, fructose or maltodextrin), about the same concentration of particles as body fluids, which makes them isotonic. They will be absorbed faster than plain water.

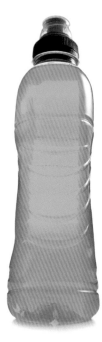

Do you need them?

They may increase your stamina and performance if you're exercising at a high intensity for longer than one hour (see page 44). The sugars in the drink help maintain blood glucose and spare muscle glycogen. As with low-calorie sports drinks, the sodium in these drinks improves palatability, increases thirst, and helps the body hold on to fluid but will not improve your performance unless you are exercising for longer than 2 hours. Drink 400–800 ml/hour, depending on your thirst, sweat rate and surrounding temperature and humidity.

Make your own: Add 100 ml cordial or 130 ml squash to a 1-litre water bottle and top up with water. Alternatively, mix 500 ml apple juice with 500 ml water. If you plan to exercise for more than 2 hours, add 0.5–0.7 g (one eighth of a tsp) of salt.

3. Dual source sports drinks

What's in them?

These contain glucose (or maltodextrin) and fructose in a 2 to 1 ratio, as well as sodium, preservatives, flavouring and colouring. They contain 7–9 g sugar/100 ml, which makes them isotonic. The dual combination of sugars (glucose and fructose) means that the body can absorb the sugar faster compared with other drinks. Studies suggest you can absorb up to 90 g/hour from dual source sports drinks compared with 60 g/hour from regular drinks.

Do you need them?

They may help increase your stamina and performance during high-intensity exercise lasting more than 3 hours, e.g. triathlon, marathon, ultra-distance events.

Make your own: Mix 60 g of glucose (or a mixture of glucose and maltodextrin) and 30 g of fructose in 1 litre of water. Add a dash of sugar-free squash to flavour, if you like.

Gels

What's in them?

Gels comprise of sugar (such as sucrose, fructose and glucose) and maltodextrin (a carbohydrate consisting of 4–20 glucose units). They may also contain sodium, potassium and, sometimes, caffeine. Most contain 18–25 g of carbohydrate per sachet.

Do you need them?

If you have access to water (e.g. at race stations or water fountains), gels are a convenient alternative to sports drinks. They may help increase your stamina and performance during high-intensity endurance exercise lasting more than an hour. How much gel you need depends on how hard and how long you're exercising. As a general rule, you'll benefit from 30–60 g sugar (one or two gels)/hour. Their caffeine content may also boost your performance by reducing the perception of effort and fatigue.

Always take gels with water to avoid gastrointestinal discomfort. There are a huge variety of textures and flavours, so experimenting with different brands and flavours is very important for this category!

Real food alternatives: Try honey energy gels, which can be found in easy to carry pouches, or honey sticks.

Sports confectionery

What's in them?

These products include beans, blocks, jellies and chews. They are essentially just sugar (sucrose, maltodextrin), but may also contain small amounts of sodium, caffeine and vitamins.

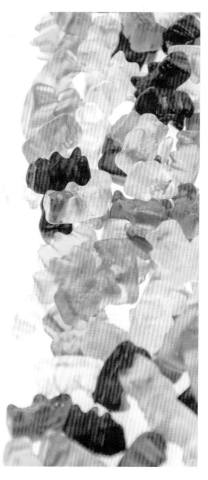

Do you need them?

If you're exercising at a high intensity for longer than an hour, then sports confectionery may be a convenient way of ingesting extra sugar to help maintain your blood sugar and spare muscle glycogen. A study funded by Jelly Bean undertaken by University College Davis in California found that Sports Beans® jelly beans were just as effective as popular carbohydrate supplements (sports drinks and gels) in maintaining blood sugar levels and improving exercise performance (Campbell *et al.*, 2008). Athletes achieved faster times in cycling trials with carbohydrate supplements than they did while consuming only water. One serving provides approximately 25 g sugar, enough fuel for 45–60 minutes of high-intensity activity. Some of the products are sticky and may adhere to your teeth. Make sure you rinse your mouth with water after eating them.

Real food alternatives: Try dried fruit such as raisins, dates, pineapple or mango. A study by researchers at the University of California Davis found that people who consumed raisins were able to complete a 5-km time trial faster than those who had only water (Too *et al.*, 2012).

Energy bars

What's in them?

Energy bars consist mainly of sugar and maltodextrin; and provide around 250 calories and 25–35 g of carbohydrate/bar. Some may also have added vitamins and minerals, cereals or soy flour to boost the nutritional content.

Do you need them?

Energy bars provide a convenient way of consuming carbohydrate before, during or after intense exercise lasting more than one hour. An Australian study compared an energy bar (plus water) with a sports drink during exercise; it was found that both boosted blood sugar levels and endurance equally (Mason *et al.*, 1993).

In a study at the University of Texas, cyclists were given either a sports drink (containing 10 per cent carbohydrate), an energy bar with water, or a placebo (Yaspelkis *et al.*, 1993). Those who consumed some form of carbohydrate managed to keep going 21 minutes 30 seconds longer before reaching exhaustion than those who only drank flavoured water. The reason? The extra carbohydrate helped fuel the cyclists' muscles, reducing the dependency on glycogen. After 3 hours in the saddle, the cyclists sipping the sports drink or eating food had 35 per cent more glycogen than those who had no carbohydrate.

The main benefit of energy bars is their convenience: they are easy to carry for eating during or after exercise. Make sure to drink water with your bar as this will aid digestion and replace fluids lost in sweat. They are an acquired taste and you may need to experiment with different flavours and brands.

Real food alternatives: Bananas, granola bars or fig rolls. An Appalachian University study found that bananas were just as effective as sports drinks in increasing performance in a 75-km cycling time trial (Kennerly *et al.*, 2011). Trained cyclists consumed 0.2 g carbohydrate/kg of body weight every 15 minutes. On one occasion the carbohydrate were given in the form of a sports drink; on the other occasion they came in the form of bananas. It made no difference where the carbohydrate came from; the cyclists performed the same.

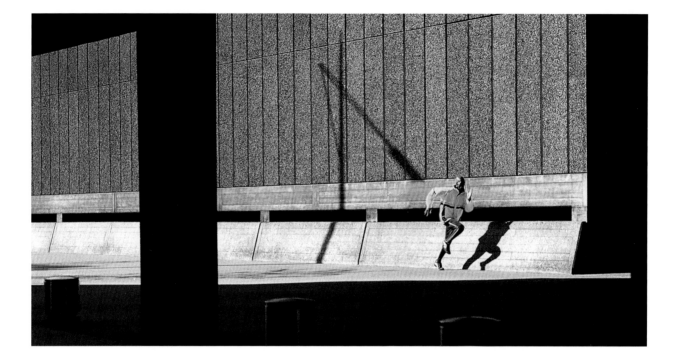

Recovery drinks

What's in them?

These contain sugar (or maltodextrin), whey protein (some may also contain casein), sodium, flavouring and sweeteners. They provide carbohydrate and protein, usually in a ratio of 3 to 1 and are formulated to promote muscle repair and glycogen replenishment after endurance exercise.

Do you need them?

These can be helpful in the post-exercise recovery period. If you're planning to exercise again within 24 hours, consuming a recovery drink within 2 hours should help kick-start recovery. Otherwise, simply ensure you get your macronutrient and micronutrient requirement within 24 hours.

Real food alternatives: Milk, flavoured milk and other milk-based drinks provide the all-important 20 g of protein/600 ml. Alternatively, opt for flavoured milk, which provides around 20 g protein and 60 g sugar in 500 ml, or mix 600 ml milk and 2 tbsp (30 g) milkshake powder.

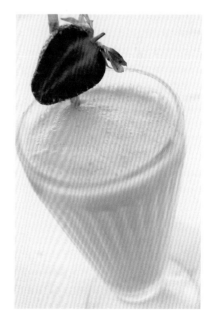

Category 2: Ergogenic aids that have a solid evidence base

Beetroot juice

What is it?

Beetroot juice (and beetroot) contains very high levels of naturally occurring nitrate. Nitrate is also found in smaller amounts in other vegetables, such as spinach, rocket, celeriac, cabbage, endive, leeks and broccoli. It is converted to nitrite by 'friendly' bacteria in the mouth and then in the stomach to nitric oxide.

What does it do?

Beetroot juice increases the amount of nitric oxide (NO) in your body. This gas has well-known cardiovascular benefits as it plays an important role in vasodilation and regulating blood pressure. Increasing NO levels prior to exercise could be an advantage, as it means blood vessels become more dilated, aiding the delivery of oxygen and nutrients to muscles during exercise.

What is the evidence?

A number of studies have shown that nitrate in the form of beetroot juice can reduce the amount of oxygen needed by exercising muscles to sustain sub-maximal exercise, thereby increasing the muscles' efficiency and tolerance of high-intensity exercise and increasing endurance.

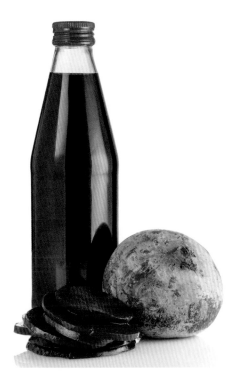

Beetroot increases average power output, exercise efficiency, and length of time to exhaustion. For example, researchers at the University of Exeter found that drinking 500 ml of beetroot juice a day for a week enabled volunteers to run 15 per cent longer before experiencing fatigue (Lansley *et al.*, 2011a). This was due to the higher levels of nitrate measured in the blood, which reduced muscle uptake of oxygen and made them more fuel-efficient. A further study by the same researchers found that cyclists given 500 ml beetroot juice 2½ hours before a time trial race improved their performance by 2.8 per cent in a 4-km race and 2.7 per cent in a 16.1-km race (Lansley *et al.*, 2011b). University of Maastricht researchers found that 170 ml of beetroot juice concentrate over 6 days improved 10-km time trial performance (by 12 seconds) and power output in cyclists (Cermak *et al.*, 2012). These results suggest that the nitrates in beetroot juice reduce maximal oxygen uptake, improve exercise economy, and allow athletes to exercise longer.

Do you need it?

Beetroot may help you sustain higher levels of power for longer before fatigue sets in. It could improve your performance during high-intensity endurance exercise lasting between 4 minutes and 30 minutes, or during intense intermittent exercise and team sports. Typical doses used in studies are 0.3–0.4 g (0.62 mg/kg body weight), equivalent to 500 ml beetroot juice, 170 ml beetroot juice concentrate, or a 70 ml shot 200 g cooked beetroot (equivalent to 300 mg nitrate).

Research at the University of Exeter suggests that 2 x 70 ml concentrated beetroot shots (with about 2 x 0.3 = 0.6 g natural dietary nitrate) is the optimal dose for high-intensity exercise (Wylie *et al.*, 2013). These 2 shots are best consumed 2–3 hours before exercise. NO levels peak 2–3 hours after consumption and then gradually fall over 12 hours. Taking more than two shots will not produce greater increases in stamina or performance. You can also 'load' for 3–7 days prior to a competition to ensure your blood levels of NO remain high (Cermak *et al.*, 2012).

Are there any side effects?
Beetroot can cause a harmless, temporary, pink colouration of urine and stools.

Real food alternatives: Whole beetroot. Athletes who consumed 200 g cooked beetroot an hour before exercise were able to run faster in the latter stages of a 5-km run (Murphy *et al.*, 2012).

Caffeine

What is it?
Caffeine is classed as a drug rather than a nutrient. However, it is often considered a dietary supplement because it is found in many everyday foods and drinks such as coffee, black and green tea, cola, chocolate, energy drinks and gels. It stimulates the central nervous system but provides no actual energy in the form of calories. Caffeine was removed from the banned substance list in January 2004. It does, however, remain on the monitoring programme and may be added to the prohibited list again if it is found to be misused.

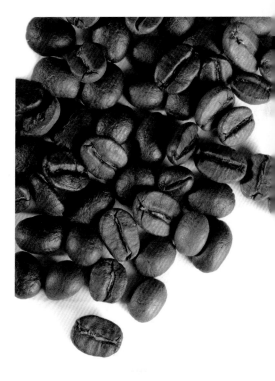

What does it do?
Caffeine acts as a neuromuscular stimulant and changes perceptions of effort or fatigue and improves fibre recruitment. In endurance events, it delays fatigue by reducing the perception of effort. Caffeine does this by increasing the concentration of hormone-like substances in the brain called ß-endorphins during exercise. The endorphins affect mood state, reduce the perception of pain, and create a sense of well-being. It may also improve alertness, reaction time and attention span. In shorter events, caffeine increases muscle recruitment, which ultimately boosts performance.

What is the evidence?

When taken 1–3 hours before exercise, caffeine has been shown to enhance performance in sprints, in high-intensity activities lasting 4–5 minutes, in intermittent activities such as team sports, and in endurance activities (Burke, 2008). Benefits occur at modest levels – 1–3 mg caffeine/kg body weight, when taken before and/or during exercise. This is a lower dose than has been quoted in the past (6–9 mg/kg has been used).

An analysis by UK researchers of 40 studies on caffeine and performance concluded that it significantly improves endurance, on average by 12 per cent (Doherty and Smith, 2004). Another study at the University of Saskatchewan found that consuming caffeine in amounts equivalent to 2 mg caffeine/kg of body weight one hour before exercise significantly increased bench press muscle endurance (Forbes *et al.*, 2007).

THE CAFFEINE CONTENT OF VARIOUS FOODS AND DRINKS	
Drink/food source	**(Caffeine content mg per cup)**
Instant coffee	60 mg
Espresso	45–100 mg
Cafetière/filter coffee	60–120 mg
Tea	40 mg
Green tea	40 mg
Energy drinks	100 mg
Cola	40 mg
Energy gel, 1 sachet	25 mg
Dark chocolate, 50 g bar	40 mg
Milk chocolate 50 g bar	12 mg

Do you need it?

Taking 1–3 mg caffeine/kg about one hour before training may boost performance. This equates to a dose of 70–210 mg caffeine (equivalent to approximately 2 cups of coffee) for a 70 kg person. Performance benefits occur soon after consumption, so caffeine may be consumed just before exercise, spread throughout exercise, or late in exercise as fatigue begins to occur. However, the only problem is that the amount of caffeine in coffee can vary, making it hard to know exactly what dose you are getting. As individual responses vary, you should experiment during training to find the dose and protocol that suits you. You may prefer to take caffeine tablets or 'shots' if you want to get a precise dose.

Sometimes, athletes cut caffeine for a few days or significantly reduce their intake prior to a competition. The idea is to reduce your tolerance so that when you reintroduce caffeine to your system, you'll get a greater response again. However, studies have found that there is no difference in the performance response to caffeine between non-users and users of caffeine, and that withdrawing athletes from caffeine does not increase the net improvement in performance achieved with caffeine supplementation

Are there any side effects?

The effect of caffeine differs between individuals. Some people do not respond to it, and others may experience negative side effects such as tremors, increased

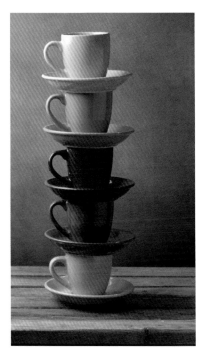

heart rate and headaches. These side effects are more common at higher doses, i.e. 6–9 mg caffeine/kg.

Other side effects caused by taking too large a dose include nausea, irritability, diarrhoea, insomnia, trembling and nervousness. High doses – above 300 mg – will have a diuretic effect, and may affect hydration status. So it is important to keep the intake below this.

Creatine

What is it?

Creatine is a protein that is made naturally in the body from three amino acids (arginine, glycine and methionine), but is also found in meat and fish or taken in higher doses as a supplement. As a supplement, creatine is most commonly taken as creatine monohydrate powder mixed with water, but capsule forms are also available.

What does it do?

Creatine combines with phosphorus to form phosphocreatine (PC) in muscle cells. This is an energy-rich compound that fuels muscles during high-intensity activities, such as lifting weights or sprinting. Boosting PC levels with supplements enables you to sustain all-out effort longer than usual and recover faster between exertions or 'sets', resulting in greater strength and improved ability to do repeated sets.

What is the evidence?

Creatine monohydrate supplements have been well researched over the years and, on balance, have proven an effective aid for increasing strength and muscle mass as well as enhancing performance in high-intensity activities (Gualano *et al.*, 2012).

Studies show significant increases in lean mass and total mass, typically 1–3 per cent lean body weight (approx 0.8–3 kg) after a 5-day loading dose, compared with controls – although not all studies show positive results (Buford *et al.*, 2007). The observed gains in weight are due partly to an increase in cell fluid volume (i.e. water weight) and partly to muscle synthesis. A review of

Q&A

Question: *Does caffeine dehydrate you?*

Answer: Although caffeine is a diuretic, studies have shown that regular but moderate caffeine intake does not dehydrate the body as was once thought. Only if caffeine is taken in large doses – equivalent to more than three cups of coffee – or infrequently is it likely to have a noticeable diuretic effect. You only need to consume it regularly to build up a tolerance to caffeine weakening its diuretic action.

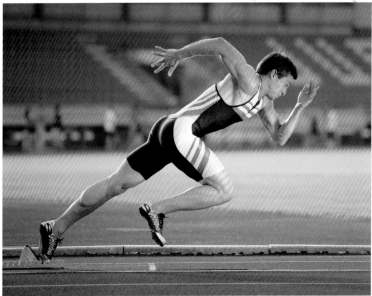

studies concluded that creatine supplements increase maximum strength (i.e. 1 rep maximum) as well as endurance strength, i.e. maximum reps at a given percentage of 1RM (Cooper *et al.*, 2012; Rawson and Volek, 2003).

Do you need it?

If you train with weights, sprint or do any sport that includes repeated sprints, jumps or throws (such as rugby and football), creatine supplements may help increase your strength, muscle mass and performance. But creatine doesn't work for everyone – several studies have found that creatine made no difference to performance, and it is unlikely to benefit endurance performance.

The quickest way of increasing your creatine stores is to use a 'loading protocol' of 0.3 g/kg of body weight for 5–7 days. For a 70 kg person, this translates to 21 g/day. Take this amount in four equally divided doses through the day, e.g. 4 x 5 g. Alternatively, you can 'load'

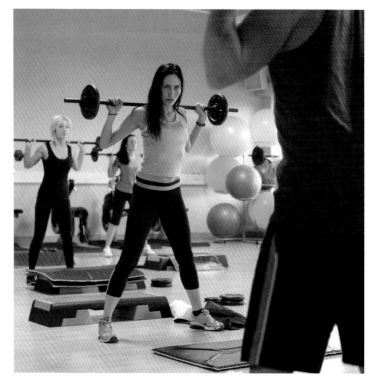

with a smaller dose of 2–3 g/day, but it will take 3–4 weeks to achieve optimal levels in your muscles. However, there is no advantage in taking more than 20 g/day, nor in loading for more than five days consecutively, as this is the time it usually takes for your muscular stores to reach their maximal capacity. After your stores are loaded, any extra creatine you ingest will not be absorbed by your muscles. Following the loading phase your creatine stores can be maintained by taking 0.03 g/kg of body weight a day for no longer than one month. For a 70 kg person, that's 2 g/day. The maintenance amount just needs to replace the amount of creatine degraded on a daily basis. As creatine is stored in the muscle it can be taken at any time of day. However, there is some evidence that it may be absorbed better when consumed along with carbohydrate immediately after training.

Creatine monohydrate has been extensively used in studies and appears to be the most effective form of creatine. However, the powder form is not very soluble and produces a chalky liquid when you mix with water. Tablets and capsules may be a good alternative. Other forms such as citrate, phosphate, malate (tri-creatine malate) and pyruvate are less effective (Cooper *et al.*, 2012).

Are there any side effects?

The main side effect is weight gain. This is due partly to extra water in the muscle cells and partly to increased muscle tissue. While this is desirable for bodybuilders and people who work out with weights, it could be disadvantageous in sports where there is a critical ratio of body weight to speed (e.g. for runners) or in weight-category sports. Some people suffer from water retention, particularly during the loading phase. As larger-than-normal amounts of creatine need to be processed by the kidneys, there is a theoretical long-term risk of kidney damage, but this has not been proven. One study found no evidence of impaired kidney function after 12 weeks of creatine supplementation (Lugaresi *et al.*, 2013).

Whey protein

What is it?

Whey protein is derived from milk (it is the by-product of cheese production) and provides a balanced source of all nine essential amino acids, including the branched chain amino acids, leucine, isoleucine and valine. Leucine is both a key signal molecule for initiation and an important substrate for new protein synthesis. Whey is digested quickly and rapidly absorbed in the intestine (vs. casein which is digested much slower). Whey protein may also help enhance the immune function thanks to its high content of glutamine. There are three types of whey supplements:

- Whey protein concentrate – produced by ultrafiltration of whey, and generally contains about 80 per cent protein (the remainder being lactose, fat and water).

- Whey protein isolate – produced by a variety of membrane filtration or ion-exchange techniques that remove almost all the lactose and fat, and generally contains more than 90 per cent protein.

- Whey protein hydrolysates – produced by enzymatic hydrolysis of whey concentrate or whey isolate, which 'pre-digests' the protein by separating peptide bonds; so it is digested and absorbed faster.

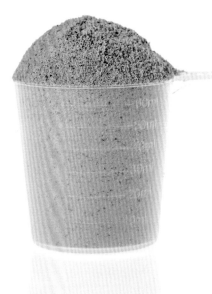

What is the evidence?

Whey supplements may help increase muscle synthesis following resistance training, but most studies have compared them with carbohydrate, casein or soy supplements, and not real food. There is no proof that they are superior to real food sources.

In one study, those consuming 20 g of whey supplement before and after resistance exercise had greater increases in muscle mass and muscle strength over 10 weeks compared with those consuming a placebo (Willoughby *et al.*,

2007). Another study found that when athletes consumed a whey supplement immediately before and after a training session they could perform more reps and lift heavier weights 24 hours and 48 hours after the workout compared with those taking a placebo (Hoffman *et al.*, 2010).

However, consuming any high-quality protein source immediately after resistance training will also promote muscle repair and growth (Tipton *et al.*, 2004). Compared with casein or soy, whey supplements may be a better option in the immediate post-exercise period as whey is absorbed quicker, but there is no evidence that it results in greater muscle growth over 24 hours (Tang *et al.*, 2009).

Additionally, whey may also help boost immunity. Researchers found that those who consumed whey supplements following a 40-km cycling time trial experienced a smaller drop in glutathione levels, which is linked with lowered immunity.

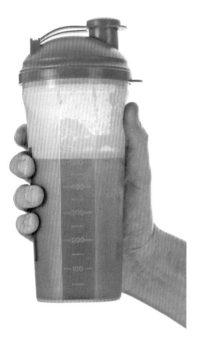

Do you need them?

Whey protein supplements represent an easy and convenient way of adding protein to your diet if you have higher-than-average requirements. They may be useful for bodybuilders and strength athletes, as well as vegetarians who do not get enough protein from food sources. Protein supplements are also a convenient way of getting enough protein when you're out and about.

As whey is quickly digested, supplements may be helpful for kick-starting recovery in those who are training twice a day. Its high leucine content also promotes rapid recovery. However, it won't necessarily produce faster or greater muscle gains than real food sources of whey, such as milk, yoghurt and cheese.

Are there any side effects?

An excessive intake of protein, whether from food or supplements, is not harmful but offers no health or performance advantage. Concerns about excess protein harming the liver and kidneys or causing calcium loss from the bones have been disproved.

Beta-alanine

What is it?

Beta-alanine is an amino acid.

What does it do?

Beta-alanine increases muscle levels of a natural substance called carnosine. These increased levels of muscle carnosine can help offset the build-up of fatiguing lactate during high-intensity exercise, which in turn can enhance sprint and short-distance performance. Normally, a build-up of acidity results in fatigue.

What is the evidence?

Beta-alanine supplementation may improve performance in high-intensity events lasting between 1 and 7 minutes. It may also be beneficial in events involving repeated sprints or lifts. In a study at Ghent University in Belgium beta-alanine supplements reduced fatigue when performing a set of knee extensions (Derave *et al.*, 2007). Another study at the College of New Jersey found that beta-alanine resulted in increased training volume and reduced subjective feelings of fatigue in football players (Hoffman *et al.*, 2008). However, the research has involved only small numbers of athletes and not all studies have found significant benefits.

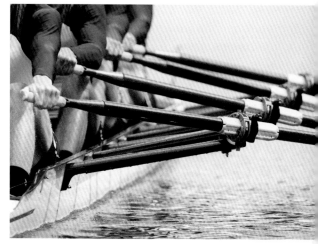

Do I need it?

Beta-alanine supplements may be beneficial if you are competing in high-intensity events such as swimming, rowing, cycling and running lasting between 1 and 7 minutes; or sports such as football and tennis that involve repeated sprints or surges of power. They may also be advantageous for bodybuilders and those following a strength-training programme. Typical doses used in studies are 3.2–6.4 g/day for 6–10 weeks.

Are there any side effects?

High doses may cause side effects such as flushing and parathesia (skin tingling). Smaller doses or sustained-release formulations are less likely to cause side effects. The long-term effects of supplements are not known.

Branched chain amino acids

What are they?

Branched chain amino acids (BCAAs) are essential amino acids: valine, leucine and isoleucine. The term 'branched chain' refers to the molecular structure.

What do they do?

BCAA supplements may have two benefits: preventing fatigue and reducing muscle breakdown. The theory is that BCAAs may reduce serotonin levels (which causes fatigue) and thus enhance exercise performance. It is claimed they also help repair damaged muscles, decrease muscle soreness, and increase muscle function.

What is the evidence?

Some data shows that BCAA supplementation before and after exercise has beneficial effects for decreasing exercise-induced muscle damage and promoting muscle-protein synthesis. A study by researchers at Florida State University found that BCAA supplementation before and during prolonged endurance exercise reduced muscle damage (Greer *et al.*, 2007). However, similar benefits were obtained following consumption of a carbohydrate drink and it is not clear whether chronic BCAA supplementation benefits performance. Studies with long-distance cyclists at the University of Virginia found that supplements taken before and during a 100-km bike performance test did not improve performance compared with a carbohydrate drink (Madsen *et al.*, 1996). In other words, BCAAs may not offer any advantage over carbohydrate drinks taken during exercise.

Do I need them?

A balanced diet with adequate protein should provide enough BCAAs. As long as you're getting enough dietary macronutrients – such as proteins, fat and carbohydrate – muscle will be spared. However, if you aren't getting sufficient protein in your diet or you're not consuming many food sources of BCAAs (e.g. dairy products), then supplements may help reduce muscle protein breakdown and promote muscle synthesis.

Are there any side effects?

BCAAs are relatively safe because they are normally found in protein in the diet. Excessive intake may reduce the absorption of other amino acids.

Vitamin D

What is it?

Vitamin D is a fat-soluble vitamin. The main source comes from exposure to ultraviolet B (UVB) radiation, but it can also be obtained from oily fish, egg yolk and fortified foods (e.g. cereals and margarine).

What does it do?

Vitamin D plays a role in muscle metabolism and immune function.

What is the evidence?

According to recent studies, a deficiency reduces muscle function and strength and may also increase the risk of injury and illness – all of which will have a detrimental effect on your training and performance (Hamilton, 2011; Larson-Meyer, 2010; Halliday *et al.*, 2011).

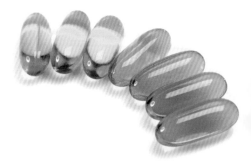

Do I need it?

As low levels may reduce performance, you should endeavour to maintain healthy blood levels of vitamin D (ideally more than 75 nmol/l) whether from sun exposure or diet. Aim for 15 minutes' sun exposure a day with face and arms uncovered, otherwise supplements may be a good idea. There's no RDA in the UK, but the USA recommend intakes of 15 µg/day (600 IU) and the EU recommend 5 µg daily. You can get this amount from 3 eggs or ½ teaspoon (2.5 ml) of cod liver oil, or 1 tin (100 g) of sardines or ½ a tin (50 g) of red salmon or 170 g tinned tuna (in oil).

Bicarbonate

What is it?
Sodium bicarbonate is a pH buffer that may help enhance performance in anaerobic and high-intensity exercise. It is a main ingredient of baking powder.

What does it do?
Supplements ('bicarbonate loading') will increase the pH of the blood and make it more alkaline. During high-intensity (anaerobic) exercise, hydrogen ions are produced, which gradually accumulate and result in fatigue ('the burn'). However, by raising the pH of the blood, hydrogen ions can pass more easily from the muscle cells to the blood, where they can be removed (buffered), which allows you to continue exercising at a high intensity for a little longer. It also means lactate is removed faster so you can recover more quickly.

What is the evidence?
Research has shown improvement in high-intensity events lasting 1–7 minutes. One meta analysis found an improvement of 1.7 per cent for events lasting about 1 minute (Carr *et al.*, 2011).

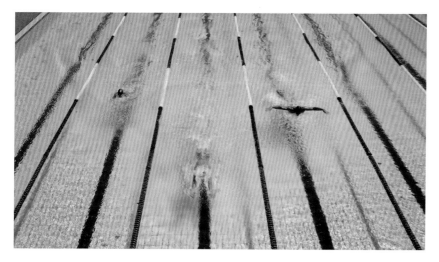

Do I need it?

You may benefit from bicarbonate if you are competing in high-intensity events lasting 1–7 minutes – e.g. sprint and middle-distance swimming, running and rowing events – or in events that involve multiple sprints, e.g. tennis, football, rugby. However, there is a high risk of side effects (see below) so you should try it first in training. The most common dose for bicarbonate loading is 0.3 g/kg (with at least 500 ml water) 60–90 minutes before the start of exercise (see below).

Are there any side effects?

Bicarbonate may cause gastrointestinal upset, nausea, stomach pain, diarrhoea and vomiting. These side effects could cancel out any performance advantage. Symptoms may be reduced by taking the loading dose in divided doses over a 2–2½-hour period before the event, along with a small carbohydrate-rich meal and plenty of water.

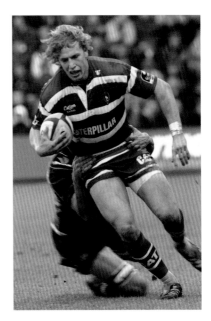

Glutamine

What is it?

Glutamine is a non-essential amino acid found abundantly in the muscle cells and blood. Glutamine supplements can be taken as powders, which are mixed with water or added to a protein shake, and as capsules.

What does it do?

Glutamine is needed for cell growth as well as serving as a fuel for the immune system. The glutamine hypothesis is that blood levels of glutamine fall during periods of heavy training or stress, potentially weakening the immune system and putting you at risk of infection. It has also been suggested that glutamine may have a protein-sparing effect during intense training.

What is the evidence?

The evidence for glutamine is divided. One study has shown that taking supplements of glutamine immediately after heavy training or an exhaustive event (such as a marathon) can help you recover faster, reduce muscle soreness and the risk of catching colds and other infections (Castell and Newsholme, 1997). However, most of the research on immune suppression has been done in the lab rather than real-life situations. Other studies have failed to show any benefits; for example, Canadian researchers found glutamine produced no increase in strength or muscle mass compared with a placebo (Candow *et al.*, 2001).

Do you need it?

Taking glutamine supplements won't do any harm, but is unlikely to be of substantial benefit in terms of preventing immune-suppression after exercise (Gleeson, 2008).

Are there any side effects?

No side effects have currently been identified.

HMB (beta-hydroxy beta-methyl butyrate)

What is it?

HMB is the by-product of the body's normal breakdown of leucine, an essential amino acid.

What does it do?

HMB is involved with the repair and growth of muscle cells. It reduces protein breakdown and increases protein manufacture. Supplements may therefore enhance recovery after intense exercise and promote muscle strength and growth.

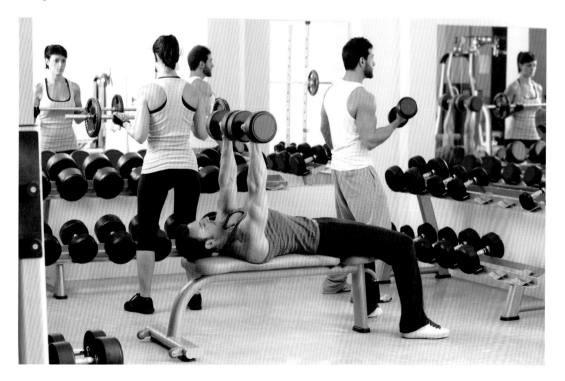

What is the evidence?

Studies have suggested that HMB may reduce muscle breakdown and damage, promote faster muscle repair, and increase muscle mass (Wilson *et al.*, 2013). But these benefits have not been found in all athletes, particularly more experienced athletes. One Australian study found that six weeks of HMB supplementation had no effect on the strength or muscle mass gains of well-conditioned athletes (Slater *et al.*, 2001).

Do you need it?

If you're new to lifting weights, HMB may help boost your strength and build muscle. Doses of 1–2 g can be taken 30–60 minutes prior to exercise if consuming HMB (free acid form) or if consuming calcium HMB, 60–120 minutes prior to exercise. Alternatively, 3 g (divided into 3 x 1 g doses)/day for two weeks can be taken prior to a major competition. However it is unlikely to be useful to more experienced gym goers. Finally, it may help prevent loss of lean body mass when dieting.

Are there any side effects?

No side effects have yet been found.

Fish oil

What is it?

Fish oil contains the two unsaturated fatty acids, eicosapentaenoic acid (EPA) and docosahexaenoic acid (DHA) derived from the tissues of oily, coldwater fish such as tuna, cod (liver) and salmon.

What does it do?

Taking supplements is a good way of boosting your intake of omega-3 fats. These may reduce your risk of heart disease, cancer of the breast and colon, type 2 diabetes, depression and degenerative diseases such as Parkinson's. They can also help reduce inflammation in the body, including post-exercise muscle soreness. Finally, fish oils may improve muscle functioning, blood vessel elasticity, delivery of oxygen to muscles, as well as speed up recovery and reduce muscle soreness after intense exercise.

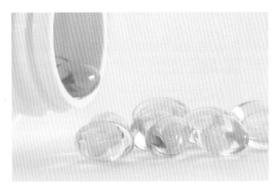

What is the evidence?

A study at the University of South Australia showed that overweight people who took fish oils in conjunction with exercise lowered their blood fats and increased HDL cholesterol levels (Hill *et al.*, 2007).

They also lost significantly more body fat compared with the control group who didn't take fish oils.

In a 2010 study, scientists at Gettysburg College in Pennsylvania supplemented diets of healthy, active adults with either safflower oil or fish oil (Noreen *et al.*, 2010). After six weeks, those taking the fish oil benefited from a significant increase in lean body mass and reduction in fat mass.

Other studies suggest that omega-3s can decrease inflammation, increase blood flow by up to 36 per cent during exercise, and decrease symptoms of rheumatoid arthritis (Calder *et al.*, 2006; Walser *et al.*, 2005). One study found that taking a supplement containing DHA for 14 days reduced levels of inflammation after intense exercise (Phillips *et al.*, 2003).

However, not all studies have produced positive results. In one, supplementation with 3.6 g fish oil/day for six weeks had no effect on delayed-onset muscle soreness compared with a placebo (Lenn *et al.*, 2002).

Do you need it?
If you don't eat oily fish regularly, 2 capsules of fish oil will provide approximately 500–600 mg of EPA and DHA, which is in line with population recommendations for heart disease risk reduction (Gebauer *et al.*, 2006). The government recommends 450–900 mg of the long-chain EPA and DHA per day, which can also be met with two portions of oily fish per week.

Are there any side effects?
Very high doses (more than 3 g/day) may increase the risk of bleeding. This is due to fish oil's ability to break down blood clots.

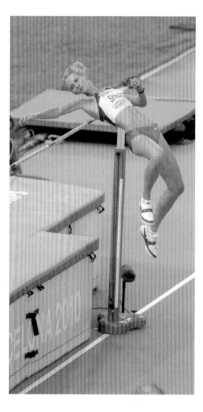

Category 3: Ergogenic aids you should avoid

Stimulants
These include ephedrine, yohimbine, synephrine and methylhexaneamine (DMAA). They are banned substances, but frequently appear in over the counter and internet-bought products. These ingredients should only be available on prescription, but they may be found in unlicensed sports supplements, including 'fat-burners' or 'diet' pills. These claim to speed your metabolism, increase alertness, and shed body fat. But these stimulants are capable of causing significant side effects, such as increased and irregular heart beat, raised blood pressure, kidney failure, seizures and heart complications. More severe consequences such as heart attack, stroke and death have been reported in the press. Several athletes have tested positive for DMAA and it has been linked to a number of fatalities.

Prohormones and steroid precursors

Prohormone supplements, including DHEA, androstenedione (or andro for short) and norandrostenedione are marketed to bodybuilders and other athletes looking to increase strength and muscle mass. Manufacturers claim the supplements will increase testosterone levels in the body and produce similar muscle-building effects to anabolic steroids, but without the side effects. However, while some may raise testosterone, studies have found that prohormones do not live up to their claims and may produce unwanted side effects.

Prohormones may increase oestrogen (which can lead to breast development) and decrease HDL cholesterol levels. Some supplements include anti-oestrogen substances such as chrysin, but there is as yet no evidence that they work.

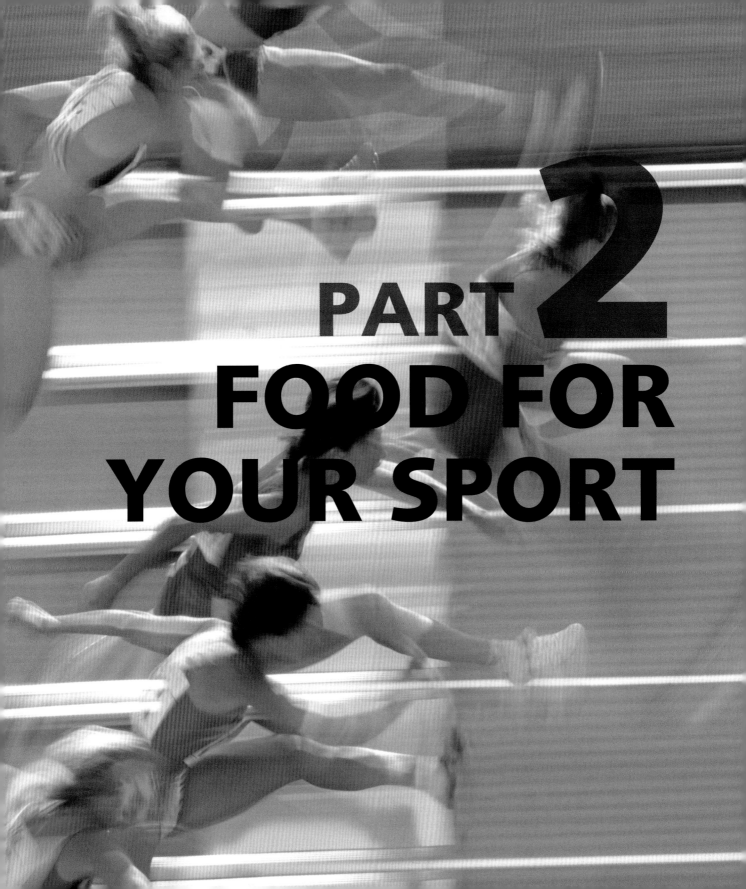

PART 2
FOOD FOR YOUR SPORT

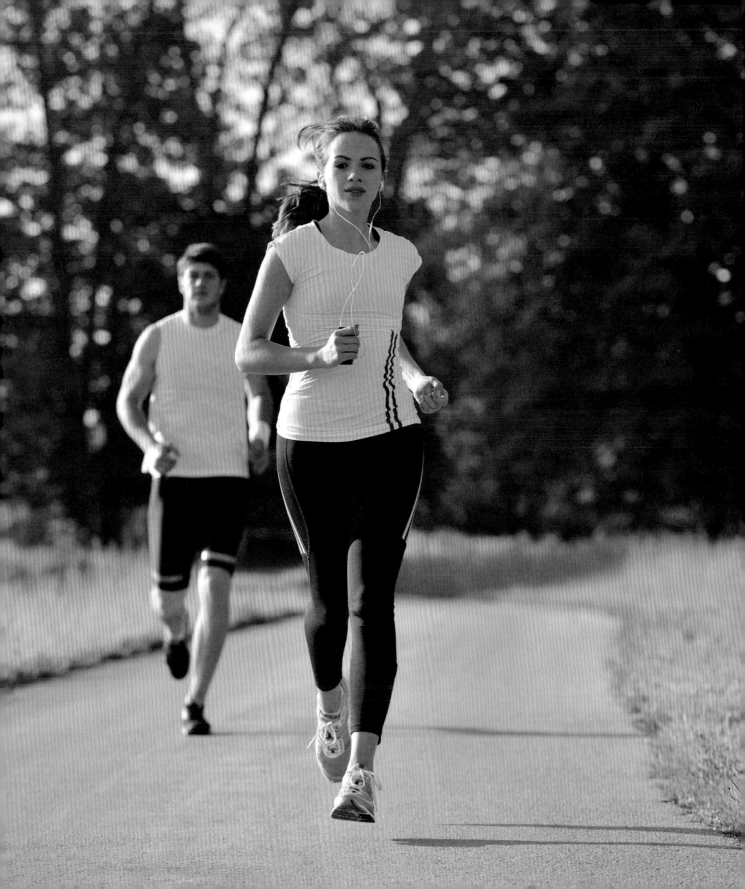

7 NUTRITION FOR RUNNING

Whether you are a competitive runner or you simply enjoy running for fitness, eating a healthy diet will help you run faster and longer. Running places high energy demands on the body so it's important to have a healthy intake of calories and nutrients to help you cope with your training programme. This chapter translates the information in Chapters 1–6 into a practical nutrition strategy to suit your daily running schedule, and covers some of the common nutritional problems and issues faced by runners. It also provides a flexible pre-race nutrition strategy for running a 5-km, 10-km, half-marathon and marathon, and a race-day nutrition and hydration plan to help you get ahead of the competition.

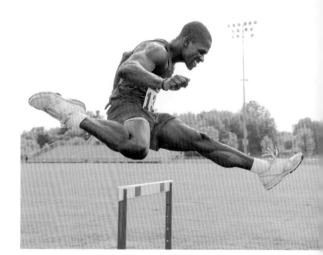

How many calories?

Running burns a lot of calories – the exact number depends on your speed, the incline, and your weight. For example, on the flat, you could burn more than 1,000 calories/hour if you weigh 70 kg. Use these values and the calculations on page 3 to help you work out how many calories you should eat each day. Table 7.1 gives some average values for people of different weights at various speeds running on level ground.

TABLE 7.1 CALORIES USED IN RUNNING

Speed	cals/kg/hour	60 kg	65 kg	70 kg	75 kg	80 kg
Jog (8.3 km/hour or 5.2 mph)	8.1	486	527	567	608	648
Fast (12.0 km/hour or 7.5 mph)	12.5	750	813	875	938	1,000
Hard (16.0 km/hour or 10.0 mph)	15.1	906	982	1,057	1,133	1,208

Fuel rules

Because they fuel workouts and promote muscle recovery, carbo-hydrate should be the backbone of a runner's diet. But some carbohydrate deliver greater nutritional value than others. Make most of your carbohydrate whole grains, fruits and vegetables. And remember: the less processing a plant receives, the more nutritious it is (think potatoes, not potato crisps).

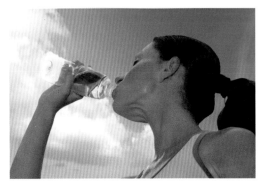

The two main causes of fatigue during endurance exercise are depletion of carbohydrate stores and dehydration. Filling your glycogen stores before training will delay the onset of fatigue. As a bonus, the run will seem easier to complete when you have enough glycogen on board. Eating a daily diet containing 5–7 g carbohydrate/kg of body weight (that's 350–490 g for a 70 kg runner) will speed your recovery from daily runs.

It's important to begin a run properly hydrated if you want to put in a good performance. Aim to drink 5–7 ml of fluid/kg of body weight about 4 hours before exercise – equivalent to 350–490 ml for a 70 kg person. That way, you'll have enough time for your body to excrete what you don't need before you begin exercising.

Short runs (<60 minutes)

During short-duration, moderate-intensity runs extra carbohydrate is not neces-sary. Provided you've consumed enough carbohydrate during the previous 24 hours, then your muscles should have stored enough glycogen to fuel your training run. If you're running for less than an hour, you won't deplete glycogen completely so there's no need to consume anything other than water during your run.

There are no hard and fast rules about how much to drink but, for most conditions, 400–800 ml/hour will prevent dehydration as well as overhydration. You should listen to your body and drink when you are thirsty.

Long runs (>60 minutes)

If you're running for longer than an hour, carbohydrate becomes an important part of your nutrition strategy as there's a higher risk of depleting your glycogen stores. This can result in early fatigue and slower performance. Consuming carbohydrate either in the form of a drink or as food provides your muscles with a ready supply of blood glucose for immediate energy, which spares glycogen stores and helps you to run longer. This should help delay fatigue and increase your endurance.

Q&A

Will I use more calories over a given distance if I run fast or slowly?

If you were to cover, say, 5 miles in 30 minutes, you would burn the same calories as you would jogging the same distance in 45 minutes. In fact, the calorie burn would be the same even if you walked the distance.

The difference comes once you have stopped. Your metabolic rate will stay higher for longer after intense exercise, whereas the metabolic boost will be far lower after moderate activity. This means that you burn more calories after you have finished a fast run than after a slow run.

However, it's important to consume the optimal amount and concentration of carbohydrate and fluid. If you over-consume carbohydrate, it will stay in your stomach longer and cause discomfort. If you under-consume carbohydrate, it may compromise your performance. For maximum performance, aim to consume 30–60 g carbohydrate/hour, depending on how hard you are exercising. That's equivalent to 400–800 ml of a 6 per cent drink (6 g sugar/100 ml), such as cordial or squash diluted 1 to 6, or an isotonic sports drink (*see* page 67).

Extra sodium in the form of sports drinks is not necessary for runs lasting less than 2 hours as it does not speed fluid delivery during exercise. It simply promotes thirst (and therefore makes you drink more) and makes the body hold on to more water.

Alternatively, you can get your carbohydrate in the form of gels, energy bars, bananas, granola bars or dried fruit (*see* page 122). Two gels/hour delivers 50 g of carbohydrate. Experimenting with different foods and products in training is important as individual responses can vary.

Drink according to your thirst and your body's sweat rate. You'll sweat more in hot and humid conditions and when working out harder/faster. It's better to drink little and often – say, 100–150 ml every 15 minutes, as this will result in greater retention and less urination.

After a run

The sooner you start to replace the fluid, the sooner you will recover. This is why you should make drinking your priority immediately after a run. The exact amount you need to drink depends on how dehydrated you are after exercising. To get an idea of how much fluid you have lost through sweat, weigh yourself before and after exercise. For each 0.5 kg (1 lb approx) of body weight lost, drink 600–750 ml of fluid, but not all in one go.

Both water and sodium need to be replaced to restore normal fluid balance after exercise. This can be achieved either by consuming a sports drink (which contains sodium) or water with food (that naturally contains sodium) if there is no urgency for recovery.

Replacing your glycogen stores after a run is crucial if you want to run well the next day. If you plan to run again within 24 hours, get into the habit of having a drink or snack containing carbohydrate and some protein, ideally in a ratio of 3 to 1, after a run. Consuming carbohydrate and protein within 2 hours of running speeds glycogen recovery and muscle repair. Suitable options include flavoured milk, fruit with yoghurt, a commercial recovery drink, or a flapjack with milk (see Table 7.2).

Q&A

I often get cramps in my calves during a run. Is there anything I can eat or drink to stop this happening?

There is no single explanation for muscle cramps – research suggests that some people are more susceptible than others (see page 67). They are most likely due to altered neuromuscular control, which can occur if you set off too fast in a training run or race or if you have muscular imbalances. There's little evidence that they are caused by dehydration or lack of sodium. If you get cramp during a run, slow down, stretch and try to relax the affected muscle(s).

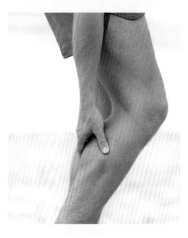

TABLE 7.2 FUELLING AND HYDRATION STRATEGY FOR RUNNING

When	Hydration	Fuel needs	Suitable foods
2–4 hours before a run	Drink 5–7 ml/kg (approx 350–500 ml)	Eat 2–4 g carbohydrate/kg (approx 100–200 g)	Pasta and chicken; rice and fish
OR <1 hour before a run	Drink approx 100–250 ml	Eat 1 g carbohydrate/kg (approx 50–70 g)	Bananas; toast and honey
During a short run (<1 hour)	According to thirst; little and often	Not needed	Water, low-calorie squash or sports drink
During a long run (1–2 hours)	Drink 400–800 ml/hour according to thirst; little and often	15–30 g carbohydrate every 15–30 minutes for a total of 30–60 g/hour	Cordial, squash, sports drink, bananas, gels, energy or granola bars, dried fruit, honey
During a long run (>2 hours)	Drink 400–800 ml/hour according to thirst; little and often	30–60 g/hour (up to 90 g if running >3 hours)	Sports drinks; dual source sports drinks; bananas, gels, energy or granola bars, dried fruit, honey
After a long run (>1 hour)	Drink 750 ml/0.5 kg weight loss	Eat a small snack with a 3:1 ratio of carbohydrate to protein	Milk (plain or flavoured) and flapjack; sandwich and yoghurt

Preparing for a race

Whether you're running a 5-km or a marathon, your nutritional intake during the days before a race, as well as on the day of the event, can have a big effect on your performance. You need to ensure that you arrive at the starting line properly hydrated and with high levels of glycogen in your muscles to fuel your event. Starting the race with high glycogen levels will help you to keep going longer before you fatigue.

5-km or 10-km

If you will be racing for less than 60 minutes, eat your normal diet for the days before the event. If you're running for less than an hour, you won't deplete glycogen completely so there's no need to consume extra carbohydrate. Your muscles should have stored enough glycogen to fuel your event. Do only very light training the day or two before so that you don't deplete your muscle glycogen.

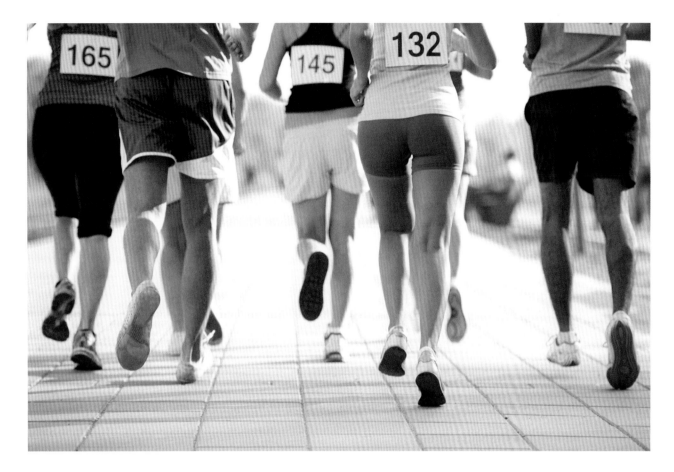

Half-marathon

For the last few days before the race, reducing your mileage and dropping your training intensity will help your muscles store more glycogen. Do only very light training or rest completely for the day or two before the race.

You'll be training less as the week progresses, so you may need to drop your calorie intake a little, you can do this by cutting down on portion sizes. You may also need to change the nutrient mix of your pre-race diet so you get more of your calories from carbohydrate (60–70 per cent) and fewer from fat (less than 15–20 per cent), with the balance coming from protein. Remember, it's the proportion of carbohydrate not the total calories that needs to go up.

Marathon

Carbohydrate loading – increasing glycogen stores above normal – may improve performance during races lasting 90 minutes or longer. It won't help you run faster in shorter runs – the heaviness associated with elevated glycogen stores may hinder your performance. You can try carbohydrate loading during the days before a marathon, but rehearse it in training several weeks beforehand.

The old regime (an exhaustive run 7 days out followed by 3 days of low carbohydrate, then 3 days of high carbohydrate) has been superseded by a newer protocol that produces the same glycogen-boosting results but without the drawbacks of the low-carbohydrate phase (lethargy, irritability, feeling unwell).

Do your last long workout (but not an exhaustive workout) a week from race day followed by increasingly shorter workouts throughout race week. Eat your normal diet until 3 days before racing, and then switch to a high-carbohydrate diet (7–10 g carbohydrate/kg of body weight) for the final 3 days, plus on race morning.

Don't increase your total calorie intake. Instead, reduce fat and protein intake in an amount that equals (or slightly exceeds) the amount of carbohydrate you add. Combining less training with more total calories could result in last-minute weight gain that will only slow you down.

The day before the race

By now, your muscle glycogen stores should be almost fully stocked and you should be feeling rested. Your goals are to top up your glycogen stores, stay well hydrated and avoid any pitfalls that may jeopardise your performance.

Eat little and often throughout the day and avoid big meals. It's not a good idea to overindulge the night before a race as this can play havoc with your digestive system and keep you awake at night. You may also feel sluggish the next day.

Stick with familiar foods. Eat only foods that you know agree with you and eat them in normal-sized amounts. Avoid gas-forming foods (or combinations of food) such as beans, lentils, cruciferous vegetables (broccoli, Brussels sprouts, cauliflower), bran cereals and spicy foods the night before the race. They may make you feel uncomfortable.

Keep a water bottle handy so you remember to drink regularly throughout the day. This is especially important if you are travelling to the race venue on this day, as it is easy to forget to drink. Because alcohol is a diuretic, it's better to avoid it completely. If you overindulge, you may feel below par the next day.

PRE-RACE MEALS IDEAS

- Eggs on toast
- Porridge with bananas, raisins and honey
- Cereal with milk and bananas
- Toast with jam, fruit and milk
- Pancakes with honey
- All-in-one shake
- Milkshake or yoghurt and fresh fruit

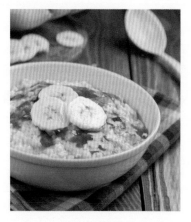

Race day nutrition

By now, your muscle glycogen stores should be fully stocked and you should feel ready to go! All that remains to be done before the race is to top up your liver glycogen stores at breakfast time (liver glycogen is normally depleted during the overnight fast), replace any fluids lost overnight, and keep your blood sugar level steady.

Schedule your pre-race meal 3–4 hours before the race start time. For example, if your race starts at 9 a.m., have breakfast at 5–6 a.m. Consume 25–50 g of carbohydrate for each hour before the start of the race, depending on your body weight and the race duration. Carbohydrate-rich foods, such as porridge, cereal, toast and fruit, are good choices. Include a little protein or healthy fat to reduce the glycaemic response and give a slow, steady energy release. If you can't eat because of pre-race nerves, have an extra bedtime snack the night before or try a liquid meal (e.g. an all-in-one shake, milkshake, smoothie or yoghurt drink) for breakfast, which will empty from your stomach faster than solid food.

Drink 350–500 ml of water or diluted fruit juice (1 part juice to 1–2 parts water) 2–4 hours before the race, then another 125–250 ml during the warm-up or just before you get to the starting line. If you decide to take caffeine, whether in the form of a drink or gel, consume this about 30–60 minutes before the race start time.

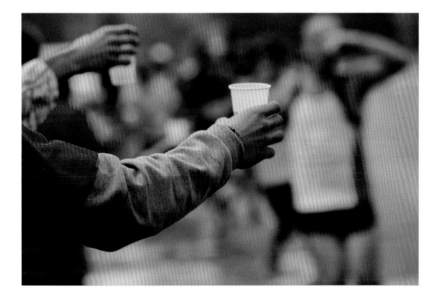

Q&A

Despite doing a lot of running, I have cellulite. Is it different from ordinary fat and is there a special diet I could follow to help get rid of it?

Cellulite is simply fat. The reason it appears dimpled and puckered is that it lies very close to the skin's surface and is criss-crossed by weak collagen strands that aren't very effective at supporting fat cells. This results in the characteristic bulging appearance of cellulite. The reason women get cellulite far more than men is the female hormone oestrogen, which favours fat storage on the thighs and bottom; hence women tend to put weight on in these areas. Inactivity, loss of muscle tone and excess calories are major contributors to the formation of cellulite. A healthy but careful calorie consumption combined with cardiovascular and resistance exercise is the only proven way to beat cellulite. There is no evidence that it is caused by 'toxins' or that following a detox diet reduces cellulite. However, cutting back on processed foods or those high in sugar, salt and fat will help reduce fat.

The sodium naturally present in your food will also help the body hold on to fluid (which may be advantageous prior to a race when it's important to avoid dehydration) so, despite the marketing hype, there's no need to consume a sports drink, i.e. a drink with sodium or electrolytes, beforehand. (See Table 7.3.)

TABLE 7.3 RACE DAY FUELLING AND HYDRATION PLAN

When	Hydration	Fuel needs	Suitable foods
4 hours before the race	Drink 5–7 ml/kg (approx 350–500 ml)	Eat 2–4 g carbohydrate/kg (approx 100–200 g)	Eggs on toast; porridge with bananas, raisins and honey; cereal with milk and bananas; toast, fruit and milk
1–2 hours before the race	Drink approx 100–250 ml	Eat 1 g carbohydrate/kg (approx 50–70 g)	Bananas; toast and honey; energy or granola bar
During 5-km or 10-km race (<1 hour)	According to thirst; little and often	Not needed	Water, low-calorie squash or sports drink
During half-marathon	Drink 400–800 ml/ hour according to thirst; little and often	15–30 g carbohydrate every 15–30 minutes for a total of 30–60 g/hour	Cordial, squash, sports drink, bananas*, gels*, energy or granola bars*, dried fruit*, honey*
During a marathon	Drink 400–800 ml/ hour according to thirst; little and often	30–60 g/hour (up to 90 g for ultra-distance events >3 hours)	Sports drinks; dual source sports drinks; bananas*, gels*, energy or granola bars*, dried fruit*, honey*
After the race	Drink 750 ml/0.5 kg weight loss	Eat a small snack with a 3:1 ratio of carbohydrate to protein	Recovery drink; flavoured milk; milk and flapjack; sandwich and yoghurt

*Accompany with water

During the race

There are no strict rules about how much to drink as this depends on how much fluid you lose through sweat (see page 63). By now you probably have a good idea how much to drink if you've practised a drinking strategy in training. As a rough guide, aim to drink 125–250 ml – about two or three swigs – every 15 to 20 minutes or according to thirst. Use whichever drinking method you have trained with. Be extra diligent in hot and humid weather.

At drinks stations, squeezing the cup into a spout makes it easier to drink. Don't be tempted to miss out the early fluid stations to gain valuable time – dehydration later on will slow you down even more. Stick with whatever you have used in training and don't try anything new.

Q&A

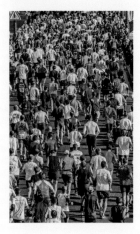

How can I avoid 'hitting the wall' during a marathon?

'Hitting the wall' occurs when the muscles run out of glycogen and blood sugar levels fall below normal. At this stage you are in real trouble. The body needs carbohydrate to burn fat, and when there is no carbohydrate the brain and nervous system can't work properly. This makes exercise difficult if not impossible. You may feel weak, dizzy, nauseous and disorientated.

Here's how to avoid hitting the wall. Consume carbohydrate at regular intervals during your run, aiming to have 30–60 g of carbohydrate for every hour of exercise, or up to 90 g if you are running longer than 3 hours. This is equivalent to drinking 400–800 ml of sports drink (containing 60 g of carbohydrate per litre) each hour. Try to take regular sips and start drinking early because it takes about 30 minutes for the carbohydrate to reach your muscles. This will help to keep your blood sugar levels steady and fuel your muscles during that last stage of the race.

After the race

You have made it past the finishing line. However, your nutrition strategy isn't over yet; you still have to replenish your fluid losses and depleted glycogen stores. This is especially important if you plan to train the next day.

Start with water or, if you have been running for longer than 60 minutes, a sports drink. You need to replace the fluid you have lost but you won't know exactly how much without a set of scales. For every 0.5 kg of body weight lost you need to drink 750 ml of fluid. Try to drink around 500 ml, little and often, in the first 30 minutes after the race, and then keep sipping every 5 to 10 minutes until you are passing pale-coloured urine again. You should be able to pass urine within 2 hours of a race. If you pass only a small volume of dark-yellow urine, or if you have a headache and feel nauseous, then you need to keep drinking. If you are dehydrated, sports drinks or diluted cordial/fruit juice with a pinch of salt added are the best options.

Have a snack containing carbohydrate and protein – ideally in a 3 to 1 ratio – within the first 30 minutes of the end of the race (when blood flow to your muscles is greater and the muscles are more receptive to carbohydrate). This will help rebuild your glycogen stores. Good options include milk-based drinks, recovery drinks, dried fruit and nuts, sandwiches, yoghurt and flapjacks.

POST-RACE SNACKS

- Milk or flavoured milk
- Recovery drink
- Flapjack, granola bar or energy bar
- Milkshake
- Bananas and other fresh fruit
- Dried fruit and nuts
- Sandwich, roll or bagel with meat, fish, egg, cheese

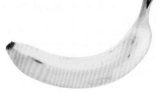

Q&A

I sometimes suffer from 'the trots' on long runs. What causes it and how can I prevent it?

The 'trots' or 'runs' is common among endurance runners. Studies have shown that as many as one in four marathon runners experience it. The most likely explanation is that the lower gut (colon) becomes starved of oxygen during a long run due to a reduced blood flow. Blood is diverted away from the gut to the muscles and the skin, where more blood is required. This can result in spasmodic contractions of the colon. Being dehydrated will make the situation worse as the reduced blood volume means that even less blood is available to the gut.

The best strategy to prevent diarrhoea is to drink plenty of water before and during a run. Make sure that you drink during the early stages. It is also a good idea to avoid eating high-fibre foods, especially bran and wholegrain cereals, pulses and dried fruit, too close to the time of your run. These may loosen the stools and trigger bowel movements, a situation made worse by pre-race nerves. Caffeine and sorbitol sometimes have a laxative effect so you may also wish to avoid drinks and foods containing them. Keeping a food and training diary can help you work out which foods you can tolerate and which you need to avoid before a run.

Continue eating a similar-sized snack every 2 hours until your proper meal. This will promote faster recovery. It takes at least 24 hours to replenish glycogen stores after a 10-km run, but up to 7 days after a marathon.

Core menu plans for running

The following two core menu plans can be used as a template for developing your individual daily eating plan. Each plan gives you the amounts of foods needed to meet your calorie and macronutrient requirements, providing approximately 3,000 and 2,500 calories. Pick the plan that most closely matches your training schedule (less than an hour or between 1 and 2 hours daily training) and energy requirement. However, if you run for longer than 2 hours, then you should increase the portion sizes to take account of your greater calorie expenditure.

Where the menu plan gives a choice of food type (e.g. carbohydrate), simply pick your preferred option (e.g. pasta or potatoes) or substitute an equivalent (high-carbohydrate) food (e.g. quinoa or noodles). Try to vary your choice of fresh

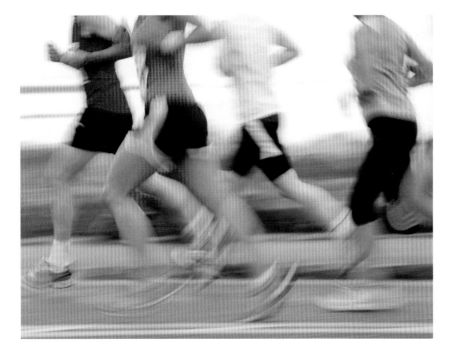

fruit and vegetables as much as possible according to what's in season as this will give you a greater range of micronutrients, antioxidants and phytonutrients. Many of the lower-carbohydrate recipes in Part 3 can be incorporated into your plan; simply use the amount of carbohydrate, protein and fat in the core menu plan as a guide.

Measure and weigh your portions carefully to start with to get an idea of what different amounts of foods look like. Thereafter, you should find it quicker and easier to judge how much to eat.

You should also adjust portion sizes according to your appetite and how energetic you feel during training. If you feel hungrier than usual, that's your body's way of signalling its needs, so you should eat more food. Similarly, if you fatigue early in training or find it harder to recover between training sessions, then you should also increase your portion sizes. Keep a check on your weight and body composition and adjust your intake accordingly.

The menu plans do not give quantities for water or other drinks as the amount you need is quite individual and will vary from day to day according to the climate and your sweat rate. Check your hydration status with the 'pee test' (*see* page 61) and ensure you drink sufficient fluids to maintain proper hydration.

Q&A

I have no appetite after a run and I certainly don't feel like eating. Should I wait until I'm hungry or force myself to eat?

A lot of runners find they have little appetite after racing. Running (along with other types of intense exercise) elevates body temperature and diverts blood away from the digestive system, which in turn depresses the appetite. If you want to recover faster, you should consume carbohydrate within the first 30 minutes after a race or, at the very least, within 2 hours. Try a liquid meal, such as a milkshake, smoothie or yoghurt. You'll feel better for it the next day.

MENU

Core menu plan for runners (1–2 hours daily training)

Breakfast	Water Porridge (75 g oatmeal plus 500 ml milk) Banana and 25 g dried fruit
Snack	25 g nuts 100 g fresh fruit Water
Lunch	Water Protein: 100 g chicken, meat, fish or 2 eggs or 50 g cheese Vegetables or salad Carbohydrate: 3 slices bread or 75 g wholegrain pasta or rice or 300 g potato Fat: 15 g olive/coconut oil or butter 100 g fresh fruit and 125 g whole-milk yoghurt
Snack	2 x bananas Water
Training (1–2h)	100 ml cordial or squash (diluted 1 to 8)
Snack	600 ml milk/flavoured milk/milkshake 50 g flapjack
Dinner	Water Protein: 100 g chicken or fish or 2 eggs or 50 g cheese Vegetables or salad Carbohydrate: 75–100 g (uncooked weight) wholegrain pasta or rice or 300 g potato Fat: olive/coconut oil or butter 100 g fresh fruit and 125 g whole-milk yoghurt

Nutritional analysis:
3,035 calories
144 g protein (19 per cent calories)
98 g fat (29 per cent calories)
422 g carbohydrate (52 per cent calories)

MENU

Core menu plan for runners (< hour daily training)

Breakfast
Water
Porridge (75 g oatmeal plus 500 ml milk)
Banana and 25 g dried fruit

Snack
25 g nuts
100 g fresh fruit
Water

Lunch
Water
Protein: 100 g chicken, meat, fish or 2 eggs or 50 g cheese
Vegetables or salad
Carbohydrate: 3 slices bread or 75 g wholegrain pasta or rice or 300 g potato
Fat: 15 g olive/coconut oil or butter
100 g fresh fruit and 125 g whole-milk yoghurt

Snack
Banana
Water

Training (<1h)
Water

Snack
600 ml milk/flavoured milk/milkshake

Dinner
Water
Protein: 100 g chicken or fish or 2 eggs or 50 g cheese
Vegetables or salad
Carbohydrate: 75–100 g (uncooked weight) wholegrain pasta or rice or 300 g potato
Fat: 15 g olive/coconut oil or butter
100 g fresh fruit and 125 g whole-milk yoghurt

Nutritional analysis:

2,581 calories

141 g protein (22 per cent calories)

85 g fat (29 per cent calories)

338 g carbohydrate (49 per cent calories)

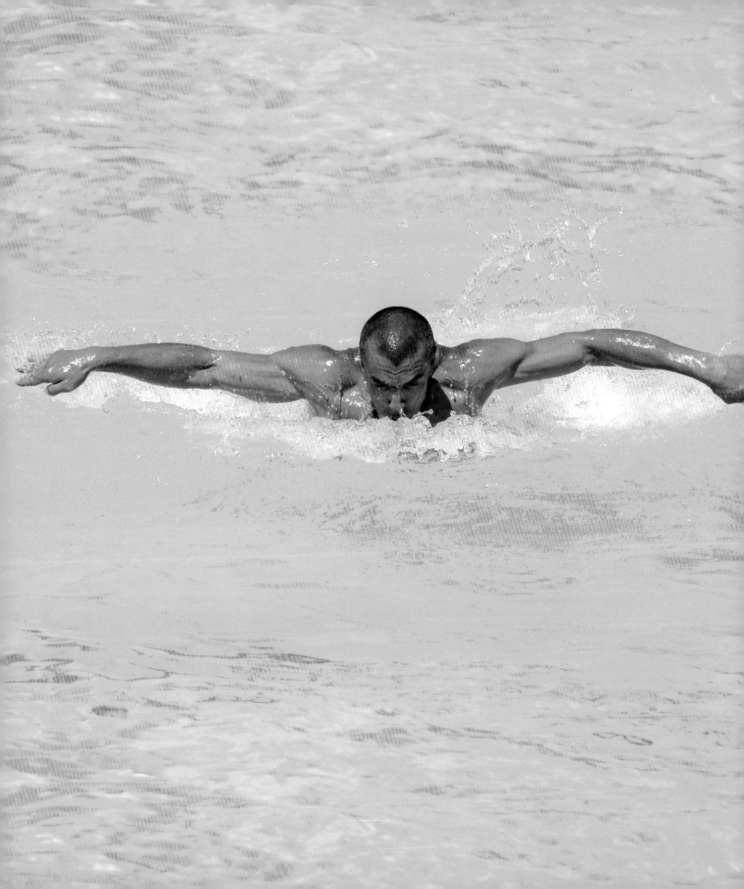

NUTRITION FOR SWIMMING

Whether you work out in the pool as part of a cross-training programme or you swim to compete, you'll benefit from a healthy nutrition plan. What you eat and drink can make a big difference to your stamina, speed and technique in the pool, as well as helping you recover between training sessions. This chapter gives you extra tips on eating for performance as well as answering nutrition questions frequently asked by swimmers. It also gives you a pre-competition nutrition and hydration strategy and a race-day plan to help you swim faster.

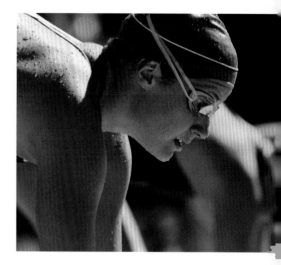

How many calories?

The number of calories you burn swimming depends on which stroke you're using and how fast you're going. Some unfit swimmers swim in such a slow relaxed fashion that their breathing rate hardly increases and they burn no more calories than if they were sitting! Hard swimming, on the other hand, can burn as many as 600 calories in half an hour. Use these values and the calculations on page 3 to help you work out how many calories you should eat each day. Table 8.1 shows you approximately how many calories you burn per hour using various strokes.

TABLE 8.1 CALORIES USED IN SWIMMING

Stroke	cals/kg/hour	Your weight				
		60 kg	65 kg	70 kg	75 kg	80 kg
Slow crawl	7.68	461	499	538	576	614
Medium crawl	9.36	562	608	655	702	749
*Fast crawl**	17.1	1,026	1,112	1,197	1,283	1,368
Breaststroke	9.72	584	632	680	729	778
Backstroke	10.14	608	659	710	760	811

*Most swimmers probably could not maintain this speed continuously for 1 hour

Fuel rules

Carbohydrate is an important fuel for competitive swimming. If you train for 1–2 hours a day you will need to eat between 5 and 7 g/kg of body weight each day (that's 300–420 g in a 60 kg swimmer). However if you spend more than 2 hours a day training (whether it's in the pool or doing other activities), you will need more like 7–10 g of carbohydrate/kg of body weight per day (that's 420–600 g for a 60 kg swimmer). If you swim for less than an hour, you'll need less carbohydrate to fuel your muscles: approximately 3–5 g/kg of body weight, which equates to 180–300 g/day for a 60 kg person.

For all swimmers, a general guideline is to have one-third of your plate as nutrient-dense ('quality') carbohydrate-rich foods (e.g. potatoes, sweet potatoes, wholegrain bread, pasta or rice); one-third protein (meat, fish, chicken, eggs, cheese, beans, lentils) and one-third vegetables (or salad). You should also include healthy fats (butter, olive oil, oily fish, nuts) in your meals and snacks, and at least 400 g (5 portions) of fruit and veg a day to ensure you get the omega-3 fats, vitamins, minerals, fibre and other protective nutrients needed to stay healthy and promote recovery.

Before swimming

The optimal time for your pre-exercise meal is 2–4 hours before training. If your training session starts at 7 p.m., have dinner at 4 or 5 p.m. Aim for 'comfortably full', not stuffed. If there isn't time for a meal, then have a smaller meal or healthy snack 30 minutes or 1 hour before training, with a drink.

Of all the foods you could have before a workout, prioritise ones rich in carbohydrate (plus protein), especially if you will be training for 2 hours or longer. Combining carbohydrate with protein produces a low to moderate glycaemic response (gradual rise blood glucose), which will provide sustained energy and maximum performance.

Before early morning swim training

If you train early in the morning, prioritise drinking first thing to ensure you arrive at the pool properly hydrated. Drink around 200–300 ml water to replace fluid lost in sweat during the night. If you plan to swim for longer than an hour, eat a mini-breakfast 30–60 minutes before training – you should never train on empty! Training on empty may result in early fatigue, low blood glucose levels, lightheadedness, nausea and a poor performance. Consume nutritious high-carbohydrate foods, such as wholegrain toast with honey, porridge, dried fruit or a banana. If a meal is out of the question, have a nutritious drink, such as milk, a

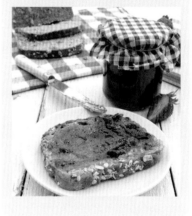

PRE-TRAINING MEAL IDEAS

- Jacket potato with cheese, tuna or beans plus veg
- Pasta with meat, cheese, tuna or chicken plus veg
- Rice with chicken, fish or beans plus veg
- One-pot dish with meat or fish or beans; potatoes or pasta and veg
- Toast (wholegrain) with honey or jam
- A banana (or other fresh fruit)
- A handful of dried fruit (e.g. raisins, apricots)
- Porridge or wholegrain breakfast cereal with milk
- Milk or an all-in-one protein/ carbohydrate shake

milkshake, hot chocolate or an all-in-one protein/carbohydrate shake. Some fuel is better than no fuel at all.

During swimming

It's hard to imagine that with so much water around, you could still get dehydrated. But you will still lose some fluid through sweating while swimming – it's just that it goes straight into the surrounding water. Fluid losses are likely to be smaller than for land-based activities, so be guided by thirst. The easiest way of preventing dehydration in swimming is by starting your session properly hydrated. If you begin training in a dehydrated state, then you won't be able to rehydrate or 'catch-up' during your session no matter how much you try to drink – your performance will suffer and you will tire quickly.

If you plan to swim for longer than 30 minutes, keep a water bottle on the poolside, and try to have a few swigs every 20 or so laps (according to your thirst), rather than a large volume in one go. For hard (elite) swimming, the general rule is to drink about 125 ml of fluid for every kilometre swum.

If you swim for longer than an hour, opt for a drink containing 4–8 g carbo-hydrate/100 ml, such as cordial or squash diluted 1 to 6 or an isotonic sports drink (*see* page 67). The extra fuel will top up blood glucose, spare glycogen in your muscles, make swimming feel easier and help you keep going longer. But you'll need to start drinking within the first 30 minutes as it takes around 30 minutes for those carbohydrate to reach your muscles. Try different drinks until you find one that you like. If some sit heavy in your stomach, you may need to reduce the strength by mixing them with extra water.

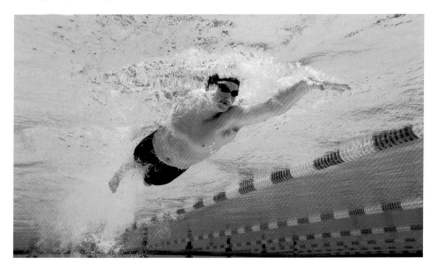

Alternatively, you may prefer to eat solid carbohydrate rather than liquid carbohydrate midway in your session if you're training for 2 hours. A banana, granola bar or a handful (40–50 g) of raisins or other dried fruit are suitable options. When eating these foods try to accompany them with a drink of water.

After swimming

After a hard session, you need to replace your energy stores by having a carbohydrate- and protein-rich snack (even if it's late in the evening). Eating around 1 g of carbohydrate/kg of your body weight (that's 60 g if you weigh 60 kg) within 30 minutes after your swim will speed glycogen recovery. This is especially important if you plan to train again within 24 hours. If you wait longer than 2 hours then you'll feel tired during swimming the following day. Include protein in your snack too as this increases glycogen storage and allows your muscles to repair faster. Aim for a ratio of about 1 g of protein to 3 g of carbohydrate.

Ironically, most snacks on offer at swimming venues are high in sugar and poor sources of micronutrients – certainly unsuitable for refuelling your muscles after swimming. Faced with a choice at the cafeteria, shun those fast foods, chips, chocolate bars and crisps in favour of milk, bananas, nuts, wholegrain sandwiches, fresh or dried fruit, granola bars, protein shakes or bars, and smoothies. If your venue doesn't provide the right food, bring your own.

AFTER-SWIMMING SNACK IDEAS

- Milk or milkshake or hot chocolate
- Milk and banana or yoghurt
- Wholegrain sandwich with chicken, fish, egg or cheese
- Flapjack and yoghurt
- Fresh fruit and yoghurt

TABLE 8.2 FUELLING AND HYDRATION STRATEGY FOR SWIMMING

When	Hydration	Fuel needs	Suitable foods
2–4 hours before swimming	Drink 5–7 ml/kg (approx 350–500 ml)	Eat 2–4 g carbohydrate/kg (approx 100–200 g)	Pasta and chicken; rice and fish; potatoes and cheese
OR <1 hour before swimming	Drink approx 100–250 ml	Eat 1 g carbohydrate/kg (approx 50–70 g)	Banana; flapjack; toast and honey
During swimming (<1 hour)	According to thirst; little and often	Not needed	Water, low-calorie squash, or sports drink
During swimming (>1 hour)	Drink 125 ml/km according to thirst; little and often	15–30 g carbohydrate every 15–30 minutes for a total of 30–60 g/hour	Cordial, squash, sports drink, banana, granola bar
After swimming (>1 hour)	Drink 750 ml/0.5 kg of weight loss	Eat a small snack with a 3:1 ratio of carbohydrate to protein	Flavoured milk; milk and flapjack; sandwich and yoghurt

Preparing for a competition

Preparing for a swimming event in which you'll be racing several times in one day requires a well-planned nutrition strategy. Depending on the number and type of races you'll be swimming (sprint, middle distance or distance) and how long the warm-ups and warm-downs will be, you may burn several hundred calories. This will take its toll on your energy reserves. By ensuring your glycogen stores are fully stocked and your body properly hydrated, you'll be able to put in your best performance on the day.

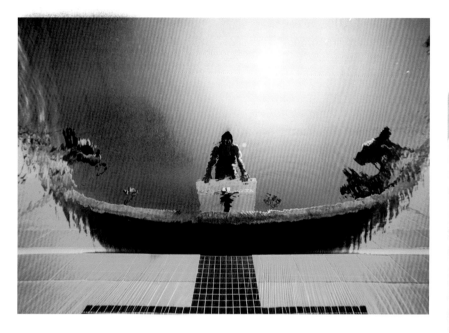

A few weeks before

If you need to shed some body fat, now is the time to adjust your diet and training. Count on losing between ½ kg (1 lb) and 1 kg (2 lb) of body fat per week and then work out how long you need to reach your target weight. Do this by cutting back on your calorie intake gradually. Save calories by cutting down on sugar and processed foods high in (low-nutrient) carbohydrate, such as biscuits, chocolate bars, puddings and savoury snacks. Include other cardiovascular activities to burn fat and include some strength training to preserve muscle.

If you are likely to be racing at an unusual time, say early in the morning, change your eating times to reflect this up to a week beforehand. This way, your body will find it easier to exercise at the new time and you'll slip into an eating

Q&A

Why do I feel ravenous after swimming? Should I follow my appetite and eat loads?

Your appetite may be bigger after swimming than after other activities because you are cooler. Other activities that make you hot for a while after exercise reduce your appetite temporarily. Swimming, on the other hand, may make you warm, but you cool down far quicker in water so by the time you're out and dressed, your body temperature is back to normal, even cooler. After swimming, eat a healthy snack if you're hungry (see p. 56), but choose wisely and don't get carried away. There's no evidence that swimmers need to eat any more food after a workout than runners, cyclists or gym-goers.

pattern that suits your exercise schedule. Practise your competition-day eating strategy in training – maybe have a simulated competition – prior to putting it in place.

The week before

Carbohydrate loading, practised by endurance athletes to increase their muscle glycogen levels above normal, is not relevant for most swimming competitions. Unless you plan to swim for more than 2 hours continuously, you are not likely to run out of glycogen. However, ensuring that you have 'normal' levels of glycogen in your muscles will help you swim faster and recover better between heats.

If you compete frequently, then you will probably 'swim through' the minor meets and only taper for major competitions. For these, you should reduce the volume of your training over a period of between a few days and two weeks, depending on your age and experience. In practice this usually means maintaining the frequency but reducing the distance and number of sets per session, together with a reduction in the amount of land-based training you do. As your training volume drops, you should also adjust your food (calorie) intake to match your energy expenditure otherwise you may end up with unwanted last-minute weight gain. Doing only very light training or resting completely for the last day or two will allow the carbohydrate you eat to be stored as glycogen and not to be burned during a workout.

Eating a balanced diet is really all you need to do during the last week. Provided that you ease back on your training, you will allow your muscles to fill out with glycogen. Focus on the nutritional quality (nutrient-density) of your diet by minimising sugar and refined carbohydrate.

The day before

Keep exercise to a minimum and plan your meals and snacks carefully, especially if you will be travelling to the venue the day before. You need to top up those muscle glycogen stores and keep properly hydrated. If travelling, it is a good idea to contact the hotel or venue beforehand to find out what kind of food will be available. If necessary, take your own food.

Have small meals every 2–4 hours to keep your blood sugar levels steady and fuel your muscles in preparation for the next day's event. Avoid big meals or over-eating during the evening, as this will almost certainly make you feel uncomfortable and lethargic the next day. If you feel nervous you probably won't have much of an appetite. Try liquid meals such as all-in-one shakes, milkshakes, milk or smoothies. Swimmers sometimes find that semi-liquid or soft-textured

Q&A

I normally swim first thing in the morning before breakfast and before work. Am I burning more fat this way or would I be better off eating something before I get to the pool?

Swimming on an empty stomach may burn slightly more fat but it won't burn more calories overall or make you lose weight faster. The downside is that you may run out of energy. If you want to increase your performance, consume a carbohydrate-rich snack or drink before you swim, this will boost your endurance. However, if you have plenty of energy for that early morning swim and you're getting results, stick with what you're doing.

foods are easier to digest when they get pre-race nerves. Try yoghurt, rice pudding, custard, pureed fruit, instant porridge or ripe bananas.

Stick to plain and familiar foods. Unless you are used to eating curries, spicy foods, baked beans and pulses they can cause gas and bloating. Make sure that you keep yourself hydrated by drinking plenty of water throughout the day. Your urine should be pale yellow (see 'pee test', page 61).

Competition day nutrition

Your aims are to keep your blood sugar levels steady, top up liver glycogen stores in the morning, and keep yourself properly hydrated. You should have rehearsed your pre-swim meal in training so you know exactly what agrees with you.

Drink approximately 350–500 ml of water, cordial, squash or diluted fruit juice (1 part juice to 1–2 parts water) 2–4 hours before the race, then another 125–250 ml just before the race. This will allow plenty of time for that fluid to get absorbed into your body and then for any excess to be excreted. Sip frequently rather than drinking it in one go. The sodium naturally present in your food will help the body hold on to fluid (which may be advantageous prior to a competition when it's important to avoid dehydration) so, despite the marketing hype, there's no need to consume a sports drink, i.e. a drink with sodium or electrolytes, beforehand. Check your urine is pale yellow in colour by the start time.

Schedule your pre-race meal approximately 4 hours before the race start time. Aim for 75–150 g carbohydrate but be guided by your appetite. Carbohydrate-rich foods such as porridge, cereal, toast and fruit are good choices. Include a little protein and healthy fat to reduce the glycaemic response and give a slow, steady energy release. Don't swim on empty. Skipping that pre-race meal may leave you low in energy during the final stages. You'll perform better if you eat something before your competition but If you are feeling too nervous, try a liquid meal instead. An all-in-one shake, milkshake, smoothie or yoghurt drink for breakfast will empty from your stomach faster than solid food.

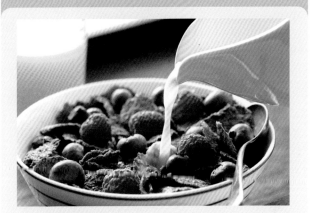

PRE-EVENT MEAL IDEAS

- Cereal with fruit and milk
- Porridge with honey
- All-in-one shake or milkshake
- Banana and yoghurt
- Toast with jam or honey
- Smoothie or milkshake
- Eggs on toast
- Pancakes with honey

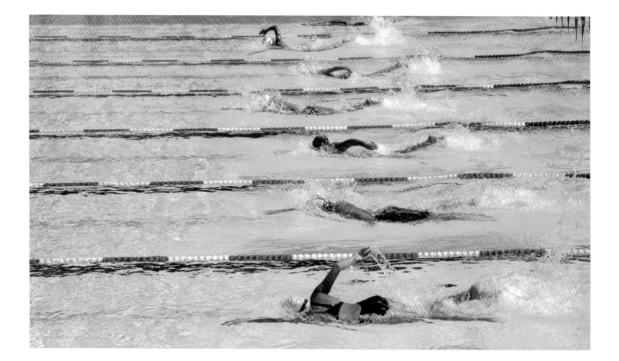

Between events

If you don't know what food will be available at the venue, take your own. Organise your food and drink the day before so that you have a supply of suitable foods and drinks for race day. Remember, don't eat anything that you haven't tried during training.

If you will be competing in several heats, you will need to rehydrate and refuel during your rest periods. It's best to eat light snacks between heats to keep your blood sugar levels steady. Try to eat and drink as soon as possible after your heat, allowing a couple of hours between eating and your next heat. Take frequent drinks of water and, if you cannot face solid food, have sports drinks or diluted cordial so at least you'll get the carbohydrate you need. Swimming venues are often hot and humid so fluid losses can be high even if you are just resting between heats.

If you will be racing later in the day, schedule a mini meal or lunch 2–4 hours before the start. It should contain carbohydrate as well as protein and fat. Sandwiches with a protein filling, a baked potato with tuna or cheese, a pasta or rice dish would be suitable options.

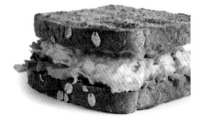

REFUELLING SNACKS BETWEEN EVENTS

- Fresh fruit (easy to eat): bananas, prepared pineapple and melon, grapes, apples, satsumas
- Dried fruit, e.g. raisins, apricots, mango
- Rice cakes or mini-pancakes
- Granola bars
- Yoghurt, milkshake

Light meals

- Pasta or rice – add any combination of vegetables (peppers, tomatoes, cucumber, sweetcorn), nuts, tuna, chicken, cheese
- Sandwiches, wraps, rolls, pitta with chicken, tuna, cheese, peanut butter

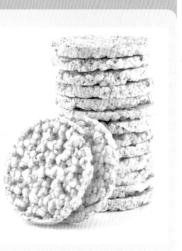

MYTH: BODY FAT IS AN ADVANTAGE FOR SWIMMING

Fact: It's a myth that extra body fat makes you a better swimmer. It may make you more buoyant (i.e. float), but it also slows you down and reduces your stroke efficiency. Research shows that swimmers with lower body fat levels (below 15 per cent for men and below 25 per cent for women) swim faster. If you can pinch more than an inch, you need to lose some body fat because it could quite literally be dragging you down (*see* page 87).

After the event

Before you begin celebrating, think about rehydrating and refuelling your body – your body will thank you for it the following day!

Major swimming competitions are often held over several days. Your preparation for your next day's events starts the moment the previous one has finished. So you must refuel and rehydrate as soon as possible. You need to replace the fluid you have lost but you won't know exactly how much without a set of scales. For every 0.5 kg of body weight lost, you need to drink 750 ml of fluid. Have at least 250–500 ml of water as soon as you've got changed, or at least within 30 minutes of finishing your event. If you are dehydrated (check your urine), a sports drink or diluted juice with a pinch of salt added will help to rehydrate you faster.

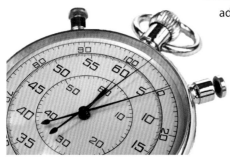

Kick-start your recovery by eating a carbohydrate-rich snack within 30 minutes of your event. Glycogen is restocked faster than normal for up to 2 hours after exercise so take advantage of this opportunity to refuel. Aim to consume around 1 g of carbohydrate/kg of body weight. If you weigh 60 kg, you will need to eat 60 g of carbohydrate. A little protein (1 g of protein for every 3 g/carbohydrate) increases glycogen storage and helps muscles repair faster. Get this either in liquid or solid form.

After you've attended to your immediate refuelling needs, you need to plan a balanced meal for about 2 hours later. It should contain a rich source of carbohydrate as well as protein and fat. Try pasta with chicken and vegetables or a jacket potato with tuna and ratatouille. Avoid the temptation to feast on fast foods, which could make you feel unwell shortly after an event. Table 8.3 gives a fuelling and hydration plan for swimming.

TABLE 8.3 RACE DAY FUELLING AND HYDRATION PLAN

When	Hydration	Fuel needs	Suitable foods
2–4 hours before the event	*Drink 5–7 ml/kg (approx 350–500 ml water)*	*Eat 2–4g carbohydrate/kg (approx 100–200 g)*	*Eggs on toast, porridge with bananas, raisins and honey, cereal with milk and bananas, toast, fruit and milk*
Warm-up			
Post-warm-up	*100–200 ml*	*Eat 1 g carbohydrate/kg (approx 50–70 g)*	*Water, squash, sports drink, bananas, fruit, dried fruit, rice cakes, energy or granola bars, yoghurt*
Race			
Between races	*Drink approx 100–250 ml immediately after the race, and then little and often*	*Eat 1 g carbohydrate/kg (approx 50–70 g)*	*Water, squash or sports drink; bananas, fruit, dried fruit, rice cakes, energy or granola bars, yoghurt*
After the event	*Drink 750 ml/0.5 kg of weight loss*	*Eat a small snack with a 3:1 ratio of carbohydrate to protein*	*Flavoured milk; milk and flapjack; recovery drink, sandwich and yoghurt*

Core menu plans for swimming

The following two core menu plans can be used as a template for developing your individual daily eating plan. Each plan gives you the amounts of foods needed to meet your calorie and macronutrient requirements, providing approximately 3,000 and 3,500 calories. Pick the plan that most closely matches your training schedule (twice a day or once a day) and energy requirement. However, if you do additional land-based training then you should increase the portion sizes to take account of your greater calorie expenditure.

Where the menu plan gives a choice of food type (e.g. carbohydrate), simply pick your preferred option (e.g. pasta or potatoes) or substitute an equivalent (high-carbohydrate) food (e.g. quinoa or noodles). Try to vary your choice of fresh fruit and vegetables as much as possible according to what's in season as this will give you a greater range of micronutrients, antioxidants and phyto-nutrients. Many of the lower-carbohydrate recipes in Part 3 can be incorporated into your plan; simply use the amount of carbohydrate, protein and fat in the core menu plan as a guide.

Measure and weigh your portions carefully to start with to get an idea of what different amounts of foods look like – you should find it quicker and easier to judge how much to eat. Also try to adjust portion sizes according to your appetite and how energetic you feel during training. If you feel hungrier than usual, that's your body's way of signalling its needs so you should eat more food. Similarly, if you fatigue early in training or find it harder to recover between training sessions, then you should also increase your portion sizes. Keep a check on your weight and body composition and adjust your intake accordingly.

The menu plans do not give quantities for water or other drinks as the amount you need is quite individual and will vary day to day according to the climate and your sweat rate. Check your hydration status with the 'pee test' (see page 61) and ensure you drink sufficient fluids to maintain proper hydration.

Q&A

Can sugar be beneficial before a race?

Many swimmers eat sweets, jellies and glucose tablets before a race in the belief that sugar will aid their performance. Sugar is a fast-acting carbohydrate so it will raise blood glucose rapidly – but this doesn't necessarily mean it will make you swim faster. It's easy to over-eat these foods. Eating too much sugar triggers high levels of insulin in the bloodstream, followed by sugar leaving the blood-stream rapidly, resulting in a sharp drop in blood sugar. This rebound effect can make you feel tired, weak and lightheaded. If you need an energy boost, eat only very small amounts of sugar (less than 25 g), but it's safer to choose slower-digesting carbohydrate, such as bananas, dried fruit and granola bars, that are less likely to spike your blood sugar levels.

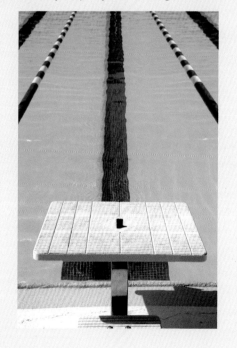

MENU

Core menu plan for swimmers (<2 hours daily training)

Breakfast	Water 2 eggs; 2 x wholegrain toast, butter Fresh fruit 300 ml milk
Snack	50 g nuts and dried fruit Water
Lunch	Water Protein: 100 g chicken, meat, fish or 2 eggs or 50 g cheese Vegetables or salad Carbohydrate: 3 slices wholegrain bread or 75 g wholegrain pasta or rice or 300 g potato Fat: 15 g olive/coconut oil or butter 100 g fresh fruit and 125 g whole-milk yoghurt
Snack	50 g flapjack Water
Dinner	Water Protein: 100 g chicken or fish or 2 eggs or 50 g cheese Vegetables or salad Carbohydrate: 75–100 g (uncooked weight) wholegrain pasta or rice or 300 g potato Fat: 15 g olive/coconut oil or butter 100 g fresh fruit and 125 g whole-milk yoghurt
Training (1–2h)	100 ml cordial or squash (diluted 1 to 8)
Post-training	600 ml milk or flavoured milk or milkshake
Post-training snack	Banana 125 g whole-milk yoghurt

Nutritional analysis:

2,867 calories

142 g protein (20 per cent calories)

116 g fat (35 per cent calories)

338 g carbohydrate (44 per cent calories)

MENU

Core menu plan for swimmers (a.m. and p.m. daily training)

Pre-training	300 ml water; 2 x wholegrain toast and honey/peanut butter
Early morning training (1–2h)	100 ml cordial or squash (diluted 1 to 8)
Post-training	600ml milk/flavoured milk/milkshake
Breakfast	Water 2 eggs; 2 x wholegrain toast, butter 100 g fresh fruit
Snack	50 g nuts and dried fruit; Water
Lunch	Water Protein: 100 g chicken, meat, fish or 2 eggs or 50 g cheese Vegetables or salad Carbohydrate: 3 slices bread or 75 g wholegrain pasta or rice Fat: 15 g olive oil or butter 100 g fresh fruit and 125 g whole-milk yoghurt
Snack	50 g flapjack Water
Dinner	Water Protein: 100 g chicken or fish or 2 eggs or 50 g cheese Vegetables or salad Carbohydrate: 75–100 g (uncooked weight) wholegrain pasta or rice Fat: 15 g olive oil or butter 100 g fresh fruit and 125 g whole-milk yoghurt
Training (1–2h)	100 ml cordial or squash (diluted 1 to 8)
Post-training	600 ml milk or flavoured milk or milkshake
Post-training	Banana 125 g whole-milk yoghurt

Nutritional analysis:

3,592 calories

175 g protein (20 per cent calories)

138 g fat (35 per cent calories)

443 g carbohydrate (46 per cent calories)

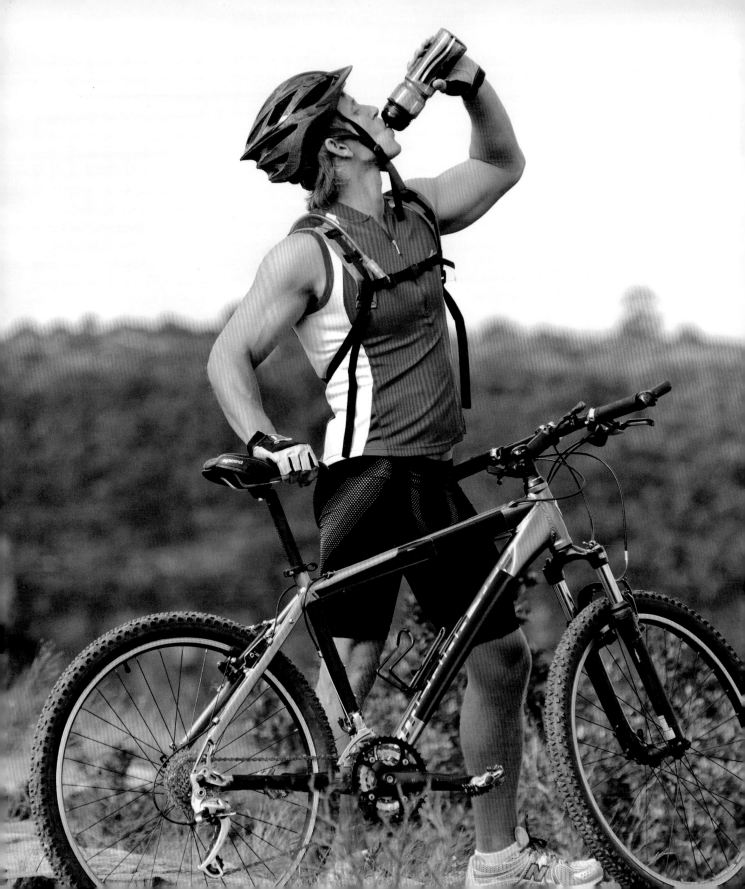

9 NUTRITION FOR CYCLING

Whether you cycle to work, cycle for fitness, or enjoy the more serious challenges of long rides and races, eating correctly will help maximise your performance. Knowing exactly what and how much to eat and drink is an important part of your day-to-day training programme, but is particularly important when it comes to preparing for a cycling event. This chapter will help you put the information in Chapters 1–6 into practice and give you a template for constructing a daily eating plan. It also provides you with a pre-race nutrition strategy and a fuelling and hydration race-day template to help you put in a winning performance – or at least make it to the finish without bonking (running out of energy, like 'hitting the wall' in running)!

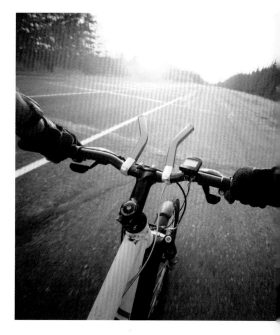

How many calories?

Cycling demands a lot of energy from your body. The number of calories you burn cycling depends on your speed, the terrain, your weight, and how long you are in the saddle. For example, cycling at a leisurely pace (11.3 km/hour or 7 mph) burns 298 calories/hour if you weigh 70 kg, while racing (25.8 km/hour or 16 mph) burns around 710 calories/hour. Table 9.1 shows you approximately how many calories you burn per hour at various speeds.

TABLE 9.1 CALORIES USED IN CYCLING

Speed	cals/kg/hour	60 kg	65 kg	70 kg	75 kg	80 kg
Leisure (11.3 km/hour or 7 mph)	4.26	256	277	298	320	341
Hard (16.1 km/hour or 10 mph)	6.42	385	417	449	482	514
Racing (25.8 km/hour or 16 mph)	10.14	608	659	710	761	811

Your daily calorie needs also depend on your weight, as well as your muscle mass, daily activity level and training frequency. To get an idea of how many calories you should be eating, *see* page 4.

Fuel rules

A carbohydrate-rich diet is essential for serious cyclists. Carbohydrate is turned into glycogen in your muscles, which then fuels your training. When your muscle glycogen stores are high, your training rides will feel easier – you'll be able to keep going longer and faster before getting tired. If you cycle for less than 2 hours per day, you'll probably need to eat 5–7 g of carbohydrate/kg of body weight per day (that's 350–490 g for a 70 kg cyclist). If you cycle up to 3–4 hours daily, you'll need more like 7–10 g of carbohydrate/kg of body weight per day (that's 490–700 g for a 70 kg cyclist).

A lot of endurance cyclists get carried away with carbohydrate and forget about protein and fat. While carbohydrate is important for fuelling your muscles, you also need protein to repair muscle fibres broken down during long hard rides. If you skimp on protein, you may lose muscle. During hard training, some protein – as well as carbohydrate and fat – is used as fuel and can make up as much as 15 per cent of the calorie mix. You need 1.2–1.4 g/kg body weight daily – that's 84–98 g if you weigh 70 kg. So include a portion (about the size of your fist) of protein with each meal – chicken, fish, lean meat, cottage cheese, tofu or Quorn™.

Eat at least five portions of fresh fruit and vegetables each day. They provide antioxidants, which not only boost your immunity but also may help counteract some of the harmful effects of pollutants you breathe in during road rides. Pollutants from traffic fumes and smog increase the number of free radicals (*see* page 29) that your body has to deal with. By stepping up your intake of antioxidant-rich foods, you'll bolster your body's natural defences against these free radicals. Choose a wide variety of fruit and vegetables – the more intensely coloured, the higher the antioxidant potential. Blueberries, blackberries, strawberries, spinach, red peppers and Brussels sprouts are richest in antioxidants.

Shorter rides (<60 minutes)

If you're cycling for less than an hour, water is all you need to maintain hydration and performance. Extra carbohydrate in the form of sports drinks, gels or bars is not necessary. You should have sufficient glycogen in your muscles to fuel your ride. Ensure that you are properly hydrated before you set off by drinking 5–7 ml of fluid/kg of body weight about 4 hours before exercise (350–490 ml for a 70 kg person). There are no hard and fast rules about how much to drink during a ride, but for most conditions 400–800 ml/hour will prevent dehydration as well as overhydration. You should listen to your body and drink when you are thirsty.

Wind chill and rapid evaporation of sweat can give you the false sense that you're not losing much fluid. Even if you don't feel hot or sweaty, you could be losing fluid so you still need to drink.

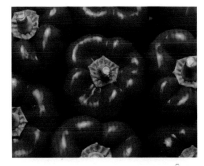

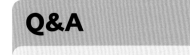

Will cola help me keep going for longer?

A lot of cyclists prefer drinking flat cola during long hard workouts and races. Much of the claimed benefits are based on hearsay handed down from one competitor to another (*see* page 71). The truth is that cola possesses no special performance-enhancing quality – it is simply a sugary drink, containing around 11 g sugar/100 ml. It can give you a quick energy boost, but won't hydrate you very fast as it is too concentrated to empty from the stomach quickly. You'll get a similar sugar 'hit' from sports drinks, bananas, energy gels or solid food. Much of the appeal of cola is probably its caffeine content (32–42 mg/330 ml can of regular or diet cola). But you would need around 200 mg of caffeine to get a performance-enhancing effect.

Longer rides (>60 minutes)

For rides longer than 60 minutes when energy demands are greater, you will certainly need something other than water to keep your blood glucose levels steady and energy output high. Take a supply of cordial or sports drinks and/or carbohydrate-rich snacks (such as dried fruit, flapjacks, energy bars, gels, bananas or granola bars) with you. You'll need to begin fuelling within the first 30 minutes as it takes a further 30 minutes for those carbohydrate to reach your active muscles. If you eat solid food, drink water rather than sports drinks. Studies have shown that consuming extra carbohydrate on rides lasting longer than 90 minutes increases endurance and performance during a race. Aim to consume around 30–60 g/carbohydrate per hour; that's 120–240 calories – equivalent to 400–000 ml/hour of a 6 per cent sugar drink, such as cordial/squash diluted 1 in 6 or an isotonic sports drink (depending on the heat, humidity and your intensity).

Be warned that some brands can 'sit heavy' in the stomach during hard rides – you may find them easier to tolerate diluted with extra water. You'll need to experiment to find the drink strength that suits you best. Try making up powdered drinks with extra water if necessary or take a bottle of sports drink and a bottle of water, alternately drinking both.

You have the advantage over other endurance athletes in that you can carry fluids and food on the bike frame or in jersey pockets. Also, it's easier to eat solid foods, as you're not bouncing around. Learning to eat during cycling without swerving can be tricky at first.

After cycling

If you plan to exercise within 24 hours, start refuelling within 30 minutes of a ride. There exists a 2-hour window when glycogen is restocked about one and a half times faster than normal. The sooner you can get carbohydrate to your muscles, the faster you will be able to recover. If you have a high-carbohydrate snack, ideally with a little protein (in a ratio of about 1 g protein/3 g carbohydrate), as soon as you have showered, you will be able to cycle better the next day and feel generally more energetic. If you leave a longer gap before eating, it will take you longer to recover and your legs won't feel as fresh the next day. Suitable options include flavoured milk, fruit with yoghurt, a commercial recovery drink or a flapjack with milk.

HOW TO EAT AND DRINK IN THE SADDLE

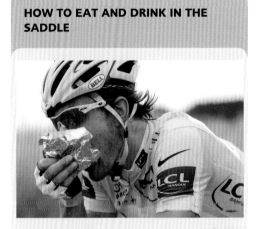

- On long rides, wearing specially designed packs that contains a plastic bladder (such as a camel pack) allows you to drink without having to take your hands off the handlebars. You can carry larger volumes of drink without needing to stop off to refill your bottle.
- In hot weather, add ice cubes to your drink or freeze half the bottle (or camel pack) overnight and top it up before you get on your bike.
- Stash small snacks in the pockets of your jersey.
- Open your bars and undo packets before you set off so the food is easy to get at with one hand during your ride.
- Peel fruit and wrap in foil for easy access.
- Wrap dried fruit and biscuits in foil or small resealable plastic bags.
- Soft-textured bars may be wrapped around your handlebars for easy access.
- Practise riding without holding on to the handlebar so that you can balance more easily while you eat and drink.

TABLE 9.2 FUELLING AND HYDRATION STRATEGY FOR CYCLING

When	Hydration	Fuel needs	Suitable foods
2–4 hours before a ride	Drink 5–7 ml/kg (approx 350–500 ml)	Eat 2–4 g carbohydrate/kg (approx 100–200 g)	Pasta and chicken, rice and fish
OR <1 hour before a ride	Drink approx 100–250 ml	Eat 1 g carbohydrate/kg (approx 50–70 g)	Bananas, toast and honey
During a shorter ride (<1 hour)	According to thirst; little and often	Not needed	Water, low-calorie squash or sports drink
During a longer ride (1–2 hours)	Drink 400–800 ml/hour according to thirst; little and often	15–30 g carbohydrate every 15–30 minutes for a total of 30–60 g/hour	Cordial, squash, sports drink, bananas, gels, energy or granola bars, dried fruit, honey
During a longer ride (>2 hours)	Drink 400–800 ml/hour according to thirst; little and often	30–60 g/hour (up to 90 g if cycling >3 hours)	Sports drinks; dual source sports drinks; bananas, gels, energy or granola bars, dried fruit, honey
After a long ride (>1 hour)	Drink 750 ml/0.5 kg weight loss	Eat a small snack with a 3:1 ratio of carbohydrate to protein	Flavoured milk, milk and flapjack, sandwich and yoghurt

Preparing for a race

What you eat and drink in the weeks and days before a race makes a big difference to your performance. Start eating a healthy diet (see Chapter 1) as early in your preparations as possible – this will help you train harder and longer – and then fine-tune your diet in the last week before the event.

A few weeks before

As you increase your weekly mileage or step up your training intensity, you'll need extra calories to fuel your body. For example, an extra 4 hours in the saddle each week burns around 1,800 extra calories if you weigh 70 kg (*see* page 4 for an idea of how many extra calories you are burning). If you don't make any adjustment to your overall calorie intake, you risk losing muscle (and fat). If you can do with shedding some body fat, the extra training will help, but make sure you step up your protein intake to 1.6–2.0 g/kg (112–140 g for a 70 kg cyclist) to preserve muscle mass (*see* page 169).

If you don't already, you'll need to practise drinking from a water bottle or eating snacks while riding. Work out how to keep your balance without swerving while you drink, or eat with one hand. Most cyclists move one hand to the centre of the handlebars.

WHAT TO EAT IN THE SADDLE

- Granola or energy bars
- Energy gels
- Fig rolls
- Bananas
- Malt loaf or fruit cake
- Raisins or sultanas

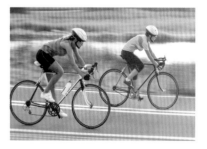

Practise your race strategy in training. Whatever you plan to do during the race, rehearse it before. Practise drinking from a water bottle, or if you plan to use a camel pack in the event, use it during your training rides. Experiment with different foods – gels, bars and bananas – to find the types and amounts that suit you best. Research the foods and drinks to be provided at the stations so you can test them out beforehand. Alternatively, take your own supplies.

The week before

What you eat and drink during the week before your long ride or race can make a big difference to your performance. You goals are to maximise your muscle glycogen stores and keep yourself well hydrated.

10- and 25-mile time trials

If you'll be racing for less than about 60 minutes, what you eat and drink before is more important than what you consume during the race. Make sure you keep hydrated – your urine should be a pale straw colour – and that you keep eating your normal diet. Your muscles will be able to store enough glycogen since you'll also be reducing your training load. You won't deplete glycogen completely so there's no need to 'carb-load'. Make sure you avoid high-intensity training the day or two before so that you don't deplete your muscle glycogen.

Long races

If you'll be racing for more than an hour, you'll need to ensure that your muscles are fully rested and stocked with glycogen before the event. Taper your training gradually. For the last few days of the week you should be cutting the time spent in the saddle by half and then resting completely for the last day or two. If you don't reduce your training you risk using the carbohydrate you're eating to fuel your training rides instead of stockpiling it for the big event.

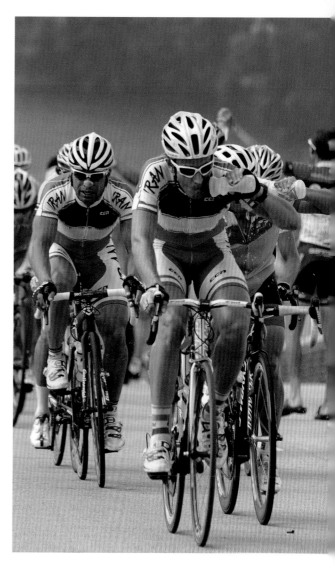

Eat your normal diet until three days before racing, and then increase your carbohydrate intake (7–10 g carbohydrate/kg of body weight) for the final three days, plus on race morning. Tipping the balance of calories a little more in favour of carbohydrate (roughly 60–70 per cent carbohydrate calories) and eating correspondingly less fat should boost your glycogen levels and give you more fuel for the event. Tapering your training along with increasing your carbohydrate intake can increase your endurance by as much as 20 per cent.

The day before the race

The day before the race is your final chance to top up your muscle glycogen stores. It's also important to keep yourself hydrated and avoid eating or drinking anything that may jeopardise your performance.

Don't try any new foods. The last thing you want before a race is a stomach upset, so play it safe by sticking to familiar foods. Choose fairly plain foods, such as fish with rice or potatoes with chicken, and avoid spicy and salty foods such as crisps, takeaways, ready-made sauces and ready-meals.

Eating small frequent meals will maximise glycogen storage without making you feel bloated and heavy. Drink plenty of fluids throughout the day to ensure you are properly hydrated. Your urine should be pale straw coloured.

Steer clear of high-fibre gas-forming foods, such as baked beans, lentils and other pulses, cauliflower, Brussels sprouts, bran cereals and spicy foods. Eating them could give you an uncomfortable ride the next day!

Do not overindulge the evening before your race. A large meal – even if it's high in carbohydrate – could make you feel sluggish the next day. Alcohol is a diuretic so it's better to avoid it completely otherwise you risk dehydration and a hangover on race day.

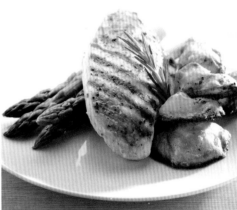

Race day nutition

On the day of the race, your muscle glycogen levels should be fully stocked and you should be feeling rested. If the event is in the morning, you'll need to get up about 4 hours before and have your pre-race meal. This should be rich in carbo-hydrate to top up the store of glycogen in your liver and keep up your blood sugar levels for the next few hours. Aim for 150–200 g of carbohydrate before a long race; for short rides under an hour, you may need only 75–150 g. If you find it difficult to eat solid food when you're feeling nervous, try a liquid meal instead (*see* page 147). Skipping that pre-race meal may leave you low in energy during the final stages.

Steer clear of bran and high-fibre cereals, *especially* if you are feeling nervous. Cereal fibre may loosen the stools and cause more bowel movements than normal. Select foods that are fairly low in fibre, such as white toast instead of brown, cornflakes instead of bran flakes.

Make sure that you are properly hydrated by drinking 350–500 ml of water, cordial, squash, a sports drink or diluted fruit juice (1 part juice to 1 or 2 parts water) about 2–4 hours before the race. Your urine should be a pale yellow colour

PRE-RACE MEAL IDEAS

- Cereal with dried fruit and milk
- Scrambled eggs on toast
- Porridge with bananas
- Toast, honey and a milky drink
- Milkshake or all-in-one shake
- Smoothie made with fruit and yoghurt

by the start time. It's also wise to top up with a further 125–250 ml in the warm-up or just before you head to the line. If you decide to take caffeine, whether in the form of a drink or gel, consume this about 30–60 minutes before the race start time. The sodium naturally present in your food will also help the body hold on to fluid (which may be advantageous prior to a race when it's important to avoid dehydration) so, despite the marketing hype, there's no need to consume a sports drink – i.e. a drink with sodium or electrolytes – beforehand.

Drink whatever you used in training. As a rule of thumb, water (or low-calorie sports drinks if you prefer the taste) is fine for 10- or 25-mile races or rides lasting less than 60–90 minutes; isotonic sports drinks, squash or cordial are better for longer races. But do not try anything different – even if it's freely provided by the organisers – in case it doesn't agree with you under race conditions.

In hot conditions, start drinking early, ideally in the first 20–30 minutes. If you pick your moment, like a steady climb, it's not much of a disruption to your rhythm. Take three or four swigs, and then according to thirst. Remember that wind chill and rapid evaporation of sweat can mask feelings of thirst.

For rides longer than 60 minutes you will need food or a sports drink to keep up your blood sugar levels. Try to consume 400–800 ml/hour. Or try gels, energy bars, granola bars, fig rolls or a banana with plenty of water. Eat little and often to save your digestive system having to work too hard.

It's easier to eat and drink when you're riding on the flat and in a straight line; climbing, descending and cornering demand your full concentration. Take advantage of the food served at the rest stops but don't eat anything you haven't used in training.

After the race
It's a great sense of accomplishment when you have completed the race and cross the finishing line. Before you load up your bike and start back home, though, start rehydrating and refuelling your body. Recovery needs to begin now to set you up for the next week's training and the next race.

Drink plenty of liquids to replace fluid losses. As a guide, have 500 ml as soon as practical, ideally within the first 30 minutes, then keep drinking small regular amounts until your urine is pale in colour. If you are dehydrated, a sports drink or diluted juice with a pinch of added salt will deliver fluid faster and the sodium they contain helps your body retain the fluid better. Alternatively, opt for a recovery drink containing carbohydrate and protein in a 3 to 1 ratio for speedy fuel and muscle recovery.

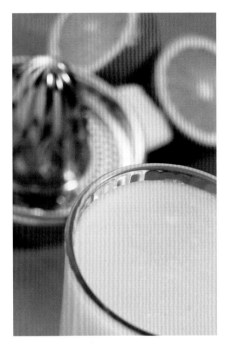

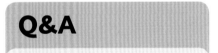

Q&A

How can I avoid the 'bonk'?

The 'bonk' is a common problem. It happens when you have used up the glycogen in your muscles and liver and have no energy left. To avoid this, drink sports drinks or eat high-carbohydrate snacks regularly during the ride. Try energy bars, bananas, energy gels, and granola or energy bars. Aim to consume 30–60 g carbohydrate/hour – that's one or two bars (depending on the size) or a couple of gel sachets, or 2–4 bananas or 400–800 ml of an isotonic sports drink (depending on the strength).

Have a carbohydrate/protein snack within the first 30 minutes (when blood flow to your muscles is greater and the muscles are more receptive to carbohydrate). This will help rebuild your glycogen stores. Suitable post-race options include milk-based drinks, recovery drinks, cheese or chicken sandwiches, yoghurt and flapjacks.

Follow your post-race snack with a carbohydrate-rich meal within 2 hours. Including protein will help replenish glycogen faster as well as help with muscle repair. Suggested meals include rice with chicken, pasta with pasta sauce and cheese, a jacket potato with steak (plus vegetables or salad).

It's tempting to head for the nearest greasy spoon café, burger van or fast food restaurant after a race. But fried, fatty or spicy foods will only sit heavily in your stomach at this time, impeding your recovery. Opt for lighter meals and save the greasy stuff for later on if you must!

Table 9.3 gives a race day fuelling and hydration plan.

RECOVERY SNACK IDEAS

- Banana and yoghurt
- Flapjack or granola bar
- Fruit cake or malt loaf
- Sandwich with meat, chicken, fish, egg or cheese
- Milk, flavoured milk, milkshake
- Dried fruit and nuts

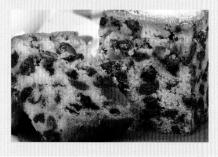

TABLE 9.3 RACE DAY FUELLING AND HYDRATION PLAN

When	Hydration	Fuel needs	Suitable foods
4 hours before the race	*Drink 5–7 ml/kg (approx 350–500 ml)*	*Eat 2–4 g carbohydrate/kg (approx 100–200 g)*	*Eggs on toast, porridge with bananas, raisins and honey, cereal with milk and bananas, toast, fruit and milk*
1–2 hours before the race	*Drink approx 100–250 ml*	*Eat 1 g carbohydrate/kg (approx 50–70 g)*	*Bananas, toast and honey, energy or granola bar*
During 40-km race (<1 hour)	*According to thirst; little and often*	*Not needed*	*Water, low-calorie squash or sports drink*
During long races (>1 hour)	*Drink 400–800 ml/hour according to thirst; little and often*	*15–30 g carbohydrate every 15–30 minutes for a total of 30–60 g/hour (up to 90 g for events >3 hours)*	*Cordial, squash, sports drink, dual source sports drinks; bananas*, gels*, energy or granola bars*, dried fruit*, honey**
After the race	*Drink 750 ml/0.5 kg of weight loss*	*Eat a small snack with a 3:1 ratio of carbohydrate to protein*	*Recovery drink, flavoured milk, milk and flapjack, sandwich and yoghurt*

*Accompany with water

Core menu plans for cycling

The following two core menu plans can be used as a template for developing your individual daily eating plan. Each plan gives you the amounts of foods needed to meet your calorie and macronutrient requirements, providing approximately 3,000 and 3,500 calories. Pick the plan that most closely matches your training schedule (up to 2 hours, or more than 2 hours a day) and energy requirement. However, if you train longer, then you should increase the portion sizes to take account of your greater calorie expenditure.

Where the menu plan gives a choice of food type (e.g. carbohydrate), simply pick your preferred option (e.g. pasta or potatoes) or substitute an equivalent (high-carbohydrate) food (e.g. quinoa or noodles). Try to vary your choice of fresh fruit and vegetables as much as possible according to what's in season as this will give you a greater range of micronutrients, antioxidants and phytonutrients. Many of the lower-carbohydrate recipes in Part 3 can be incorporated into your plan; simply use the amount of carbohydrate, protein and fat in the core menu plan as a guide.

Measure and weigh your portions carefully to start with to get an idea of what different amounts of foods look like. Thereafter, you should find it quicker and easier to judge how much to eat.

You should also adjust portion sizes according to your appetite and how energetic you feel during training. If you feel hungrier than usual, that's your body's way of signalling its needs, so you should eat more food. Similarly, if you fatigue early in training or find it harder to recover between training sessions, then you should also increase your portion sizes. Keep a check on your weight and body composition and adjust your intake accordingly.

The menu plans do not give quantities for water or other drinks as the amount you need is quite individual and will vary day to day according to the climate and your sweat rate. Check your hydration status with the 'pee test' (*see* page 61) and ensure you drink sufficient fluids to maintain proper hydration.

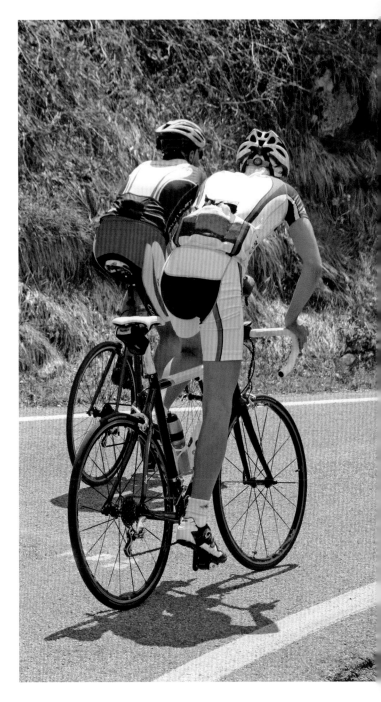

MENU

Core menu plan for cyclists (1–2 hours training)

Breakfast	Water Porridge (75 g oatmeal plus 500 ml milk) 25 g honey, 1 banana and 25 g dried fruit
Training (1–2h)	100 ml cordial or squash (diluted 1 to 8) Water 50 g granola bar
Snack	600 ml milk/flavoured milk/milkshake
Lunch	Water Protein: 100 g chicken, meat, fish or 2 eggs or 50 g cheese Vegetables or salad Carbohydrate: 3 slices bread or 75 g wholegrain pasta or rice or 300 g potato Fat: 15 g olive/coconut oil or butter 100 g fresh fruit and 125 g whole-milk yoghurt
Snack	25 g nuts 100 g fresh fruit Water
Dinner	Water Protein: 100 g chicken or fish or 2 eggs or 50 g cheese Vegetables or salad Carbohydrate: 75–100 g (uncooked weight) wholegrain pasta or rice or 300 g potato Fat: 15 g olive/coconut oil or butter 100 g fresh fruit and 125 g whole-milk yoghurt

Nutritional analysis:

2,917 calories

142 g protein (19 per cent calories)

98 g fat (30 per cent calories)

395 g carbohydrate (51 per cent calories)

MENU

Core menu plan for cyclists (>2 hours training)

Breakfast	Water Porridge (100 g oatmeal plus 600 ml milk) 25 g honey, 1 banana and 25 g dried fruit
Training (>2h)	1 litre sports drink or dual source sports drink Water 50 g granola bar and 2 gels
Snack	600 ml milk/flavoured milk/milkshake Banana
Lunch	Water Protein: 100 g chicken, meat, fish or 2 eggs or 50 g cheese Vegetables or salad Carbohydrate: 4 slices bread or 100 g wholegrain pasta or rice or 400 g potato Fat: 15 g olive/coconut oil or butter 100 g fresh fruit and 125 g whole-milk yoghurt
Snack	25 g nuts 100 g fresh fruit Water
Dinner	Water Protein: 100 g chicken or fish or 2 eggs or 50 g cheese Vegetables or salad Carbohydrate: 75–100 g (uncooked weight) wholegrain pasta or rice or 300 g potato Fat: 15 g olive/coconut oil or butter 100 g fresh fruit and 125 g whole-milk yoghurt

Nutritional analysis:

3,481 calories

157 g protein (18 per cent calories)

102 g fat (27 per cent calories)

518 g carbohydrate (55 per cent calories)

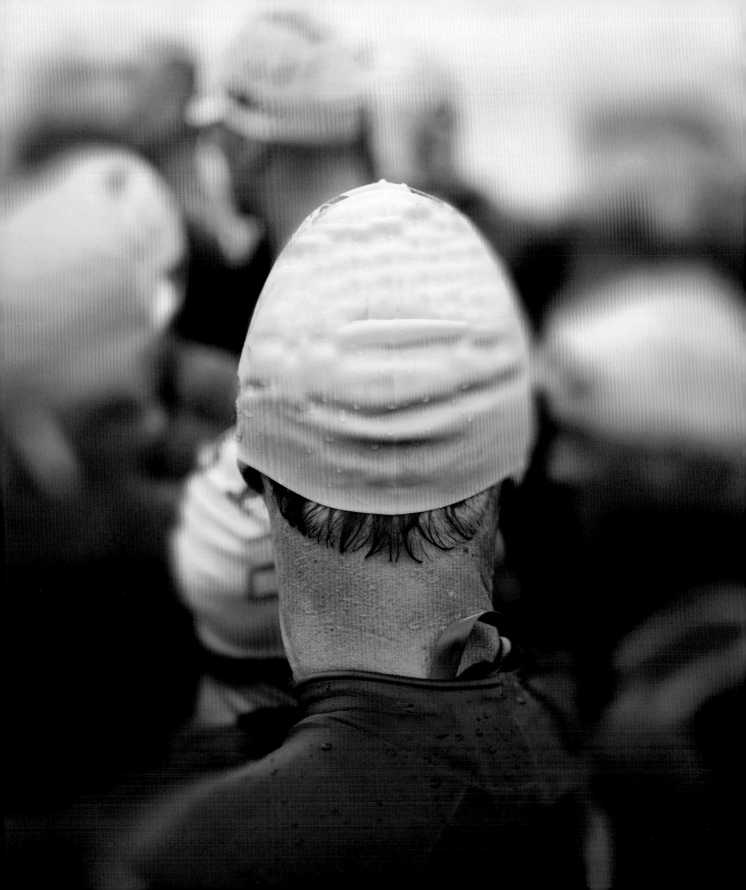

10 NUTRITION FOR TRIATHLON

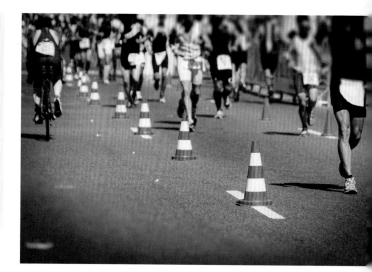

Nutrition and hydration play a large part of your training and recovery whether you compete in sprint, Olympic, Half Ironman or Ironman triathlons. But they become even more important in the run-up to competitions and also on race day for fuelling performance, avoiding stomach discomfort, and recovering from your efforts. This chapter condenses the information in Chapters 1–6 into a pre-race nutrition strategy and a race-day template to help you achieve your best triathlon performance.

How many calories?

Swimming, cycling and running all place high energy demands on your body. The number of calories you burn will depend on your speed, the terrain, your weight and how long you are training. Table 10.1 shows you approximately how many calories you burn per hour in the different activities.

TABLE 10.1 CALORIES USED IN TRIATHLON

Activity	cals/kg/hour	60 kg	65 kg	70 kg	75 kg	80 kg
Cycling (16.1 km/hour or 10 mph)	6.42	385	417	449	482	514
Cycling (25.8 km/hour or 16 mph)	10.14	608	659	710	761	811
Running (12.0 km/hour or 7.5 mph)	12.5	750	813	875	938	1,000
Running (16.0 km/hour or 10.0 mph)	15.1	906	982	1,057	1,133	1,208
Swimming (slow crawl)	7.68	461	499	538	576	614
Swimming (medium crawl)	9.36	562	608	655	702	749
Swimming (fast crawl)	17.1	1,026	1,112	1,197	1,283	1,368

Preparing for an event

A few weeks before

Make any nutritional changes as early in your preparations as possible – this will help you train harder and longer – and then fine-tune your diet in the last week before the event. Match your calorie intake with your training load; if you increase your weekly mileage or training intensity, you'll need extra calories to fuel your body. When you reduce your training load during your taper, then you'll need to consume fewer calories.

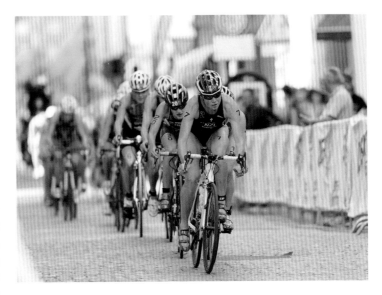

Test in training what you plan to do during the race. Practise drinking from a water bottle on the bike. Or, if you plan to use a camel pack in the event, use it during your training rides. Practise grabbing cups and drinking on the move without spilling or choking. Experiment with different foods – gels, bars and bananas – to find the types and amounts that suit you best. Research the foods and drinks to be provided at the stations so you can test them out beforehand. Alternatively, take your own supplies.

Follow the nutrition and hydration strategies for running (page 141), cycling (page 169) and swimming (page 155) according to your training programme.

The week before the event

In the last few days before the race, your goals are to maximise muscle glycogen stores and keep yourself hydrated.

Sprint triathlon

A sprint triathlon, which comprises a 400–750-m swim, a 20-km bike ride, and a 5-km run, can take between 1 and 2 hours. Whether you're a novice or a more experienced triathlete, you'll be taxing your body and using considerable amounts of muscle glycogen. However, it's not necessary to increase your usual carbohydrate intake or carb-load – your muscle glycogen stores will increase once you cut back on your training. Eat your normal diet during the last week and make sure you keep hydrated – your urine should be pale. Just avoid depleting your glycogen with high-intensity training during the final few days before the race.

Olympic, Half Ironman and Ironman

An Olympic distance triathlon, which has a 1500-m swim, 40-km bike ride, and a 10-km run can take anything between 2 and 3½ hours, depending on your level. An Ironman triathlon consists of a 2.4-mile swim, a 112-mile bike ride, and a marathon (26.2-mile run) and has a cut-off time of 17 hours. Both require considerable endurance and require careful nutrition preparation. Tapering your training along with increasing your carbohydrate intake will boost glycogen levels and give you more fuel for the event.

Do your last long training session (but not an exhaustive workout) a week from race day followed by increasingly shorter workouts throughout race week. Eat your normal diet until 3 days before racing, and then increase your carbohydrate intake (7–10 g carbohydrate/kg body weight) for the final 3 days, plus race morning.

Don't increase your total calorie intake. Instead, reduce fat and protein intake in an amount that equals (or slightly exceeds) the amount of carbohydrate you add. Combining less training with more total calories could result in last-minute weight gain that will only slow you down. Make sure you drink plenty of water each day to ensure you are properly hydrated.

The day before the event

Complete your taper today – perform only very light exercise.

The day before the race is your final chance to top up your muscle glycogen stores. It's also important to keep yourself hydrated and avoid eating or drinking anything that may jeopardise your performance.

Get organised for the next day. Don't rely on finding nutritious foods at outlets en route or at the venue – healthy choices are often limited at these places. It is always best to take your own food supplies for the journey as well as for race day. Take extra water in case of delays – it's easy to become dehydrated when you're travelling.

Eat a relatively early supper, no later than 12 hours before your race start if possible. This will allow your body enough time to digest the food. Make carbohydrate (pasta, rice or potatoes) the focal point of your meal, but don't over-eat otherwise you may feel heavy and sluggish the next day. Play it safe by sticking to plain and familiar foods that you know agree with you. Don't try anything that you wouldn't normally eat or drink or risk an upset stomach – steer away from anything spicy or salty, and avoid meat or fish that may be undercooked. Avoid gas-forming foods (or combinations of food) such as baked beans and other pulses, cruciferous vegetables (broccoli, Brussels sprouts, cauliflower),

EATING AND DRINKING IN THE SADDLE

- Many triathletes use specially designed packs containing a plastic bladder (such as a camel pack). This will allow you to carry larger volumes of drink without needing to stop off to refill your bottle.
- For a cooler drink, add ice cubes to your drink or freeze half the bottle (or camel pack) overnight, then top it up before you get on your bike.
- Carry small snacks in the pockets of your jersey.
- Wrap dried fruit and biscuits in foil or small resealable plastic bags.
- Soft-textured bars may be wrapped around your handlebars for easy access.
- Practise riding without holding on to the handlebars so that you can balance more easily while you eat and drink.

bran cereals and spicy foods the night before the race. These can make you feel uncomfortable. Avoid alcohol as it's a diuretic – failing this, limit yourself to a single unit.

Race day nutrition

Your pre-race breakfast is key to ensuring that your muscles and liver are fully stocked up with glycogen. Skipping breakfast may leave you low in energy during the final stages.

Eat a moderate-sized carbohydrate-rich breakfast about 4 hours before competing to top up the store of glycogen in your liver and keep up your blood sugar levels for the next few hours. This ensures the body has enough time to empty the stomach and digest the food. Aim for 150–200 g of carbohydrate before a long race. For sprint races you may need only 75–150 g. Your breakfast can also contain a little fat and protein, e.g. eggs and milk. If you find it difficult to eat solid food when you're feeling nervous, try a liquid meal instead (*see* page 147). Avoid bran and high-fibre cereals as they may loosen the stools and cause more bowel movements than normal.

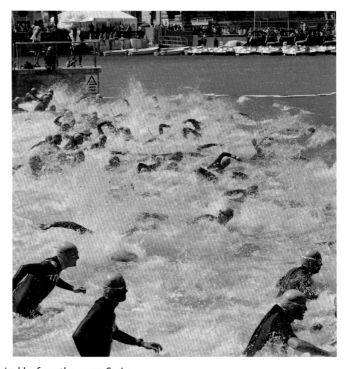

Starting the swim part of your race properly hydrated is key to performance, particularly for Olympic and Ironman triathlons. Have 350–500 ml of water, cordial, squash, a sports drink or diluted fruit juice (1 part juice to 1–2 parts water) during the 2–4-hour period before the race. Swig frequently rather than drinking it in one go. The sodium naturally present in your food will also help the body hold on to fluid (which may be advantageous prior to a race when it's important to avoid dehydration) so, despite the marketing hype, there's no need to consume a sports drink, i.e. a drink with sodium or electrolytes, beforehand.

Consuming a small carbohydrate-rich snack or drink about 1–2 hours before the start of the race will help maintain blood sugar levels. This should supply about 1 g carbohydrate/kg body weight (70 g for a 70 kg athlete). Suitable options include a sports drink, energy drink or cordial, a banana, rice cakes or a gel.

Drink a further 125–250 ml in the warm-up or just before you head to the line. If you decide to take caffeine, whether in the form of a drink or gel, consume this about 30–60 minutes before the race start time.

PRE-RACE MEAL IDEAS

- Cereal with dried fruit and milk
- Scrambled eggs on toast
- Porridge with bananas
- Toast, honey and milky drink
- Milkshake or all-in-one shake
- Smoothie made with fruit and yoghurt

During the race

You will not be able to drink during the swim, but start drinking as soon as you get on the bike. In sprint triathlons the bike and run tend to be relatively flat so you can carry a bottle on your bike without adversely affecting your time. Drink little and often according to thirst and sweat rate. Two or three swigs at a time suits many triathletes. Stick to whatever fluids you drank during your training. This should provide you with enough energy to see you through the 5-km run.

For longer events (more than 90 minutes), you will need to consume extra carbohydrate in the form of sports drinks, energy gels, bars or fruit; these should be taken with sufficient water to maintain hydration and blood sugar levels. Take advantage of the food served at the rest stops, but don't eat anything you haven't previously eaten in training. It is easier to eat and drink when you're riding on the flat and in a straight line; climbing, descending and cornering demand your full concentration.

You may benefit from a sports drink containing sodium (electrolytes) during Olympic distance and Ironman triathlons when you'll be competing for longer than 2 hours. The sodium helps the body retain fluid. For events longer than 3 hours, dual source sports drinks that supply a higher amount of carbohydrate than regular isotonic drinks will help spare your muscle glycogen stores and increase your endurance.

After the race

The key to fast recovery is food and drink, so the sooner you eat and drink the better. Make sure you are rehydrated before embarking on a celebratory drink. You should drink about 500 ml of water, sports drink or recovery drink within the first 30 minutes of completing the event, then keep drinking small regular amounts until your urine is pale in colour. If you are dehydrated, a sports drink or diluted juice with a pinch of salt added will deliver fluid faster, and the sodium they contain will help your body retain the fluid better. Alternatively, opt for a recovery drink containing carbohydrate and protein in a 3 to 1 ratio for speedy fuel and muscle recovery.

Eat a carbohydrate-rich snack within the first 30 minutes of completing the event, when blood flow to the muscles is greater and glycogen storage is 1½ times faster than normal. This will help rebuild your glycogen stores. Suitable post-race options include milk-based drinks, recovery drinks, cheese or chicken sandwiches, yoghurt and flapjacks.

WHAT TO EAT IN THE SADDLE

- Energy bars, granola bars, flapjacks
- Gels
- Bananas
- Malt loaf or fruit cake
- Dried fruit
- Fig rolls
- Rice cakes
- Sandwiches

RECOVERY SNACKS

- Bananas and yoghurt
- Flapjack or granola bars
- Fruit cake or malt loaf
- Sandwich with meat, chicken, fish, egg or cheese
- Milk, flavoured milk, milkshake
- Dried fruit and nuts

Eat a carbohydrate-rich meal within 2 hours of finishing the race. This should also include a portion of lean protein, to help replenish glycogen faster and aid muscle repair.

Table 10.2 gives a race day fuelling and hydration plan.

TABLE 10.2 RACE DAY FUELLING AND HYDRATION PLAN

When	Hydration	Fuel needs	Suitable foods
4 hours before the race	*Drink 5–7 ml/kg (approx 350–500 ml)*	*Eat 2–4 g carbohydrate/kg (approx 100–200 g)*	*Eggs on toast; porridge with bananas, raisins and honey; cereal with milk and bananas; toast, fruit and milk*
1–2 hours before the race	*Drink approx 100–250 ml*	*Eat 1 g carbohydrate/kg (approx 50–70 g)*	*Bananas; toast and honey; energy or granola bar*
During sprint triathlon (<2 hours)	*Drink 400–800 ml/ hour according to thirst; little and often*	*15–30 g carbohydrate every 15–30 minutes for a total of 30–60 g/hour*	*Water; cordial, squash, sports drink, bananas*, gels*, energy or granola bars*, dried fruit*, honey**
During Olympic distance or Ironman triathlon (>2 hours)	*Drink 400–800 ml/ hour according to thirst; little and often*	*30–60 g/hour (up to 90 g for races >3 hours)*	*Sports drinks, dual source sports drinks; bananas*, gels*, energy or granola bars*, dried fruit*, honey**
After the race	*Drink 750 ml/0.5 kg weight loss*	*Eat a small snack with a 3:1 ratio of carbohydrate to protein*	*Recovery drink; flavoured milk; milk and flapjack; sandwich and yoghurt*

*Accompany with water

Core menu plans for triathlon

The following two core menu plans can be used as a template for developing your individual daily eating plan. Each plan gives you the amounts of foods needed to meet your calorie and macronutrient requirements, providing approximately 2,500 and 3,500 calories. Pick the plan that most closely matches your training schedule (twice a day or once a day) and energy requirement. However, if you do additional land-based training then you should increase the portion sizes to take account of your greater calorie expenditure.

Where the menu plan gives a choice of food type (e.g. carbohydrate), simply pick your preferred option (e.g. pasta or potatoes) or substitute an equivalent (high-carbohydrate) food (e.g. quinoa or noodles). Try to vary your choice of fresh fruit and vegetables as much as possible according to what's in season as this will give you a greater range of micronutrients, antioxidants and phytonutrients.

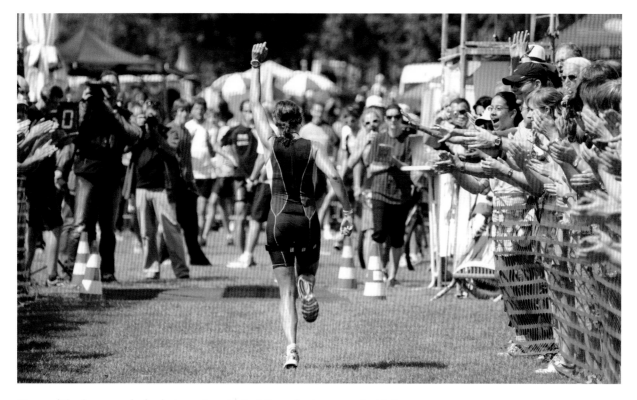

Many of the lower-carbohydrate recipes in Part 3 can be incorporated into your plan; simply use the amount of carbohydrate, protein and fat in the core menu plan as a guide.

Measure and weigh your portions carefully to start with to get an idea of what different amounts of foods look like. Thereafter, you should find it quicker and easier to judge how much to eat.

You should also adjust portion sizes according to your appetite and how energetic you feel during training. If you feel hungrier than usual, that's your body's way of signalling its needs so you should eat more food. Similarly, if you fatigue early in training or find it harder to recover between training sessions, then you should also increase your portion sizes. Keep a check on your weight and body composition and adjust your intake accordingly.

The menu plans do not give quantities for water or other drinks as the amount you need is quite individual and will vary from day to day according to the climate and your sweat rate. Check your hydration status with the 'pee test' (see page 61) and ensure you drink sufficient fluids to maintain proper hydration.

MENU

Menu plan for sprint triathletes (<1 hour daily training)

Breakfast	Water 2 eggs; 2 x wholegrain toast, butter 100 g fresh fruit
Snack	25 g nuts 125 g whole-milk yoghurt Water
Snack	600 ml milk/flavoured milk/milkshake
Lunch	Water Protein: 100 g chicken, meat, fish or 2 eggs or 50 g cheese Vegetables or salad Carbohydrate: 3 slices bread or 75 g wholegrain pasta or rice or 300 g potato Fat: 15 g olive/coconut oil or butter 100 g fresh fruit and 125 g whole-milk yoghurt
Snack	50 g flapjack Banana Water
Training (<1h)	Water
Post-training	600 ml milk/flavoured milk/milkshake
Dinner	Water Protein: 100 g chicken or fish or 2 eggs or 50 g cheese Vegetables or salad Carbohydrate: 75–100 g (uncooked weight) wholegrain pasta or rice or 300 g potato Fat: 15g olive/coconut oil or butter 100 g fresh fruit and 125 g whole-milk yoghurt

Nutritional analysis:

2,555 calories

143 g protein (22 per cent calories)

101 g fat (35 per cent calories)

291 g carbohydrate (43 per cent calories)

MENU

Menu plan for Olympic and Ironman triathletes (a.m. and p.m. training)

Pre-training	300 ml water 2 x wholegrain toast and honey/peanut butter
Early morning training (1–2h)	100 ml cordial or squash (diluted 1 to 8)
Post-training	600 ml milk/flavoured milk/milkshake
Breakfast	Water 2 eggs; 2 x wholegrain toast, butter 100 g fresh fruit
Snack	50 g nuts and dried fruit; water
Lunch	Water Protein: 100 g chicken, meat, fish or 2 eggs or 50 g cheese Vegetables or salad Carbohydrate: 3 slices bread or 75 g wholegrain pasta or rice or 300 g potato Fat: 15 g olive/coconut oil or butter 100 g fresh fruit and 125 g whole-milk yoghurt
Snack	50 g flapjack; water
Dinner	Water Protein: 100 g chicken or fish or 2 eggs or 50 g cheese Vegetables or salad Carbohydrate: 75–100 g (uncooked weight) wholegrain pasta or rice or 300 g potato Fat: 15 g olive/coconut oil or butter 100 g fresh fruit and 125 g whole-milk yoghurt
Training (1–2h)	100 ml cordial or squash (diluted 1 to 8) Water; 1–2 bananas or gels
Post-training	600 ml milk/flavoured milk/milkshake
Post-training snack	125 g whole-milk yoghurt

Nutritional analysis:

3,592 calories

175 g protein (20 per cent calories)

138 g fat (35 per cent calories)

443 g carbohydrate (46 per cent calories)

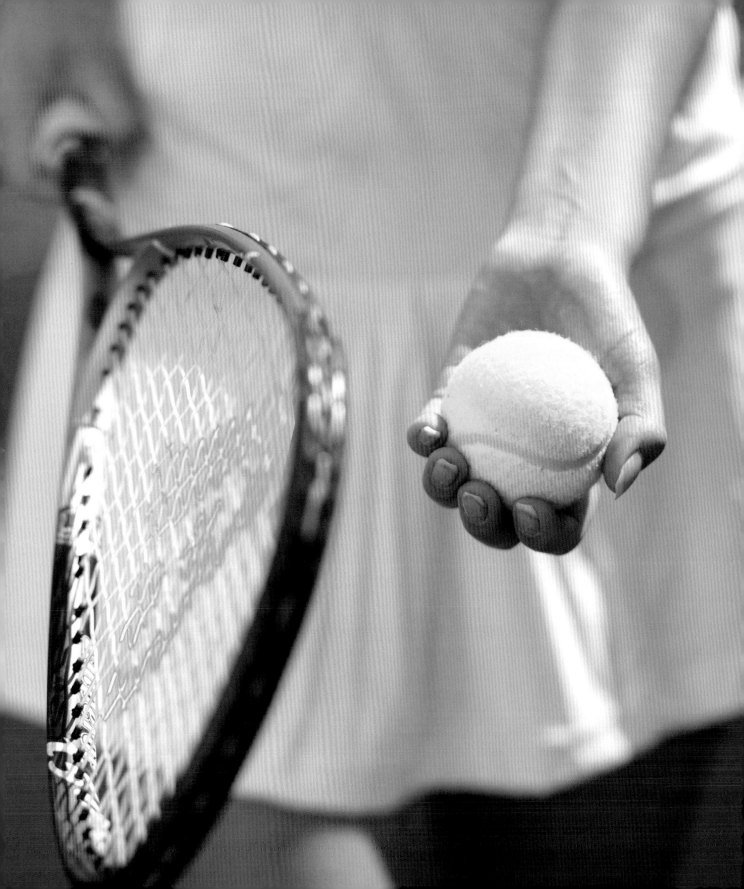

11 NUTRITION FOR TEAM AND RACKET SPORTS

Team sports such as rugby, football, hockey, netball and basketball, as well as racket sports such as tennis and squash, involve lots of short bursts of all-out effort, such as sprints, throws and jumps, interspersed with longer periods of lower-intensity activities such as jogging, walking or standing. Although you may not be running continuously, during a game lasting 60–90 minutes, you can easily deplete your leg-muscle glycogen stores – more than enough to cause fatigue and dramatically reduce running speeds. This chapter draws together the information in Chapters 1–6 into a pre-match nutrition strategy and a match-day template to help you play well and stay on the winning side.

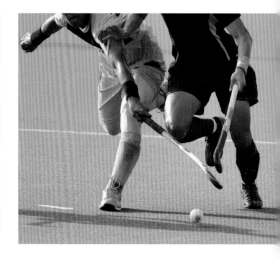

Fuel rules

A healthy daily diet helps your body adapt to the training you do, and ensures that you're well fuelled for training and fast recovery. In a nutshell, you need carbohydrate to fuel working muscles, protein to promote training adaptations, and high-quality fats necessary for health.

It's difficult to give blanket recommendations for carbohydrate intake as type, intensity and duration of training vary greatly between different sports but, as a rough guide, if you're training hard for 1–2 hours daily you'll need 5–7 g/kg of body weight carbohydrate daily – that's 350–490 g for a 70 kg person. If you're training for less than 2 hours, then a slightly lower carbohydrate intake is recommended (3–5 g/kg).

There's no need to consume anything other than water for resistance-based sessions and/or shorter lower-intensity field sessions. But for hard field-based sessions lasting more than one hour, consuming extra carbohydrate in the form of squash, cordial, sports drinks, bananas or gels will help maintain training intensity.

Immediately post-training, the timing of food intake is important. Consuming 20–25 g of protein post-resistance training will speed muscle repair and recovery. After tough game-conditioning field-based sessions, combining this protein with 70–100 g of carbohydrate will also support a fast recovery process and help facilitate improvements in fitness. Whether the protein and carbohydrate is consumed as a drink (e.g. milk or a recovery drink) or food is up to you.

Table 11.1 gives a fuelling and hydration strategy for team sports.

TABLE 11.1 FUELLING AND HYDRATION STRATEGY FOR TEAM AND RACKET SPORTS

	Hydration	Fuel needs	Suitable foods
2–4 hours before training	*Drink 5–7 ml/kg (approx 350–500 ml)*	*Eat 2–4 g carbohydrate/kg (approx 100–200 g)*	*Pasta and chicken; rice and fish; potatoes and cheese*
OR <1 hour before training	*Drink approx 100–250 ml*	*Eat 1 g carbohydrate/kg (approx 50–70 g)*	*Banana; flapjack; toast and honey*
During training (<1 hour)	*According to thirst, little and often*	*Not needed*	*Water, low-calorie squash or sports drink*
During training (>1 hour)	*Drink 125 ml/km according to thirst, little and often*	*15–30 g carbohydrate every 15–30 minutes for a total of 30–60 g/hour*	*Cordial, squash, sports drink, banana, granola bar*
After training (>1 hour)	*Drink 750 ml/0.5 kg weight loss*	*Eat a small snack with a 3:1 ratio of carbohydrate to protein*	*Flavoured milk; milk and flapjack; sandwich and yoghurt*

The week before the match

What you eat and drink in the days and weeks before a match makes a big difference to your performance. A healthy nutrition programme will help you train harder and recover faster and ensure you are match fit on the day.

For weekly matches there is no need to taper your training other than avoiding exhaustive exercise the day before. A good recovery eating plan after each training session, together with proper rehydration, should restore glycogen levels within 24–48 hours. Doing only very light training or resting completely the day before a match will allow the carbohydrate you eat to be stored as glycogen and not to be burned during training.

It is important to drink plenty of fluids in the pre-match week – dehydration is cumulative and can hinder your performance.

The day before the match

Plan to rest today so that you do not deplete glycogen stores. You should also aim to top up glycogen stores and stay well hydrated. Dividing your food intake into several small meals and avoiding eating big meals will encourage your muscles to turn all the carbohydrate you eat into glycogen. Avoid over-eating – a big meal the night before will sit heavily in your stomach and probably keep you awake at night. You may also feel sluggish the next day.

Stick with familiar foods. Opt for plain and simple foods otherwise you risk an upset stomach on match day. If travelling to a match, find out what food will be provided in advance and be prepared to take your own supplies.

Keep a water bottle handy and remember to drink regularly throughout the day, especially if you are travelling.

On match day

By now, your muscle glycogen stores should be fully stocked. All that remains to be done before the race is to replenish liver glycogen stores following the overnight fast and keep blood sugar levels up.

Have your pre-match meal approximately 4 hours before the start. This allows enough time for the food to empty from your stomach and get digested so that your muscles can use the available fuel. Your pre-match meal should be high in carbohydrate, but also contain some protein and fat to provide satiety and sustained energy. Work on the basis of 25–50 g of carbohydrate for each hour before the start of the match, depending on your body weight and the match duration. So that's 100–200 g carbohydrate 4 hours beforehand or 25–50 g if you eat a snack (or drink) one hour before the match.

For morning matches, carbohydrate-rich foods such as porridge, cereal, toast and fruit are good choices. Pasta with chicken or rice with fish would be suitable meals before an afternoon match. Aim for approximately 500–600 calories. During the 2–4 hours before the match, drink approximately 350–500 ml of water, cordial, squash or a sports drink containing 6 g of carbohydrate/100 ml, or diluted fruit juice (equal parts juice and water). Take frequent swigs rather than downing it in one go as this promotes better fluid retention. Then drink another 125–250 ml just before the start.

The sodium naturally present in your food will also help the body hold on to fluid (which may be advantageous prior to a match when it's important to avoid dehydration) so, despite the marketing hype, there's no need to consume a sports drink, i.e. a drink with sodium, beforehand.

During the match

During matches lasting less than an hour, you don't need to take on extra liquid or carbohydrate, and the chances of you being able to do that are limited anyway. However, it certainly wouldn't hurt to take a few swigs at half-time.

For longer matches lasting over an hour, fuelling and hydration are more important. The fact that your carbohydrate energy stores may run out means you

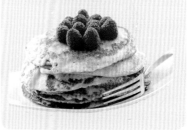

PRE-MATCH MEAL IDEAS

- Porridge with raisins and honey
- Cereal with milk and bananas
- Toast with jam and a milky drink
- Pancakes with fruit
- Pasta with chicken and salad
- Rice with beans or grilled fish and vegetables
- Spaghetti bolognese with vegetables

need to make full use of any stoppages and the half-time break to take on water, squash, cordial, a sports drink, an energy gel or whatever you're used to as your carbohydrate source. Aim for at least 30 g of carbohydrate/hour.

Swig cordial, a sports drink (6 g of carbohydrate/100 ml) or diluted juice (equal parts juice and water) at half-time and during injury time-outs. This will help avoid dehydration – you can lose as much as 1–2 litres of fluid through sweating during a match. Such losses can reduce performance and increase fatigue. Stick with whichever drink you have used in training and don't try anything new.

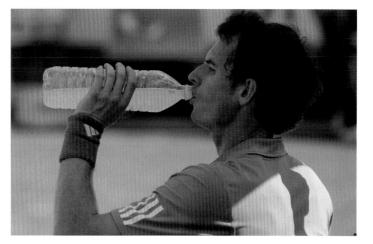

After the match

The game may be over, but your recovery strategy starts now. This is important if you want to train or have enough energy to move about in the next few days.

Start drinking as soon as possible after the match, i.e. before you shower. It is vital that you begin to replace the fluid you've lost. Try to drink around 500 ml of a sports drink or diluted juice in the first 30 minutes after the match, little and often, then keep gulping every 5 or 10 minutes until you are passing clear urine. Make sure you are rehydrated before embarking on a celebratory drink. The best alcoholic drinks are lager, beer and shandy (the extra fluid will reduce further dehydration) – or alternate water with an alcoholic drink.

The match will have depleted glycogen stores in your leg muscles, so your mission is to restock those stores immediately. Eat a high-carbohydrate snack (1 g of carbohydrate/1 kg of body weight) within the first 30–60 minutes of the match ending. This can be solid food or a drink – whatever feels right. Including a little protein with the carbohydrate (approx 1 part protein to 3 parts carbohydrate) will speed glycogen recovery.

POST-MATCH MEALS

- Pasta with tomato pasta sauce, cheese and vegetables
- Jacket potato with tuna, sweetcorn and salad
- Chicken with roast vegetables and rice
- Turkey and vegetable kebabs with pitta bread
- Baked or grilled salmon, rice and salad

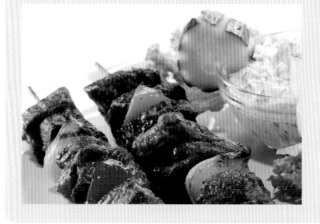

Resist the temptation to celebrate your match result with fatty foods and alcohol. Burgers, chips, kebabs and curries will sit heavily on the stomach, slow your recovery and leave you feeling bloated and sluggish. Choose plainer options, e.g. noodles, rice dishes or cheese and tomato pizza, or smaller portions with extra vegetables.

Table 11.2 gives a match day fuelling and hydration plan.

TABLE 11.2 MATCH DAY FUELLING AND HYDRATION PLAN

When	Hydration	Fuel needs	Suitable foods
4 hours before the match	Drink 5–7 ml/kg (approx 350–500 ml)	Eat 2–4 g carbohydrate/kg (approx 100–200 g)	Eggs on toast; porridge with bananas, raisins and honey; cereal with milk and bananas; toast, fruit and milk
1–2 hours before the match	Drink approx 100–250 ml	Eat 1 g carbohydrate/kg (approx 50–70 g)	Bananas; toast and honey; energy or granola bar
During shorter matches (<1 hour)	According to thirst	Not needed	Water, low-calorie squash or sports drink
During longer matches (>1 hour)	According to thirst	30–60 g/hour	Cordial, squash, sports drink, bananas*, gels*, energy or granola bars*, dried fruit*, honey*
After the race	Drink 750 ml/0.5 kg weight loss	Eat a small snack with a 3:1 ratio of carbohydrate to protein	Recovery drink; flavoured milk; milk and flapjack; sandwich and yoghurt

*Accompany with water

Core menu plan for team and racket sports

The following core menu plan can be used as a template for developing your individual daily eating plan. It gives you the amounts of foods needed to meet your calorie and macronutrient requirements, providing approximately 3,000 calories. However, if you train for longer than an hour then you should increase the portion sizes to take account of your greater calorie expenditure.

Where the menu plan gives a choice of food type (e.g. carbohydrate), simply pick your preferred option (e.g. pasta or potatoes) or substitute an equivalent (high-carbohydrate) food (e.g. quinoa or noodles). Try to vary your choice of fresh fruit and vegetables as much as possible according to what's in season as this will give you a greater range of micronutrients, antioxidants and phytonutrients.

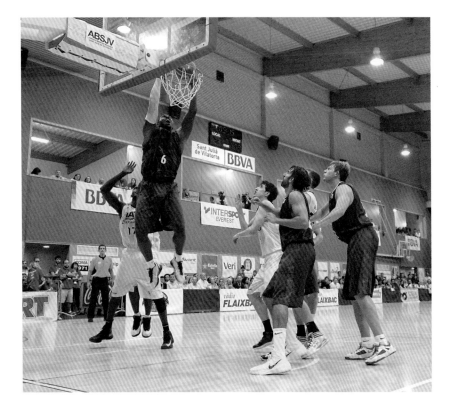

Many of the lower-carbohydrate recipes in Part 3 can be incorporated into your plan; simply use the amount of carbohydrate, protein and fat in the core menu plan as a guide.

Measure and weigh your portions carefully to start with to get an idea of what different amounts of foods look like. Thereafter, you should find it quicker and easier to judge how much to eat.

You should also adjust portion sizes according to your appetite and how energetic you feel during training. If you feel hungrier than usual, that's your body's way of signalling its needs so you should eat more food. Similarly, if you fatigue early in training or find it harder to recover between training sessions, then you should also increase your portion sizes. Keep a check on your weight and body composition and adjust your intake accordingly.

The menu plan does not give quantities for water or other drinks as the amount you need is quite individual and will vary from day to day according to the climate and your sweat rate. Check your hydration status with the 'pee test' (*see* page 61) and ensure you drink sufficient fluids to maintain proper hydration.

MENU

Core menu plan for team and racket sports (1 hour training)

Breakfast	Water 2 x toast with honey 125 g whole-milk yoghurt 250 ml milk-based drink
Snack	25 g nuts 100 g fresh fruit Water
Lunch	Water Protein: 100 g chicken, meat, fish or 2 eggs or 50 g cheese Vegetables or salad Carbohydrate: 3 slices bread or 75 g wholegrain pasta or rice or 300 g potato Fat: 15 g olive/coconut oil or butter 100g fresh fruit and 125 g whole-milk yoghurt
Snack	2 x bananas Water
Training (1h)	Water or 100 ml cordial or squash (diluted 1 to 8)
Snack	600 ml milk/flavoured milk/milkshake 50 g flapjack
Dinner	Water Protein: 100 g chicken or fish or 2 eggs or 50 g cheese Vegetables or salad Carbohydrate: 75–100 g (uncooked weight) wholegrain pasta or rice or 300 g potato Fat: 15 g olive/coconut oil or butter 100 g fresh fruit and 125 g whole-milk yoghurt

Nutritional analysis:

2,853 calories

139 g protein (20 per cent calories)

105 g fat (33 per cent calories)

362 g carbohydrate (48 per cent calories)

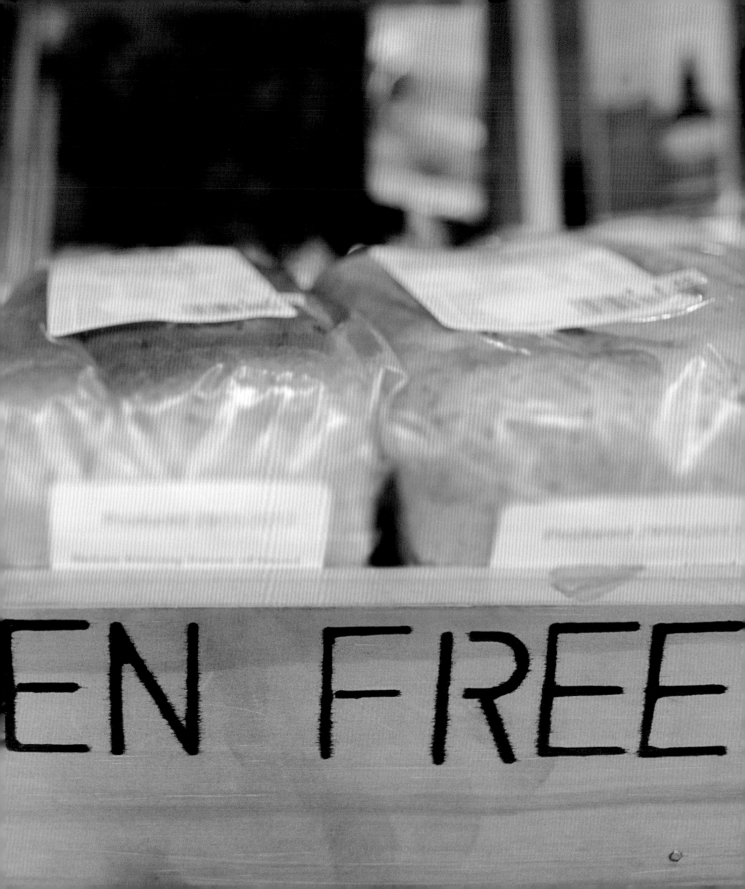

SPECIAL DIETS: VEGETARIAN, DIABETIC AND GLUTEN FREE

The vegetarian athlete

The nutrition rules for vegetarian athletes are not that different from those for non-vegetarians, apart from the meat of course. Follow the advice in Chapters 1–6 and make sure you include some protein at every meal. If you eat a wide variety of unprocessed or 'real' foods (fruit, vegetables, whole grains, dairy products and eggs), the chances are you'll be getting all the nutrients you need.

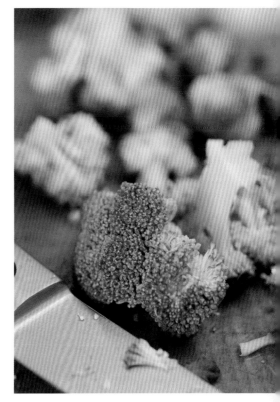

Can a vegetarian diet support athletic performance?

Lots of people imagine that, without meat, athletes can't get enough protein to train hard and build muscle. But there's no evidence for this whatsoever. In fact, there are plenty of highly successful vegetarian athletes. Protein isn't only available from meat. A report from the American Dietetic Association and American College of Sports Medicine published in 2000 stated that meat and fish are not essential for athletic performance. Many scientific studies have shown that a vegetarian diet can meet the needs of competitive athletes (Craig et al., 2009).

A review of studies on vegetarian athletes concluded that well-planned and varied vegetarian diets don't hinder athletic potential and do indeed support athletic performance (Barr and Rideout, 2004). Several studies have found no significant differences in performance, physical fitness (aerobic or anaerobic capacities), limb circumference and strength between vegetarian and non-vegetarian athletes (Williams, 1985).

In a German study, runners completed a 1,000-km race after consuming either a vegetarian or non-vegetarian diet containing similar amounts of carbohydrate (60 per cent energy) (Eisinger, 1994). There was no difference in performance between the vegetarians and the non-vegetarians.

Together, these studies suggest that a vegetarian diet, even when followed for several decades, is compatible with successful athletic performance.

How to get the key nutrients

- Protein – pulses (beans, lentils, peas); tofu and soya products; Quorn™; eggs and dairy products such as milk, cheese, yoghurt as well as nuts and seeds.

- Iron and zinc – leafy green vegetables, wholegrain bread and pasta; nuts, seeds, pulses, dried fruit, eggs and dairy products.

- Vitamin B12 – eggs and dairy products; fortified yeast extract and cereals.

- Vitamin D – fortified dairy products, breakfast cereal, eggs, and from sunlight on the skin.

- Essential fats – nuts and seeds such as walnuts, linseed, hemp, rapeseed and flaxseed, as well as omega 3-enriched eggs.

What are the health benefits?

A study at Oxford University that tracked nearly 45,000 people over ten years found that the vegetarians had a 32 per cent lower chance of dying from heart disease compared to non-vegetarians. This was due largely to their lower blood pressure and cholesterol levels as well as higher intakes of fruit, vegetables and fibre.

How can I get enough protein?

Although most vegetarians get the recommended protein intake, vegetarian diets tend to contain less protein than omnivorous diets. If you don't eat meat or fish, then you need to ensure that you include some protein with each meal. Vegetarian sources include dairy products, eggs, beans, lentils, nuts, seeds, grains, soya and Quorn™. The proteins in dairy products and eggs are all high quality (i.e. they provide a good balance of essential amino acids), but plant sources are limiting in one or more essential amino acids. The idea is to eat a combination of proteins so that the shortfall of amino acids in one food (e.g. lysine in cereals) is complemented by the higher amounts found in another (e.g. beans or lentils). So, rice with lentils (or even beans on toast) would provide a perfect profile of amino acids.

The key is to include a variety of different protein foods throughout the day in order to get a better overall balance of amino acids. This is called 'protein complementation'. For example, combining rice with lentils gives a better overall ratio of amino acids needed to make new body proteins than eating either of these foods on their own. You can achieve protein complementation by combining plant foods from two or more of the following categories:

1. pulses: beans, lentils and peas

2. grains: bread, pasta, rice, oats, breakfast cereals, corn and rye

3. nuts and seeds: peanuts, cashews, almonds, sunflower seeds, sesame seeds and pumpkin seeds

4. Dairy products: milk, cheese, yoghurt; and eggs

5. Quorn™ and soya products

Protein combinations

If low in lysine – combine with beans, lentils, cheese, eggs, soy
If low in methionine – combine with nuts, grains, dairy or eggs

Examples of suitable food combinations include:

Vegetarian chilli with rice
Vegetarian pasta bolognese
Dahl with chappati
Tofu with noodles
Toast with peanut butter

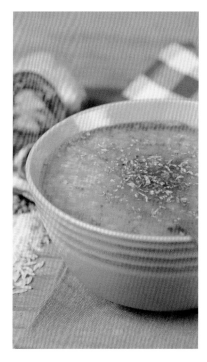

The American College of Sports Medicine advise vegetarian athletes to eat around 10 per cent more protein than non-vegetarians because plant proteins are less well digested than animal proteins (Rodriquez *et al.*, 2009).

Table 12.1 lists the protein content and the main limiting amino acid of various vegetarian protein sources within different food groups. Use this information to devise suitable food combinations that provide a good balance of amino acids.

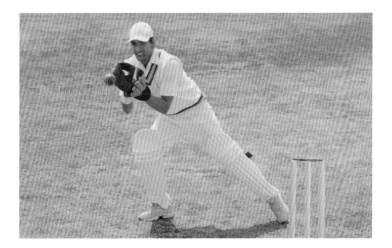

TABLE 12.1 PROTEIN AND AMINO ACID CONTENT OF VARIOUS FOODS

Food	Portion size	Protein	Limiting amino acid (aa)
Nuts and seeds			
Pumpkin seeds	25 g	6 g	All aa in good ratio
Walnuts	25 g	4 g	Lysine
Almonds	25 g	5 g	Lysine, methionine
Pistachios	25 g	5 g	All aa in good ratio
Peanuts	25 g	6 g	Lysine
Cashews	25 g	4 g	All aa in good ratio
Dairy products			
Cheddar cheese	25 g	6 g	All aa in good ratio
Mozzarella	25 g	5 g	All aa in good ratio
Parmesan	25 g	9 g	All aa in good ratio
Eggs	1	8 g	All aa in good ratio
Milk	300 ml	11 g	All aa in good ratio
Yoghurt	125 g	7 g	All aa in good ratio
Pulses			
Soya beans	150 g	21 g	Methionine
Tofu	150 g	12 g	Methionine
Red kidney beans	150 g	13 g	Methionine
Lentils	150 g	11 g	Methionine
Vegetables			
Broccoli	100 g	4 g	Methionine + cysteine
Potatoes	150 g	3 g	
Spinach	100 g	2 g	methionine + cysteine
Grains			
Oats	25 g	3 g	Lysine
Pasta (cooked)	200 g	4 g	Lysine
Noodles (cooked)	200 g	4 g	Lysine
White rice(cooked)	200 g	4 g	Lysine
Brown rice(cooked)	200 g	5 g	Lysine
Wholemeal bread	40 g slice	4 g	Lysine
White bread	40 g slice	3 g	Lysine

What are the pitfalls?

Weight loss

Some athletes may struggle to maintain their weight on a vegetarian diet if they give up meat and increase their training at the same time. That's likely to be the case if you start training for an event or race, but don't step up your calorie intake or pay attention to protein and carbohydrate intake. Tiredness or weight loss are often blamed on the vegetarian diet rather than a failure to eat enough calories. If you fail to adjust your diet when you add extra training, you will lose excessive weight, feel very tired and find recovery takes longer.

As with any dietary change, it is important to plan your diet well and gain as much knowledge about vegetarian diets as possible. Some athletes adopt a vegetarian or vegan diet in order to lose body fat in the belief that such diets are automatically lower in calories. Many do not substitute suitable foods in place of meat and fail to consume enough protein and other nutrients to support their training.

Iron and zinc

Omitting meat may result in lower intakes of iron and zinc and, theoretically, an increased risk of iron-deficiency anaemia. However, there is evidence that the body adapts over time by increasing the percentage of minerals it absorbs from food. Lowered levels of iron and zinc in the diet result in increased absorption.

Despite iron from plants being less readily absorbed, research has shown that iron-deficiency anaemia is no more common in vegetarians than in meat eaters. Even among female endurance athletes, vegetarians are not at greater risk of iron deficiency. Researchers have found that blood levels of haemoglobin and running performance are very similar between non-vegetarian and vegetarian female runners.

Eating vitamin C-rich food (e.g. fruit and vegetables) at the same time as iron-rich foods greatly improves iron absorption. Citric acid (found naturally in fruit and vegetables) and amino acids also promote iron absorption. Good sources of iron for vegetarians include wholegrain cereals, wholemeal bread, nuts, pulses, green vegetables (broccoli, watercress and spinach), fortified cereals, seeds and dried fruit. Table 12.2 shows the iron content of various vegetarian foods.

The absorption of zinc and other trace minerals, such as copper, manganese and selenium, can be reduced by bran and other plant compounds (phytates, oxalic acid), but most studies have failed to show that vegetarians have lower blood levels of these minerals. Whole grains, pulses, nuts, seeds and eggs are good sources of zinc.

Omega-3s

Oily fish are rich in long-chain omega-3 fatty acids, so vegetarians who don't eat fish will need to obtain them from other foods. One of the main omega-3 fatty acids, alpha-linolenic acid (ALA), is found in certain plant foods such as pumpkin

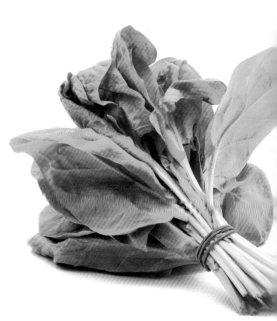

seeds and flaxseed oil (see Table 12.3, which gives the omega-3 fatty acid content of various foods). In the body it is converted to eicosapentanoic acid (EPA) and docosapentanoic acid (DHA) – the two fatty acids that are found in plentiful amounts in oily fish but not in other foods, and that offer greater cardio-protective benefits than the parent ALA.

The Vegetarian Society recommends an ALA intake of 1.5 per cent of energy, or roughly 4 g/day. This should provide sufficient of the parent omega-3 fatty acid

TABLE 12.2 VEGETARIAN FOODS CONTAINING IRON

Sources of iron			
Good sources	*(Iron, mg)*	*Fair sources*	*(Iron, mg)*
Chick peas or red kidney beans (140 g)	4.3 mg	Egg, boiled	1.3 mg
Bran flakes (45 g)	5.3 mg	Avocado (75 g)	1.1 mg
Spinach, boiled (100 g)	4.0 mg	Asparagus (125 g)	1.1 mg
Baked beans (225 g)	3.2 mg	1 slice wholemeal bread (40 g)	1.0 mg
Black treacle (35 g)	3.2 mg	Broccoli, boiled (100 g)	1.0 mg
Muesli (60 g)	2.7 mg	Brown rice (200 g)	0.9 mg
4 Dried figs (60 g)	2.1 mg	Peanut butter (20 g)	0.5 mg
8 Dried apricots (50 g)	2.1 mg		

TABLE 12.3 VEGETARIAN SOURCES OF OMEGA-3 FATTY ACIDS

Sources of Omega-3 fatty acids			
	g/100 g	*Portion*	*g/portion*
Flaxseed oil	57 g	1 tbsp (14 g)	8.0 g
Flaxseeds (ground)	16 g	1 tbsp (24 g)	3.8 g
Rapeseed oil	9.6 g	1 tbsp (14 g)	1.3 g
Walnuts	7.5 g	1 tbsp (28 g)	2.6 g
Walnut oil	11.5 g	1 tbsp (14 g)	1.6 g
Peanuts	0.4 g	Handful (50 g)	0.2 g
Broccoli	0.1g	3 tbsp (125 g)	1.3 g
Pumpkin seeds	8.5 g	2 tbsp (25 g)	2.1 g
Omega-3 eggs	0.8 g	One egg	0.4 g

to ensure enough EPA and DHA are formed by the body (conversion rates are around 5–10 per cent for EPA and 2–5 per cent for DHA). Include some of the foods listed in Table 12.3 in your daily diet.

You should also aim to achieve a LA to ALA ratio of around 4 to1 or slightly lower since a high intake of LA interferes with the conversion process of ALA to EPA and DHA. Replace fat high in omega-6 oils (such as sunflower or corn oil) with fats higher in monounsaturated oils (such as olive oil and nuts), which do not disrupt the formation of EPA and DHA.

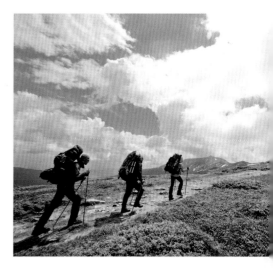

The diabetic athlete

Being diabetic does not mean you cannot exercise or play sport. There are many successful sportspeople who are diabetic – including Sir Steve Redgrave, the Olympic gold medal-winning rower. Keeping active can help avoid complications associated with diabetes, such as heart disease. Your nutrient requirements are the same as those for non-diabetics, but there may be some considerations to take into account with your diabetes before taking up a new exercise regime. You should talk to your healthcare team for more information.

What is the difference between type 1 and type 2 diabetes?

Type 1 diabetes is a condition where the body is unable to produce any insulin and is therefore unable to use glucose properly as a fuel source. It starts to rely on fat and protein as fuel. This means blood glucose levels can rise excessively and toxic by-products from fat metabolism (ketones) can build up in the blood. Type 1 diabetes is treated with regular insulin injections, diet and physical activity. It usually affects people under 40.

Type 2 diabetes develops when the body can still make some insulin, but not enough, or when the insulin that is produced does not work properly (insulin resistance). It is usually associated with being overweight and is found mostly in adults – although more children are being diagnosed with the condition. It can be treated with diet and physical activity, although you may also need tablets or injections

Can diabetes be treated?

Type 1 diabetes is treated by insulin injections as well as a healthy diet, and regular exercise. People with this type of diabetes usually take two or four injections of insulin each day.

Type 2 diabetes is treated with lifestyle changes such as a healthier diet, weight loss and increased physical activity. Tablets and/or insulin may also be required to achieve normal blood glucose levels in some people. The main aim of treatment of both types of diabetes is to achieve blood glucose, blood pressure and cholesterol levels as near to normal as possible. This, together with a healthy lifestyle, will help to improve your diabetes and protect against long-term damage to the eyes, kidneys, nerves, heart and major arteries.

What dietary changes do I need to make?

Eating a low-GI diet can help with blood glucose control so you should focus mainly on low-GI foods (*see* page 14) and combinations of foods that produce a low glycaemic (blood glucose) response. Foods with a high protein content (e.g. meat, fish, eggs, cheese, yoghurt, milk) and a high fat content (e.g. nuts, seeds, butter, olives, avocado, olive and coconut oils) have the lowest GI. When they are eaten with carbohydrate (e.g. cheese on toast) they will reduce the overall GI of the dish. For further information about low-GI diets, you should speak to your diabetes specialist or dietitian.

The sports nutrition advice is similar for diabetics and non-diabetics, particularly with regard to nutrient timing, recovery and hydration. You should follow the advice in this book, but you may need to experiment with the amount and timing of foods and fluids around exercise to achieve perfect blood glucose control. It's a good idea to keep a training and food diary so you can monitor how your body responds to exercise. You should consult your diabetes specialist if you have any concerns.

Before exercise

You'll need to get into the routine of monitoring your blood glucose before exercise. It is important to ensure your blood glucose level is within the recommended range (usually 4–8 mmol/l or 80–120 mg/dl) before you begin exercising. If it is below this range, you should consume a snack containing 15–30 g carbohydrate (e.g. a banana). If it is above this range, then it could climb even higher once you start exercising, which can be dangerous, so wait until it comes down.

As with non-diabetics, aim to have a low-GI meal about 2–4 hours before exercise. A low-GI meal will not only help avoid problems of high blood glucose levels but may also improve your endurance. It will produce a lower rise in blood glucose. Ideally, this meal should include protein and fat as well as carbohydrate as they slow the digestion of carbohydrate and produce a more gradual rise in blood glucose. Include fruit or vegetables in this meal as their high fibre content will also slow the delivery of carbohydrate to your bloodstream and avoid rapid rises in blood glucose. Suitable pre-exercise meals include porridge with fruit (for morning workouts), chicken with rice, or pasta with fish.

During exercise

If you're exercising for longer than an hour, then you may benefit from extra carbohydrate during your workout. Follow the same advice for non-diabetics, which is to consume 30–60 g/hour either in the form of a drink (e.g. squash, cordial or sports drink) or solid food (e.g. bananas, gels, bars or dried fruit). Drink or eat little and often, instead of consuming a large amount in one go.

Should you experience hypoglycaemia during exercise (shakiness, confusion and numbness in the arms and hands) consume some rapidly absorbing carbohydrate, such as glucose tablets, squash, sweets, jellies or gels.

High-intensity (e.g. weight training or sprinting) and intermittent high-intensity exercise may affect insulin levels and cause blood glucose to rise during or after exercise, so you may need to avoid carbohydrate or consume less during these activities.

Also, during the competition when adrenaline levels will be higher than normal, you need to be extra vigilant for symptoms of high blood glucose. Adrenaline can result in fluctuating blood glucose so you may need to devise a more intensive insulin routine, e.g. frequent and small doses of short-acting insulin, in conjunction with your diabetes specialist.

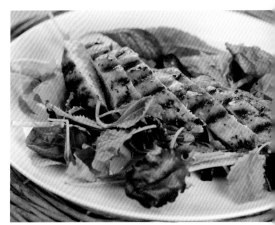

LOW-CARBOHYDRATE HIGH-FAT DIETS AND TYPE 2 DIABETES

A growing body of scientific opinion suggests that a low-carbohydrate high-fat diet may help improve blood glucose control and symptoms in those with insulin resistance (pre-diabetes) or type 2 diabetes (*see* page 205). If you are insulin resistant, it means your cells are less sensitive to the actions of insulin and your body is not able to process carbohydrate into fuel efficiently. Some scientists advise a minimal intake of carbohydrate, around 50 g per day, in order to keep insulin levels low. This is below the level generally recommended for diabetics, but may suit some individuals. Try reducing your carbohydrate intake gradually and monitor your energy, symptoms and exercise performance. Minimise your intake of sugar, sugary drinks (including sports drinks), fruit juice, confectionery, cakes, desserts, refined cereals (white bread, pasta, rice and breakfast cereals) and potatoes; and focus instead on getting calories from protein and fat: meat, fish, poultry, nuts, eggs and dairy products. You should include plenty of non-starchy vegetables. If you have excess fat to lose, a low-carbohydrate high-fat/protein diet could help you achieve a healthier body composition and, therefore, better blood glucose control and reduced diabetic symptoms. High fat and protein intakes are more satiating than carbohydrate so you may find it easier to control your appetite.

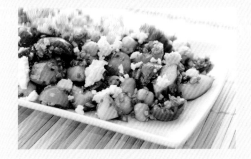

After exercise

Check your blood glucose level after exercise to make sure it is within the recommended range. If it is, then simply follow the same recovery strategy as non-diabetics. Ensure that you replace fluids as soon as practical after exercise, and if you will be exercising within 24 hours, then consume a carbohydrate/protein snack within 2 hours to speed recovery. However, the body cells are more sensitive to insulin for several hours after exercise and glycogen is replenished more rapidly, so there is a greater risk of delayed hypoglycaemia during this time. Eating a small carbohydrate-based snack (e.g. a banana or dried fruit) may help reduce this risk but you should monitor your blood glucose levels carefully. Check your blood glucose levels – you may also need to reduce your insulin dose.

The gluten-free athlete

A gluten-free diet is the treatment for coeliac disease. This is an autoimmune condition, which means the body's immune system attacks its own tissues. In people with coeliac disease this immune reaction is triggered by a protein, gluten. Gluten damages the surface of the intestines and reduces the body's ability to absorb nutrients from food. There is no cure for coeliac disease, but switching to a gluten-free diet prevents further damage to the lining of your intestines and allows your gut to heal.

If you have been diagnosed with this condition, then you must avoid gluten in all its various forms. However, this can present an extra challenge for athletes with high carbohydrate requirements as many staple foods contain gluten: bread, pasta and most breakfast cereals. It can also be difficult getting enough fibre and iron. It is important to make sure your gluten-free diet is healthy and balanced.

What is gluten and how do I avoid it?

Gluten is a type of protein found in wheat, barley and rye. Many people think they simply need to cut wheat from their diets – or even just bread – in order to go gluten-free. But it's unfortunately a lot more complicated than that. Gluten appears in pasta, cakes, breakfast cereals and bread as well as many processed foods such as soups, sauces, sausages, ready meals, cakes, biscuits and puddings.

There are many basic foods, such as meat, fish, eggs, fruit, vegetables, cheese, potatoes and rice, which are naturally gluten-free so you can still include them in your diet. You can also buy gluten free products, including pasta, pizza bases and bread, in supermarkets and healthfood shops. If you're just starting a gluten-free diet, you should consult a dietitian who can help you identify which foods are safe to eat and which are not. However, if you are unsure, use the lists in the box as a general guide.

TOP 5 TIPS FOR GLUTEN-FREE COOKS

- Have separate areas for food preparation, or make sure you thoroughly clean the area if you have used gluten-containing food beforehand.
- Store wheat, barley or rye flour and oats away from gluten-free flours.
- Use separate utensils for gluten-free cooking, e.g. chopping board, whisk, knives, sieve, rolling pin, pastry brush.
- Use separate tubs of margarine or butter or always put a clean knife into the tub.
- Use a separate toaster for gluten-free bread.

READING THE LABEL

It is important to always check the labels of the foods you buy. Look for the crossed grain symbol on packaging, which means the food is gluten free. Many foods, particularly those that are processed, contain gluten in additives, such as malt flavouring and modified food starch. If a cereal containing gluten is used as an ingredient it must be listed on the ingredients list. Coeliac UK provides a directory of gluten-free food and drink, which is updated monthly.

THE GLUTEN-FREE DIET

You can eat the following foods which are naturally gluten free (make sure that they are not processed or mixed with gluten-containing ingredients):

- Most dairy products, such as cheese, butter and milk
- Eggs
- Fruit and vegetables
- Meat, poultry and fish (although not breaded or battered)
- Potatoes
- Rice
- Gluten-free flours, including rice, corn, soy, and potato
- Buckwheat
- Corn and cornmeal
- Millet
- Sorghum
- Soy
- Quinoa

Here's what you have to avoid (unless labelled gluten free):

- Wheat
- Barley
- Rye
- Bulgur
- Bread
- Pasta
- Breakfast cereals
- Croutons
- Biscuits and crackers
- Cakes and pastries
- Pies
- Gravies and sauces
- Salad dressings
- Soups
- Processed meats
- Processed cheese
- Ready-made pie fillings
- Condiments and sauces
- Frozen potatoes with flavoured coatings
- Flavoured crisps
- Ready meals
- Sausages
- Stock cubes
- Gravy powders, granules
- Stuffing
- Beer – gluten-free beers are now available

TOP 5 TIPS FOR GLUTEN-FREE ATHLETES

- Focus on fresh produce. If you cook with naturally gluten-free foods like unprocessed fresh fruits, vegetables, eggs, meats, fish and poultry, gluten-free cooking becomes easier and healthier.
- Eat as simply as you can, using only fresh herbs, salt and pepper to season your foods. Try grains such as corn in moderation, and don't introduce packaged foods until you have a better feel for the diet and how it affects your system.
- Scrutinise the menu when eating out. Gluten-free restaurant dining can be tricky – many chefs aren't very familiar with the gluten-free diet, and mistakes are pretty common. Call ahead and speak to the chef or waiter – highlight which foods are gluten free and provide specific examples of what is not safe for you (e.g. wheat flour in sauces, breadcrumbs, croutons). If there is nothing suitable on the menu, ask if the chef could cook something else gluten free. Many restaurant chefs are happy to do this once they know the reason for the request.
- Check the label for oats. Oats do not contain gluten, but many people with coeliac disease avoid eating them because they can become contaminated with other cereals that do contain gluten during growing and processing. For this reason, doctors and dietitians usually recommend avoiding oats unless they are specifically labelled gluten free.
- Get enough fibre. To ensure you are getting enough fibre and B vitamins, eat a wide variety of gluten-free grains, fruit and vegetables. Opt for wholegrain gluten-free flour mixes that contain more fibre than the highly refined tapioca, white rice and cornstarch flours.

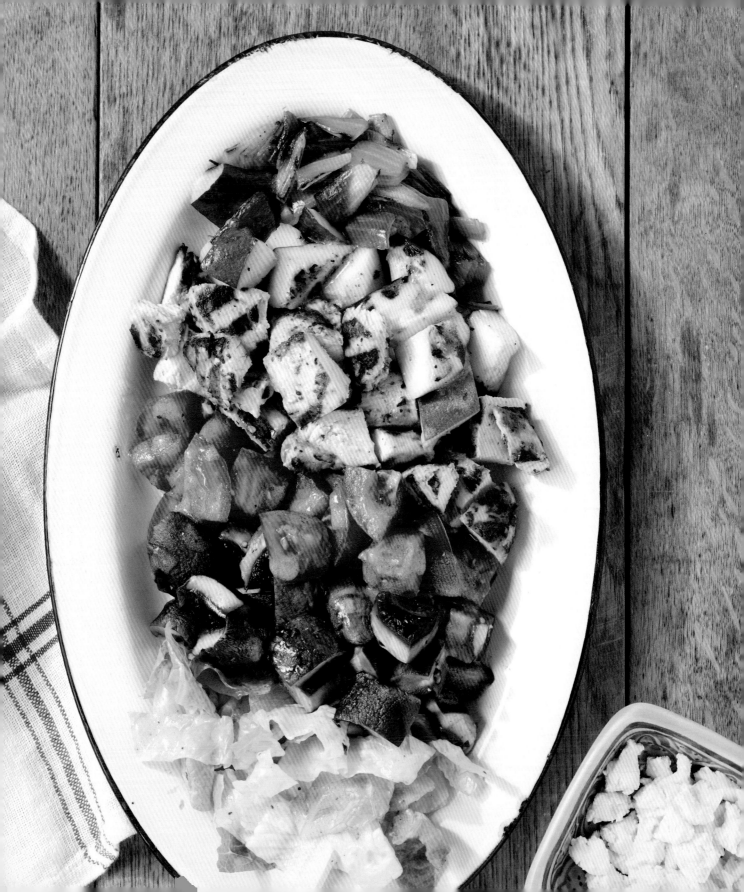

PART 3
THE RECIPES

Eating healthily for your sport or fitness regime need not be complicated, time-consuming or expensive. When it comes to preparing everyday meals, the key is to focus on simple fresh ingredients that are in season. That way, you'll be getting maximum nutritional benefits and maximum taste. I'm a great believer in simple fuss-free cooking that fits into your lifestyle, whether you're cooking for just yourself or for the entire family. The recipes in this section require no special cooking skills, are super quick to make (most can be prepared in less than 15 minutes), and will help you put the nutritional principles outlined in Parts 1 and 2 into practice. They are divided into four sections: breakfasts (Chapter 13), main meals (Chapter 14), vegetarian meals (Chapter 15) and sports snacks (Chapter 16). Each recipe provides a quick nutritional overview as well as a detailed nutritional analysis – that way, you'll know exactly what you're eating. So whether you are a culinary novice or an experienced cook looking for a bit of extra inspiration in the kitchen, here are 60 winning recipes that will help you achieve peak performance. Where salt is mentioned in a recipe, try to use low-sodium salt.

13 BREAKFASTS

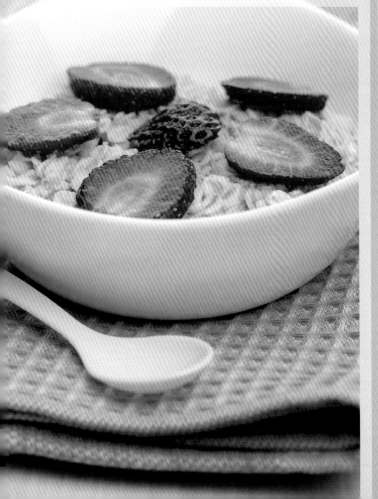

Power porridge

Starting the day with a bowl of porridge gives you a fantastic energy boost. You can use any kind of fresh fruit, such as blueberries or strawberries, or dried fruit to boost the fibre and vitamin content.

SERVES 1

554 calories, 10 g fat, of which 5 g saturates, 96 g carbohydrate, of which 66 g sugars, 19 g protein, 0.4 g salt, 6 g fibre

50 g (2 oz) porridge oats
350 ml (12 fl oz) milk
25 g (1 oz) raisins or dates
1 banana, sliced
Drizzle of honey or maple syrup

1 *Put the oats in a saucepan; add the milk and dried fruit. Bring to the boil and simmer for 4–5 minutes, stirring from time to time.*
2 *Alternatively, cook in a microwave on medium power for approximately 4–5 minutes, stirring halfway through.*
3 *Serve topped with banana slices and drizzle with honey or maple syrup.*

Apple and cinnamon porridge

The apple and cinnamon add natural sweetness to the porridge while the flaxseed oil delivers heart-healthy alpha-linolenic acid (ALA), a short-chain omega-3 fatty acid, which the body converts to EPA and DHA that can be more readily used.

SERVES 1

448 calories, 13 g fat, of which 5 g saturates, 66 g carbohydrate, of which 39 g sugars, 17 g protein, 0.4 g salt, 6 g fibre

50 g (2 oz) porridge oats
300 ml (½ pint) milk
1 apple, peeled and grated
Pinch of ground cinnamon
1 tsp flaxseed oil
2 tbsp whole-milk yoghurt
Drizzle of honey or maple syrup

1 *Put the oats, milk, apple and cinnamon into a saucepan. Bring to the boil and simmer for 4–5 minutes, stirring from time to time.*
2 *Alternatively: mix the oats, apple, cinnamon and milk and microwave on medium power for 5 minutes.*
3 *Stir in the flaxseed oil.*
4 *Pour into a bowl, spoon yoghurt on top, and drizzle with honey.*

Fig and walnut porridge

This delicious porridge, enriched with figs and nuts, is rich in soluble fibre, protein and alpha-linolenic acid (ALA) from the flaxseeds and walnuts. ALA is converted into the long-chain omega-3 fats, DHA and EPA, which are useful for promoting oxygen delivery during exercise.

SERVES 1

574 calories, 22 g fat, of which 5 g saturates, 73 g carbohydrate, of which 45 g sugars, 21 g protein, 10 g fibre, 0.4 g salt

50 g (2 oz) porridge oats
300 ml (½ pint) milk
1 tsp ground flaxseeds
Pinch of ground cinnamon
2 ready-to-eat figs, roughly chopped
1 tbsp walnuts, roughly chopped
1 tsp honey

1 *Put the oats, milk, flaxseeds, cinnamon, figs and walnuts in a saucepan. Bring to the boil and simmer for 4–5 minutes, stirring from time to time.*
2 *Alternatively, cook in a microwave on medium power for approximately 4–5 minutes, stirring halfway through.*
3 *Pour into a bowl and serve drizzled with a little honey*

Apricot and pear porridge

This truly tasty combination of apricots and pears is a super way of adding antioxidant vitamins to your breakfast. Dried apricots are rich in beta-carotene (a powerful antioxidant that also converts to vitamin A) and has a high ORAC (antioxidant) value.

SERVES 1

426 calories, 10 g fat, of which 4 g saturates, 67 g carbohydrate, of which 40 g sugars, 18 g protein, 11 g fibre, 0.4 g salt

50 g (2 oz) porridge oats
300 ml (½ pint) milk
2 ready-to-eat dried apricots, chopped
Pinch of ground cinnamon plus extra for sprinkling
A few drops of vanilla extract
½ pear, sliced
1 tsp maple syrup

1 *Put the oats, milk, apricots and cinnamon in a saucepan. Bring to the boil and simmer for 4–5 minutes, stirring from time to time.*
2 *Alternatively, cook in a microwave on medium power for approximately 4–5 minutes, stirring halfway through.*
3 *Stir in the vanilla. Pour into a bowl, top with the sliced pear, maple syrup and an extra sprinkling of cinnamon.*

Banana and chia porridge

Bananas are a natural partner for porridge, adding extra sweetness as well as potassium, fibre, vitamin C and vitamin B6. Here, I've also added chia seeds, which are packed with fibre, alpha-linolenic acid (an omega-3 fat) and protein. They can substantially lower the GI of the dish (thanks to their high soluble fibre content), so will help sustain your energy for several hours.

SERVES 1

465 calories, 15 g fat, of which 4 g saturates, 66 g carbohydrate, of which 40 g sugars, 18 g protein, 5 g fibre, 0.3 g salt

40 g (1½ oz) porridge oats
250 ml (8 fl oz) milk
1 tbsp chia seeds
1 tbsp honey
½ tsp ground cinnamon
Pinch of ground nutmeg
A few drops of vanilla extract
½ banana, sliced
Drizzle of maple syrup

1 *Put the oats and milk in a saucepan, bring to the boil, and simmer for 5 minutes.*
2 *Alternatively, cook in a microwave on medium power for approximately 4–5 minutes, stirring halfway through.*
3 Add the *chia seeds, honey, cinnamon and nutmeg and vanilla extract. Spoon into a bowl and serve topped with* banana slices and a drizzle of maple syrup.

Muesli with fruit and nuts

This muesli is very easy to make. I like to soak the oats overnight – they're nicer when they're soft and have absorbed the flavours of the dried fruit. Oats are rich in soluble fibre, which helps regulate blood sugar and insulin levels as well as reduce cholesterol levels. They also supply B vitamins, iron, magnesium and zinc. Nuts are rich in vitamin E, essential fatty acids and protein.

SERVES 1

385 calories, 16 g fat, of which 5 g saturates, 48 g carbohydrate, of which 26 g sugars, 12 g protein, 7 g fibre, 0.3 g salt

40 g (1½ oz) porridge oats
125 ml (4 fl oz) milk
25 g (1 oz) raisins (or other dried fruit such as figs)
15 g (about 2) chopped Brazil nuts or walnuts
1 tbsp ground linseeds (optional)
50 g (2 oz) blueberries, raspberries or strawberries

1 In a large bowl, mix together the oats, milk, dried fruit, nuts and, if using, ground linseeds. Cover and leave overnight in the fridge.
2 Serve in individual bowls, topped with the fresh berries.

Granola

Oats are rich in soluble fibre and provide slow-release energy as well as plenty of B vitamins and iron. Almonds and hazelnuts supply protein, calcium, zinc and healthy monounsaturated oils.

SERVES 4

Per serving: 504 calories, 25 g fat, of which 3 g saturates, 54 g carbohydrate, of which 21 g sugars, 16 g protein, 7 g fibre, trace salt

225 g (8 oz) oats
50 g (2 oz) pumpkin seeds
50 g (2 oz) flaked almonds
50 g (2 oz) hazelnuts, crushed
2 tbsp (30 ml) clear honey
2 tbsp (30 ml) coconut or rapeseed oil
85 ml (3 fl oz) water
1 tsp vanilla extract
1 tsp ground cinnamon
1 tsp ground ginger
A pinch of ground allspice (optional)
75 g (3 oz) chopped dates, raisins or apricots (or a mixture)

1 Heat the oven to 150C°/130°C fan/Gas 2.
2 Mix the oats, pumpkin seeds, almonds and hazelnuts together in a bowl.
3 In a separate bowl, combine the honey, oil, water, vanilla and cinnamon, ginger and, if using, allspice. Add to the oat mixture and mix well.
4 Spread out on a non-stick baking tray and bake in the oven for 30–40 minutes, stirring occasionally until evenly browned.
5 Remove from the oven and allow to cool. Mix in the dried fruit.
6 Serve with milk or natural yoghurt and/or fresh fruit. The granola can be stored in an airtight container for up to a month.

Breakfast bars

For a tasty energy boost, try these simple bars. They are rich in soluble fibre and packed with B vitamins and beta-carotene.

MAKES 12 BARS

Per bar: 103 calories, 2 g fat, of which 1 g saturates, 19 g carbohydrate, of which 12 g sugars, 3 g protein, 2 g fibre, 0.1g salt

125 g (4 oz) ready-to-eat dried apricots, chopped
125 g (4 oz) ready-to-eat dried dates, chopped
1 egg, lightly beaten
1 tbsp coconut oil
125 ml (4 fl oz) plain yoghurt
50 g (2 oz) sugar
50 g (2 oz) self-raising wholemeal flour
4 Weetabix, crumbled
Splash of milk (if needed)

1 *Heat the oven to 180°C/160°C fan/Gas 5.*
2 *Combine the apricots, dates, egg, coconut oil and yoghurt in a bowl. Mix well. Stir in the sugar, flour and Weetabix. Add a splash of milk if the mixture is too stiff.*
3 *Spoon into a lightly oiled non-stick 20 cm (8 in) square baking dish.*
4 *Bake for 20–25 minutes.*
5 *Remove from the oven and allow to cool. Cut into bars.*

Breakfast pancakes

These pancakes contain oatmeal for added fibre, and iron as well as eggs and milk, both excellent sources of protein. Milk is also rich in calcium, while the fruit fillings provide vitamin C, beta-carotene and fibre.

MAKES 6 PANCAKES

Per pancake (excludes toppings): 105 calories, 4 g fat, of which 1 g saturates, 13 g carbohydrate, of which 3 g sugars, 6 g protein, 1 g fibre, 0.1g salt

50 g (2 oz) plain white flour
50 g (2 oz) oatmeal or porridge oats
2 eggs
300 ml (½ pint) milk
A little butter or coconut oil for frying
Optional fruit fillings: sliced bananas, sliced strawberries, apple puree with raisins, lightly crushed raspberries, frozen berry mixture (thawed), chopped mango
Whole-milk yoghurt to serve

1 *Place all of the pancake ingredients apart from the fruit fillings in a food processor and blend until smooth. Alternatively, mix the flour and oatmeal in a bowl. Make a well in the centre. In a separate bowl, beat the eggs and milk together. Add the liquid mix to the flour gradually, beating to make a smooth batter.*
2 *Place a non-stick frying pan over a high heat. Add a little butter or oil.*
3 *Pour in enough batter to coat the pan thinly and cook for 1–2 minutes until golden brown on the underside.*
4 *Turn the pancake and cook the other side for a further minute.*
5 *Turn out on to a plate, cover, and keep warm in a low oven, while you make the other pancakes.*
6 *Serve with any of the suggested fresh fruit fillings and whole-milk yoghurt.*

Turkey bolognese

Turkey is loaded with B vitamins, phosphorus, potassium, iron, selenium and zinc – those are some serious nutrients. Plus it contains large amounts of beta-alanine, which can reduce fatigue and improve performance in both anaerobic and aerobic exercise.

SERVES 4

Per serving: 530 calories, 11 g fat, of which 2 g saturates, 70 g carbohydrate, of which 12 g sugars, 39 g protein, 7 g fibre, 0.3 g salt

350 g (12 oz) pasta shapes
1 tbsp olive oil
350 g (12 oz) turkey mince
1 onion, finely chopped
3 celery stalks, finely chopped
2 carrots, finely chopped
400 g (14 oz) tin chopped tomatoes in juice
2 tbsp tomato puree
1 tsp mixed herbs
Salt and pepper

1 *Cook the pasta in plenty of boiling water according to the directions on the packet.*
2 *Meanwhile, heat the oil in a large non-stick frying pan. Add the turkey mince and cook, stirring occasionally for approximately 4–5 minutes until it is browned.*
3 *Add the vegetables. Cook for 5 minutes until just tender.*
4 *Stir in the chopped tomatoes, tomato puree, herbs and seasoning to taste. Heat through.*
5 *Drain the pasta and return to the pan. Add the bolognese mixture to the drained pasta. Mix well to combine, then serve.*

Tomato and tuna pasta

This simple pasta dish can be prepared in just 10 minutes. Tinned tomatoes are a great source of the antioxidant nutrient lycopene, which helps protect against cancer, lower LDL cholesterol and promote healthy bones. The tuna supplies high levels of protein to help recovery after exercise.

SERVES 4

Per serving: 492 calories, 8 g fat, of which 1 g saturates, 76 g carbohydrate, of which 20 g sugars, 29 g protein, 8 g fibre, 1.1 g salt

350 g (12 oz) pasta shapes
2 tbsp olive oil
1 onion, chopped
2 garlic cloves, crushed
400 g (14 oz) tin chopped tomatoes in juice
1 tbsp tomato puree
125 g (4 oz) vegetables of choice (e.g. mushrooms, courgettes), chopped
200 g (7 oz) tin tuna in water or brine, drained and flaked
1 tsp dried basil

1 *Cook the pasta in plenty of boiling water according to the directions on the packet.*
2 *Meanwhile, sauté the onion and garlic in the olive oil in a large non-stick frying pan for 5–10 minutes until the onion is soft.*
3 *Stir in the tinned tomatoes, tomato puree and vegetables and cook for 5 minutes, or until tender.*
4 *Add the tuna and basil and heat through.*
5 *Drain the pasta and return to the pan. Add the tuna mixture, combine well, then serve.*

One-pot pasta with chicken and mushrooms

This simple one-pot pasta meal provides a good balance of protein, carbohydrate and fat. The peppers also deliver lots of vitamin C and other powerful antioxidant nutrients. Add tinned beans, such as red kidney beans, for extra fibre and iron.

SERVES 4

Per serving: 494 calories, 12 g fat, of which 2 g saturates, 70 g carbohydrate, of which 12 g sugars, 27 g protein, 7 g fibre, 0.5 g salt

4 skinless chicken drumsticks or thighs
2 tbsp olive oil
1 onion, sliced
2 green or red peppers, sliced
225 g (8 oz) mushrooms, sliced
450 ml (15 fl oz) passata
350 g (12 oz) small pasta shapes
300 ml (½ pint) stock or water

1 *Sauté the chicken drumsticks in the oil over a high heat until they are browned. Remove from the pan and set aside on a plate.*
2 *Add the onion, peppers and mushrooms to the pan and cook for 5–10 minutes.*
3 *Add the passata, chicken, pasta and stock or water. Bring to the boil and simmer until the pasta is tender and the chicken cooked through, about 10 minutes.*

Chicken and pepper risotto

This is a cheat's risotto as everything is cooked together to save time. However, the result is tasty and the peppers provide an excellent source of vitamin C and beta-carotene.

SERVES 4

Per serving: 494 calories, 10 g fat, of which 2 g saturates, 79 g carbohydrate, of which 7 g sugars, 22 g protein, 3 g fibre, 1.0 g salt

1 onion, chopped
2 garlic cloves, crushed
2 tbsp olive oil
1 red and 1 yellow pepper, cut into thin strips
2 litres (3½ pints) chicken or vegetable stock
350 g (12 oz) risotto rice
225 g (8 oz) cooked leftover chicken, chopped
25 g (1 oz) Parmesan, grated
Handful of fresh, chopped chives or parsley

1 *Heat the oil in a large non-stick pan and sauté the onion, garlic and peppers for about 5 minutes.*
2 *Add the stock and rice, bring to the boil, and simmer for 20–25 minutes until the rice is tender and the liquid has been absorbed.*
3 *Stir in the cooked chicken and the Parmesan. Heat through for a few minutes.*
4 *Stir in the herbs and serve with extra Parmesan.*

Salmon with noodles

This easy-to-make complete meal comes in a neat packet; you just pop in the ingredients and put it in the oven. Meanwhile all the flavours blend together as the ingredients cook in their own steam.

SERVES 1

402 calories, 20 g fat, of which 4 g saturates, 17 g carbohydrate, of which 8 g sugars, 39 g protein, 4 g fibre, 0.3 g salt

85 g (3 oz) cooked ('straight-to-wok') egg noodles
1 carrot, peeled and thinly sliced
2 spring onions, sliced
4 mushrooms, sliced
1 salmon steak (about 175 g/6 oz)
Fresh chopped parsley
Olive oil, to serve
Salt and pepper

1 *Heat the oven to 180°C/160°C fan/Gas 4.*
2 *Place the noodles on to the centre of a piece of oiled foil approx 50 x 30 cm (20 x 12 in).*
3 *Lay the vegetables and salmon on top. Sprinkle with salt, pepper and parsley. Fold the foil over to enclose the salmon and seal the edges. Place on a baking tray.*
4 *Bake in the oven for 15 minutes.*
5 *Open the parcel and check the salmon is cooked (the flesh should be pale pink and flake). Serve on to plates with a drizzle of olive oil.*

Fish and bean cassoulet

This highly nutritious low-carbohydrate dish is packed with protein, vitamins and fibre. Substitute other types of white fish for haddock, if you prefer. Try adding courgettes, red peppers,or aubergine if you like.

SERVES 4

Per serving: 352 calories, 8 g fat, of which 1 g saturates, 25 g carbohydrate, of which 9 g sugars, 43 g protein, 8 g fibre, 1.0 g salt

750 g (1½ lb) skinless haddock fillets
1 litre (1¾ pints) stock or water
1 bay leaf
2 tbsp olive oil
1 onion, chopped
2 celery sticks, chopped
2 carrots, peeled and chopped
4 tbsp white wine or water
400 g (14 oz) tin haricot beans, drained
1 tsp mixed herbs
4 tomatoes, chopped
4 tbsp fresh breadcrumbs
2 tbsp fresh chopped parsley
Salt and pepper

1 *Heat the oven to 190°C/170°C fan/Gas 5.*
2 *Cook the fish in the stock or water with the bay leaf for approximately 10–15 minutes. Drain, reserving 1 pint of the liquid. Flake the fish, removing any bones.*
3 *Heat the oil in a pan and fry the onion, celery and carrots for approximately 5 minutes.*
4 *Pour in the reserved fish liquid, wine or extra water, beans and herbs and cook for approximately 10 minutes until the liquid has been reduced.*
5 *Add the cooked fish and tomatoes. Check the seasoning and transfer to a shallow baking dish.*

cont.

6 *Mix the breadcrumbs and parsley together and scatter over the top.*

7 *Bake for 30–35 minutes until the top is crisp and golden.*

Stir-fried chicken with broccoli

Chicken provides protein and B vitamins. Broccoli is rich in sulphoramine, a powerful antioxidant that helps combat cancer, as well as vitamin C and folate.

SERVES 4

Per serving: 187 calories, 8 g fat, of which 2 g saturates, 3 g carbohydrate, of which 1 g sugars, 25 g protein, 2 g fibre, 0.8 g salt

2 tbsp extra virgin olive oil
300 g (10 oz) chicken breasts cut into thin strips
1 onion, thinly sliced
1 garlic clove, crushed
2.5 cm (1 in) piece fresh ginger, peeled and finely chopped
225 g (8 oz) broccoli florets
1 tsp cornflour blended with 1 tbsp water
1 tbsp light soy sauce
Handful of fresh chives, chopped
Cooked rice or noodles, to serve

1 *Heat the olive oil in a wok, add the chicken and stir-fry for 2–3 minutes until the chicken is lightly browned. Remove from the wok, place on a plate and keep warm.*

2 *Add the onion, garlic and ginger and stir-fry for 1 minute. Add the broccoli, then return the chicken to the wok.*

3 *Stir in the cornflour mixture and soy sauce. Toss in the pan and stir continuously until the mixture thickens.*

4 *Serve with cooked rice or noodles.*

Home-made beef burgers

These home-made beefburgers are packed with protein and ideal for promoting muscle growth after an intense gym workout. They are simple to make and quick to cook – and at least you know exactly what's in them!

MAKES 4 BURGERS

Per serving: 231 calories, 13 g fat, of which 4 g saturates, 11 g carbohydrate, of which 2 g sugars, 17 g protein, 1 g fibre, 0.4 g salt

250 g (9 oz) good-quality beef mince
1 small onion, finely chopped
1 egg
50 g (2 oz) fresh white breadcrumbs
2 tbsp chopped fresh sage or parsley (or 1 tbsp dried)
2 tbsp olive oil
Salt and pepper

1 *Put the mince into a large bowl and mix in the chopped onion, egg, breadcrumbs, herbs and salt and pepper.*

2 *Divide the mixture into four balls and use your hands to flatten them into burgers.*

3 *Heat the oil in a large frying pan over a medium-high heat and fry the burgers for 8 minutes, turning once, until each side is well browned. Alternatively, place the burgers on a baking sheet and cook in the oven at 200°C/180°C fan/Gas 6 for 10–15 minutes depending on the size of the burgers. Test by inserting a skewer into the middle of a burger – there should be no trace of pink in the meat and the juices should run clear.*

Chicken burgers

Chicken is a great source of protein, B vitamins and selenium. Plus it contains high levels of tryptophan, an amino acid that increases serotonin levels in the brain, enhancing your mood and combating stress.

MAKES 4 BURGERS

Per serving: 240 calories, 12 g fat, of which 2 g saturates, 12 g carbohydrate, of which 2 g sugars, 21 g protein, 1 g fibre, 0.4 g salt

1 onion, finely chopped
1 stick celery, finely chopped
1 clove garlic, crushed
2 tbsp olive oil
2 skinless, boneless chicken breasts
2 tbsp chopped fresh parsley (or 1 tbsp dried parsley)
50 g (2 oz) fresh breadcrumbs
1 egg yolk
Flour, for coating
1 tbsp olive oil
Salt and pepper

1 *Sauté the onion, celery and garlic in the olive oil for 5 minutes. Meanwhile, mince or finely chop the chicken in a food processor.*
2 *Combine the onion mixture, chicken, parsley and breadcrumbs in a bowl. Season with salt and pepper and bind the mixture together with the egg yolk.*
3 *Form into four burgers and roll in a little flour.*
4 *Heat the olive oil in a large pan over a medium-high heat and cook the burgers until golden and cooked, turning halfway through (approximately 5–6 minutes each side).*

Mackerel with fresh coriander and chilli dressing

This recipe is ultra-quick to make and full of healthy omega-3 fatty acids.

SERVES 4

Per serving: 485 calories, 41 g fat, of which 7 g saturates, 1 g carbohydrate, of which 1 g sugars, 29 g protein, 0.5 g fibre, 0.2 g salt

4 mackerel, each weighing about 250 g (9 oz), cleaned and gutted
Olive oil for brushing
Salt and freshly ground black pepper

For the dressing:
2 shallots, very finely chopped
2 plump garlic cloves, crushed
1 fresh red chilli, deseeded and chopped
6 tbsp extra virgin olive oil
Juice of 1 lemon
4 tbsp chopped fresh coriander

1 *Put all the dressing ingredients into a small bowl and mix well. Set aside until ready to use.*
2 *Make 3–4 deep slashes on each side of the mackerel. Brush with a little oil and season the inside and outside.*
3 *Grill on a barbecue or under a hot conventional grill for 8–10 minutes, turning once halfway through cooking.*
4 *Put the fish on a warm dish, pour over the dressing, and leave for 5 minutes before serving to let the flavours infuse.*

Barbecued chicken with courgettes

Infusing chicken thighs in this tasty citrus marinade helps reduce the formation of potentially carcinogenic chemicals during barbecuing.

SERVES 4

Per serving: 248 calories, 15 g fat, of which 3 g saturates, 2 g carbohydrate, of which 2 g sugars, 27 g protein, 1 g fibre, 0.4 g salt

Zest and juice of 1 unwaxed lemon
2 tbsp olive oil
½ tsp salt
¼ tsp coarsely ground black pepper
4 medium skinless, boneless chicken thighs
4 courgettes, each cut lengthwise into 4 wedges
Small handful of fresh chives, snipped
Grilled lemon slices, for garnishing

1 *In a medium bowl, whisk together the lemon zest and juice, oil, salt and pepper. Reserve 2 tablespoons in a cup.*
2 *Add the chicken thighs to the bowl of marinade. Cover and leave to stand for 15 minutes at room temperature or 30 minutes in the fridge.*
3 *Discard the chicken marinade. Place the chicken and courgettes on a hot barbecue grill rack. Cover the grill with a lid or foil, and cook for 10–12 minutes or until the juices run clear when the thickest part of the thigh is pierced with the tip of knife, and the courgettes are tender and lightly browned. Turn the chicken and vegetables over once and remove the pieces as they are done.*
4 *To serve, toss the courgettes with reserved lemon juice marinade, then combine with chicken and sprinkle with chives. Garnish with grilled lemon slices.*

Salmon with roasted root vegetables

Salmon is a concentrated source of omega-3 fatty acids, which help reduce the risk of heart attacks and strokes, as well as benefiting the skin, reducing the appearance of wrinkles, and helping to control blood pressure.

SERVES 4

Per serving: 542 calories, 28 g fat, of which 5 g saturates, 36 g carbohydrate, of which 20 g sugars, 38 g protein, 14 g fibre, 0.3 g salt

4 carrots, peeled and halved
2 parsnips, peeled and cut into quarters
2 red onions, cut into wedges
2 leeks, trimmed and thickly sliced
½ butternut squash, peeled and thickly sliced
1 garlic clove, crushed
A few sprigs of fresh or 1 tsp dried rosemary
2 tbsp olive oil
2 x 300 g (10 oz) skinless salmon fillets
4 tbsp porridge oats
2 tbsp sesame seeds
Lemon wedges to serve
Salt and pepper

1 *Heat the oven to 200°C/180°C fan/Gas 6.*
2 *Prepare the vegetables and place in a large roasting tin. Scatter over the crushed garlic, rosemary, salt and black pepper. Drizzle over the oil. Roast in the oven for 30–40 minutes until tender.*
3 *Meanwhile, cut the salmon fillets in half. Mix the porridge oats, sesame seeds, salt and black pepper. Coat the salmon pieces in the oat mixture, evenly.*

4 *Brush a non-stick frying pan or griddle with a little olive oil, heat, then add the salmon. Cook over a moderate heat for 3 minutes on each side, covering with a lid. The salmon should be light brown and crispy on the outside.*

5 *Divide the roasted vegetables on to four plates, place a salmon fillet on top, and serve with the lemon wedges.*

Lamb kebabs with a caper dip

Lamb is an excellent source of readily absorbed iron, as well as zinc, protein and B vitamins.

MAKES 4 KEBABS

Per serving: 376 calories, 26 g fat, of which 11 g saturates, 6 g carbohydrate, of which 4 g sugars, 31 g protein, 1.6 g fibre, 0.6 g salt

450 g (1 lb) lean lamb leg steaks, cut into 2.5cm cubes
2 red onions, cut into chunks
25 g (1 oz) butter
A few sprigs of fresh rosemary

For the caper dip:
2 tbsp capers, drained and rinsed
3 pickled gherkins, chopped
1 tbsp wholegrain mustard
1 tbsp white wine vinegar
1 tbsp chopped fresh mint
1 tbsp chopped fresh parsley
2 tbsp mayonnaise

1 *Thread the lamb pieces on to skewers with the red onion chunks.*

2 *Melt the butter in the microwave and add the fresh rosemary leaves, brush over the skewers. Cook under a pre-heated grill for 12–15 minutes, turning occasionally.*

cont.

3 *Meanwhile, make the caper dip: in a bowl mix together the capers, gherkins, mustard, vinegar, fresh mint, parsley and mayonnaise.*

4 *Serve the kebabs with the caper dip alongside rice and a green leafy salad.*

Chicken casserole with lentils and leeks

Chicken is a rich source of protein as well as B vitamins, iron and zinc. In this healthy casserole, it is slow-cooked with Puy lentils, which provide extra protein as well as soluble fibre, iron, B vitamins, zinc and magnesium.

SERVES 4

Per serving: 387 calories, 11 g fat, of which 2 g saturates, 25 g carbohydrate, of which 9 g sugars, 47 g protein, 9 g fibre, 0.8 g salt

2 tbsp olive oil
4 chicken breasts
2 leeks, trimmed and thickly sliced
1 onion, sliced
2 large carrots, peeled and sliced
4 sage leaves, roughly chopped
125 g (4 oz) Puy lentils
500 ml (18 fl oz) chicken stock
2 tbsp chopped fresh parsley
Salt and pepper, to taste

1 *Heat the oven to 190°C/170°C fan/Gas 5.*

2 *Heat the oil in a flameproof casserole dish on top of the stove and brown the chicken.*

3 *Add the leeks, onions and carrots and continue to cook for a few minutes.*

cont.

4 Now add the sage, lentils and stock and bring to the boil. Season with salt and black pepper.

5 Cover and transfer to the oven for 1 hour or until the chicken is very tender, stirring halfway through cooking. Stir in the parsley just before serving.

Pan-fried salmon with vegetables and rice

Salmon is rich in heart-healthy omega-3 oils as well as protein and vitamin E. This dish also provides carbohydrate, vitamin C, beta-carotene, fibre and iron.

SERVES 4

Per serving: 555 calories, 21 g fat, of which 3 g saturates, 53 g carbohydrate, of which 8 g sugars, 39 g protein, 5 g fibre, 0.9 g salt

1 tbsp olive oil
1 onion, chopped
1 garlic clove, crushed
2 courgettes, diced
1 red or yellow pepper, chopped
225 g (8 oz) brown basmati rice
900 ml (1 ½ pints) vegetable stock
125 g (4 oz) frozen peas
4 x 150 g (5 oz) salmon fillets
Handful of rocket leaves
Salt and pepper, to taste

1 Heat the oil in a large pan and sauté the onion, garlic, courgettes and peppers for 5 minutes.

2 Add the rice and stir over the heat for a further 2–3 minutes.

3 Add the stock, bring to the boil, then reduce the heat and simmer for 25–30 minutes until the liquid has been absorbed and the rice is tender.

cont.

4 Add the peas during the final 3 minutes of cooking. Season to taste.

5 Brush each salmon fillet with a little olive oil. Heat a non-stick pan until hot. Add the salmon fillets and fry for 4–5 minutes, turn them over, and cook the other side for 3 minutes. Remove from the heat.

6 Serve onto plates, scatter with rocket and place a salmon fillet on top.

Stir-fried Indonesian prawns with peanut sauce

SERVES 4

Per serving: 299 calories, 18 g fat, of which 8 g saturates, 8 g carbohydrate, of which 4 g sugars, 27 g protein, 2 g fibre, 1.4 g salt

225 g (8 oz) green beans, trimmed
450 g (1 lb) raw, shelled king prawns
75 g (3 oz) crunchy peanut butter
150 ml (¼ pint) coconut milk
1 tbsp soy sauce
2 tsp curry powder
A few spring onions, chopped

1 Place a wok over a high heat. Add the green beans and prawns and stir fry for 3 minutes.

2 In a small bowl, whisk together the peanut butter, coconut milk, soy sauce, curry powder and 175 ml (6 fl oz) of water. Pour over the beans and prawns. Stir for 1–2 minutes.

3 Add the spring onions. Stir and cook for a few minutes until warmed through and the sauce has thickened. Serve with noodles or rice.

Grilled coconut fish

SERVES 4

Per serving: 203 calories, 8 g fat, of which 4 g saturates, 1 g carbohydrate, of which 1 g sugars, 34 g protein, 0 g fibre, 0.4 g salt

4 fillets firm white fish, e.g. halibut, haddock, monkfish or Icelandic cod
2 tsp green curry paste
1 tsp grated fresh ginger
3 tbsp chopped fresh parsley
3 tbsp coconut cream

1 *Pre-heat the grill to a high temperature. Place the fish fillets on a lightly oiled baking tray. Grill for about 4 minutes.*
2 *Meanwhile, make a paste by combining the green curry paste, ginger, parsley and coconut cream.*
3 *Turn the fish fillets over and brush the paste over each one. Return to the grill and cook for about 5–7 minutes or until the paste is slightly coloured.*
4 *Serve with lemon or lime wedges.*

Chicken with butternut squash

SERVES 4

Per serving: 278 calories, 10 g fat, of which 2 g saturates, 10 g carbohydrate, of which 5 g sugars, 39 g protein, 3 g fibre, 0.2 g salt

1 butternut squash
2 tbsp extra virgin olive oil
4 chicken breasts on the bone
2 tbsp chopped fresh thyme leaves (or 2 tsp dried thyme)
Salt and pepper

cont.

1 *Heat the oven to 200°C/180°C fan/Gas 6.*
2 *Peel the butternut squash and cut the flesh into 5 mm slices. Cover the base of a baking tray with the squash slices, drizzle over a little oil, then scatter with thyme and season with salt and black pepper.*
3 *Place the chicken breasts over the squash, drizzle over a little more olive oil, and turn so that they are well coated with oil.*
4 *Cook the chicken and the squash in the oven for 20–30 minutes, depending on the size of the chicken breasts, or until the chicken is golden. The squash should be soft but not mushy.*

Trout with roasted Mediterranean vegetables

SERVES 4

Per serving: 388 calories, 18 g fat, of which 3 g saturates, 12 g carbohydrate, of which 11 g sugars, 35 g protein, 6 g fibre, 0.8 g salt

2 small bulbs fennel
2 red peppers
2 courgettes
1 red onion
200 g (7 oz) cherry tomatoes
About 12 black olives
3 tbsp (45 ml) extra virgin olive oil
2 garlic cloves, crushed
A few sprigs of fresh rosemary
2 lemons, cut into wedges
4 medium trout, cleaned, gutted and heads removed if preferred
250 ml (8 fl oz) white wine
Salt and vinegar

1 *Pre-heat the oven to 200°C/180°C fan/Gas 6.*
2 *Trim the the fennel bulbs and cut into halves or quarters, depending on size. Remove the seeds from*

cont.

the peppers and cut them into wide strips. Cut the red onion into wedges.

3 Place the prepared vegetables, tomatoes and olives in a large roasting tin with the garlic, rosemary and lemon wedges. Drizzle over the olive oil and toss lightly so that the vegetables are well coated in the oil. Place the trout on top of the vegetables.

4 Pour the wine over the trout and vegetables and season with salt and black pepper. Cover the dish with foil and roast in the oven for about 30 minutes until the vegetables are slightly charred on the outside and tender in the middle.

Thai fish curry

SERVES 4

Per serving: 303 calories, 17 g fat, of which 9 g saturates, 11 g carbohydrate, of which 4 g sugars, 27 g protein, 4 g fibre, 0.5 g salt

2 tbsp coconut or olive oil
1 onion, chopped
1 tbsp Thai green curry paste
200 ml (7 fl oz) coconut milk
200 ml (7 fl oz) water
200 g (7 oz) raw, shelled king prawns
300 g (11 oz) white skinless fish (such as cod, haddock, coley or pollock) cut into 2.5 cm (1 in) cubes
200 g (7 oz) frozen peas

1 Heat the oil in a large pan or wok over a low-medium heat. Add the onions and sauté for about 5 minutes until soft and translucent. Stir in the curry paste, and cook for a further 2–3 minutes.

2 Pour in the coconut milk and water, and simmer for 5 minutes. Mix in the prawns, fish and peas, then cook for 10 minutes, stirring carefully to prevent the fish from breaking up, or until the prawns are bright pink and the fish is opaque.

3 Serve alongside cooked rice

Chicken with lemon and herb couscous

SERVES 4

Per serving: 360 calories, 11 g fat, of which 2 g saturates, 34 g carbohydrate, of which 5 g sugars, 34 g protein, 5 g fibre, 0.1 g salt

400 g (14 oz) chicken breast fillets
3 tbsp olive oil
1 garlic clove, crushed
Zest and juice of 2 unwaxed lemons
1 tbsp chopped fresh rosemary
1 tsp paprika
225 g (8 oz) wholewheat couscous
1 red pepper, deseeded and sliced
1 yellow pepper, deseeded and sliced

1 Place the chicken breasts in a large, clean plastic food bag, seal, then beat them with a rolling pin to flatten out to about 1 cm thickness.

2 Place 2 tbsp of the oil, the garlic, zest and juice of the lemons, the rosemary and paprika in a shallow dish. Add the chicken and turn to coat. Cover and place in the fridge and marinate for 3–4 hours.

3 Heat a large, heavy-based frying pan until very hot. Add the chicken with the marinade and cook for 6–7 minutes on each side until thoroughly cooked. Remove from the pan and keep warm.

4 Meanwhile, cook the couscous according to the packet instructions.

5 Heat the remaining oil and stir-fry the peppers until just starting to soften. Remove and mix with the couscous. Serve the chicken with the couscous.

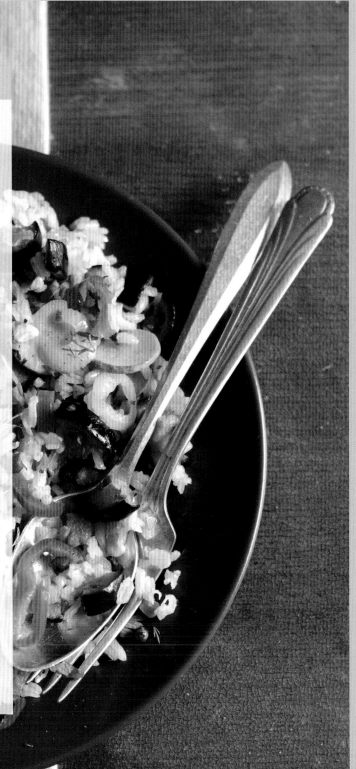

15 VEGETARIAN MEALS

VEGETARIAN MEALS

Dahl with sweet potatoes

Red lentils are an excellent source of protein, complex carbohydrate, fibre, iron, zinc and B vitamins. They have a low GI, which makes them a great base for pre-workout meals. Sweet potatoes have a slightly lower GI than ordinary potatoes and provide higher amounts of beta-carotene and vitamin C.

SERVES 4

Per serving: 262 calories, 7 g fat, of which 1 g saturates, 38 g carbohydrate, of which 8 g sugars, 12 g protein, 6 g fibre, 0.7 g salt

2 tbsp olive or rapeseed oil
2 onions, chopped
2 garlic cloves, crushed
1 tsp ground cumin
2 tsp ground coriander
1 tsp turmeric
175 g (6 oz) red lentils
750 ml (1 ¼ pints) vegetable stock
200 g (7 oz) sweet potato, peeled and diced
1 tbsp lemon juice
A small handful of fresh coriander, finely chopped
Salt

1 Heat the oil in a heavy-based pan and sauté the onions for 5 minutes. Add the garlic and spices and continue cooking for 1 minute while stirring continuously.
2 Add the lentils, stock and sweet potato. Bring to the boil. Cover and simmer for approximately 20 minutes.
3 Add the lemon juice and salt. Finally, stir in the fresh coriander.

Bean and pasta salad with pumpkin seeds and feta

SERVES 4

Per serving: 563 calories, 27 g fat, of which 9 g saturates, 58 g carbohydrate, of which 6 g sugars, 26 g protein, 11 g fibre, 1.8 g salt

200 g (7 oz) wholewheat pasta shapes
75 g (3 oz) pumpkin seeds
400 g (14 oz) tin red kidney beans in water, rinsed and drained
150 g (5 oz) baby plum tomatoes, halved
1 yellow pepper, deseeded and chopped
1 bunch salad onions, trimmed and finely sliced
200 g (7 oz) feta cheese, crumbled
40 g (1½ oz) chopped flat-leaf parsley
Zest and juice of 1 unwaxed lemon
2 tbsp (30 ml) olive oil
Salt and pepper

1 Pre-heat the oven to 220°C/200°C fan/Gas 7.
2 Cook the pasta shapes according to the packet instructions. Drain.
3 Place the pumpkin seeds on a baking tray lined with baking parchment and place in the oven for 8–10 minutes, turning once, until light brown.
4 Place the beans in a large serving bowl with the pasta.
5 Add the tomatoes, pepper, salad onions, feta, parsley and toasted pumpkin seeds.
6 In a small bowl, use a fork to whisk together the lemon juice, zest, olive oil and seasoning. Drizzle over the salad and mix well to combine.

Vegetarian chilli

Vary this classic vegetarian dish with different varieties of beans. Try borlotti beans or flageolet beans for an exciting twist. The chilli provides a good balance of protein, complex carbohydrate, fibre and plenty of vitamins A and C.

SERVES 4

Per serving: 287 calories, 5 g fat, of which 1 g saturates, 47 g carbohydrate, of which 20 g sugars, 16 g protein, 21 g fibre, 2.3 g salt

1 tbsp olive oil
1 large onion, chopped
2–3 garlic cloves, crushed
Pinch of chilli powder, according to your taste
1 tbsp tomato puree
1 tbsp paprika
400 g (14 oz) tinned chopped tomatoes
400 g (14 oz) tinned red kidney beans, drained
400 g (14 oz) tinned cannellini beans, drained
500 g (1 lb) vegetables (e.g. carrots, peppers, courgettes, etc.), chopped

1 *Heat the oil in a large pan. Add the onion, garlic and chilli powder and sauté for 5 minutes.*
2 *Add the tomato puree and paprika and cook for 2 minutes.*
3 *Add the tomatoes, beans and vegetables. Stir and bring to the boil. Simmer for 20 minutes until the vegetables are tender. Serve with rice or salad.*

Bean Provençal

Cannellini beans are rich in protein, low-GI carbohydrate and soluble fibre, which helps to control blood sugar and insulin levels. The peppers deliver vitamin C, a powerful antioxidant that helps speed recovery after exercise.

SERVES 4

Per serving: 144 calories, 4 g fat, of which 1 g saturates, 19 g carbohydrate, of which 7 g sugars, 8 g protein, 9 g fibre, 1.1 g salt

1 tbsp olive oil
1 onion, sliced
1 red pepper, deseeded and sliced
1 green pepper, deseeded and sliced
1 garlic clove, crushed
2 courgettes, trimmed and sliced
400 g (14 oz) tinned chopped tomatoes
400 g (14 oz) tinned cannellini beans or butter beans
1 tbsp tomato puree
1 tsp dried oregano or basil
Salt and pepper

1 *Heat the olive oil in a heavy-based pan and sauté the onion and peppers over a moderate heat until soft. Add the garlic and courgettes and continue cooking for a further 5 minutes, stirring occasionally.*
2 *Add the tomatoes, beans, tomato puree and dried oregano or basil. Cover and simmer for 15–20 minutes. Season with salt and black pepper.*

Lentil burgers

These highly nutritious burgers are easy to make and packed with protein, iron and fibre.

MAKES 4 BURGERS

Per burger: 247 calories, 4 g fat, of which 1 g saturates, 38 g carbohydrate, of which 4 g sugars, 14 g protein, 6 g fibre, 1.1 g salt

1 tbsp oil, plus extra for brushing
1 onion, finely chopped
1 tbsp curry powder
175 g (6 oz) red lentils
600 ml (1 pint) vegetable stock
125 g (4 oz) fresh wholemeal breadcrumbs
Salt and pepper, to taste

1 *Heat the oven to 200°C/180°C fan/Gas 6.*
2 *Heat the oil in a large pan and cook the onion for 5–10 minutes until softened. Stir in the curry powder and cook for a further 2 minutes.*
3 *Add the lentils and stock. Bring to the boil and simmer for 20–25 minutes. Alternatively, cook in the pressure cooker for 3 minutes and turn off the heat.*
4 *Allow to cool slightly and mix in the breadcrumbs. Shape into 4 burgers. Place on a lightly oiled baking tray and brush with a little oil.*
5 *Bake for 7–10 minutes until golden and firm. Serve with a leafy green salad and a dollop of Greek yoghurt or tomato salsa.*

Walnut and rosemary burgers

These burgers are really easy to make if you have a food processor. Not only are they super-nutritious, but they are also perfect for vegetarian guests at a barbecue. Walnuts are a great source of heart-healthy alpha-linolenic (ALA), an omega-3 oil, which the body converts to long-chain omega-3 oils, important for healthy joints and oxygen delivery during exercise.

MAKES 8 BURGERS

Per burger: 221 calories, 17 g fat, of which 2.2 g saturates, 9 g carbohydrate, of which 3 g sugars, 8 g protein, 3 g fibre, 0.3 g salt

175 g (6 oz) walnuts
125 g (4 oz) fresh wholemeal breadcrumbs
1 large red onion, finely chopped
1 garlic clove, crushed
1 tsp dried rosemary
1 tsp lemon zest
2 eggs, lightly beaten
Olive oil, for brushing
Salt and pepper

1 *Heat the oven to 190°C/170°C fan/Gas 5.*
2 *Place the walnuts in a food processor and ground finely.*
3 *Add the breadcrumbs with the onion, garlic, rosemary, lemon zest, salt and pepper. Process the mixture for about 30 seconds until it is evenly combined.*
4 *Add the eggs and process until it holds together firmly. If it is too wet, add a few more breadcrumbs.*
5 *Form the mixture into 8 burgers 1.5 cm (½ in) thick.*
6 *Place on an oiled baking tray then brush with olive oil. Bake in the oven for 25–30 minutes until lightly crisped on the outside.*

Chickpeas with butternut squash

This delicious recipe is one of my favourite winter meals. Chickpeas are an excellent source of fibre, protein and iron. They also contain fructooligosaccharides, a type of fibre that maintains healthy gut flora.

SERVES 4

Per serving: 242 calories, 9 g fat, of which 1 g saturates, 29 g carbohydrate, of which 12 g sugars, 11 g protein, 10 g fibre, 1.4 g salt

2 tbsp olive oil
1 onion, chopped
1–2 garlic cloves, crushed
1 yellow pepper, chopped
1 red pepper, chopped
200 g (7 oz) butternut squash, peeled and diced
1 courgette, trimmed and sliced
400 g (14 oz) tinned chopped tomatoes
400 g (14 oz) tinned chickpeas, drained and rinsed
1 tsp vegetable bouillon powder
½ tsp dried thyme
A handful of fresh basil leaves

1 *Heat the oil in a large heavy-based saucepan and add the onion, garlic and peppers. Cook over a moderate heat for 5 minutes.*
2 *Add the butternut squash and courgette and continue cooking for a further 5 minutes until the vegetables have softened.*
3 *Add the tomatoes, chickpeas, vegetable bouillon and thyme. Bring to the boil, and then simmer for 10 minutes.*
4 *Stir in the fresh basil just before serving.*

Roast vegetable lasagne

This tasty vegetarian lasagne contains a perfect balance of protein, low-GI carbohydrate, fat, fibre as well as vitamin C, vitamin A and calcium. The beans provide low-GI carbohydrate as well as fibre, iron, zinc and B vitamins. The cheeses supply calcium.

SERVES 4

Per serving: 588 calories, 25 g fat, of which 9 g saturates, 64 g carbohydrate, of which 19 g sugars, 27 g protein, 16 g fibre, 1.5 g salt

250 g (about ½ large) butternut squash, peeled and diced
½ red pepper, cut into strips
½ yellow pepper, cut into strips
2 courgettes, trimmed and thickly sliced
1 small red onion, roughly sliced
½ aubergine, cut into 2 cm (1 in) cubes
125 g (4 oz) cherry tomatoes
A few sprigs of fresh rosemary
1 garlic clove, crushed
4 tbsp olive oil
2 x 400 g (14 oz) tinned chopped tomatoes or passata
400 g (14 oz) tinned red kidney beans, drained
175 g (6 oz) lasagne sheets (no pre-cook type)
350 g (12 oz) ricotta cheese
40 g (1½ oz) mozzarella cheese, grated
Salt and pepper

1 *Heat the oven to 200°C/180°C fan/Gas 6.*
2 *Place all the vegetables in a large roasting tin. Put the rosemary sprigs between the vegetables and scatter over the crushed garlic. Drizzle with the olive oil.*
3 *Roast in the oven for approximately 30 minutes until the vegetables are slightly charred on the outside and tender in the middle.*

cont.

4 *Remove the vegetables from the oven and add the tomatoes or passata and the red kidney beans, then stir to combine. Season with salt and black pepper.*
5 *Place a layer of lasagne sheets in a lightly oiled baking dish. Cover with one-third of the vegetable mixture, then one-third of the ricotta. Continue with the layers, finishing with the ricotta. Finally, scatter over the mozzarella and bake for 40–45 minutes until the topping is golden.*

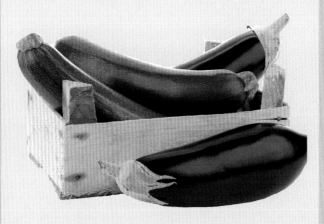

Ratatouille with flageolet beans

This Mediterranean-inspired dish is super-rich in anti-oxidant nutrients: vitamin C (from the peppers and green beans), nasuin (from the aubergine), lycopene (from the tomatoes) and quercetin (from the onions). The flageolet beans provide extra soluble fibre, protein and iron.

SERVES 4

Per serving: 220 calories, 7 g fat, of which 1 g saturates, 28 g carbohydrate, of which 15 g sugars, 11 g protein, 14 g fibre, 1.2 g salt

2 tbsp olive oil
1 onion, chopped
1 each of red, yellow and green peppers, deseeded and sliced
2 garlic cloves, crushed
2 courgettes, trimmed and sliced
1 aubergine, diced
700 g (1½ lb) tomatoes, skinned and chopped (or use 400 g/14 oz tinned tomatoes)
420 g (15 oz) tinned flageolet beans, drained
2 tbsp chopped basil leaves or parsley
Salt and pepper

1 *Heat the oil in a large saucepan. Add the chopped onion and peppers and cook gently for 5 minutes.*
2 *Add the garlic, courgettes, aubergine, tomatoes and flageolet beans. Stir then cover, and cook over a low heat for 20–25 minutes until all the vegetables are tender.*
3 *Season to taste with salt and pepper and stir in the fresh herbs. Serve hot or cold.*

Roasted peppers with lentils and goat's cheese

Peppers are packed with vitamin C as well as many other phytonutrients that support the immune system and protect the body from free radical damage. Roasting them in a small quantity of olive oil minimises any destruction of vitamins.

SERVES 4

Per serving: 218 calories, 13 g fat, of which 5 g saturates, 15 g carbohydrate, of which 5 g sugars, 12 g protein, 5 g fibre, 0.4 g salt

2 Romano red peppers
2 tbsp extra virgin olive oil
250 g (9 oz) pack ready-cooked Puy or beluga lentils (e.g. Merchant Gourmet)
85 g (3 oz) baby plum tomatoes, halved
100 g (3½ oz) goat's cheese, sliced
A handful of fresh basil leaves, roughly torn

1 *Heat the oven to 190°C/170°C fan/Gas 5.*
2 *Cut the peppers in half lengthways, keeping the stalk attached, and remove the seeds. Brush the outsides with a little of the extra virgin olive oil, then place them, skin-side down, in a roasting tin, packing quite tightly so they don't roll over.*
3 *Spoon the lentils into the 4 pepper halves and top with the tomatoes and mozzarella pieces. Drizzle over the remaining olive oil and season. Bake in the oven for 20–25 minutes, or until the peppers are tender. Scatter over the basil leaves and serve immediately.*

Tofu and vegetable kebabs with thyme and garlic

Tofu is a rich source of protein and calcium and the vegetables provide extra fibre, vitamin C and potassium. Delicious if accompanied with a tomato salsa.

SERVES 4

Per serving: 124 calories, 9 g fat, of which 1 g saturates, 4.2 g carbohydrate, of which 3.8 g sugars, 7 g protein, 2 g fibre, trace salt

250 g (9 oz) plain firm tofu, cut into 16 cubes
1 red pepper, halved and deseeded
2 small courgettes, cut into thick slices
8 large mushrooms, halved
8 cherry tomatoes
100 ml olive oil
2 tbsp chopped fresh thyme
1 garlic clove, chopped
Freshly ground black pepper

1 *Cut the tofu into 16 cubes. Place in a shallow dish.*
2 *Cut the red pepper into 2.5 cm (1 in) squares. Add to the dish, along with the courgettes, mushrooms and tomatoes.*
3 *In a small glass jug, mix together the olive oil, thyme, garlic and freshly ground pepper. Pour over the vegetables. Turn gently to coat. Cover and refrigerate, ideally for 2 hours.*
4 *Thread the tofu and vegetables on skewers, reserving the remaining marinade for basting.*
5 *Cook on the rack of a barbecue or under a hot grill for approximately 8 minutes, turning occasionally and brushing with the reserved marinade.*

Pasta with tomato and vegetable sauce

This basic pasta recipe takes less than 15 minutes to prepare, making it ideal for quick nutritious suppers. Simply add whatever fresh or frozen vegetables you have handy to the pasta pot. Any leftovers are also good served cold as a salad.

SERVES 4

Per serving: 365 calories, 10 g fat, of which 2 g saturates, 52 g carbohydrate, of which 8 g sugars, 16 g protein, 4 g fibre, 0.3 g salt

350 g (12 oz) dried pasta of your choice
2 tbsp olive oil
1 onion, chopped
2 garlic cloves, crushed
400 g (14 oz) tin chopped tomatoes
2 tbsp tomato puree
225 g vegetables, e.g. asparagus, chopped into 4 cm (1½ in) lengths; sliced courgettes; chopped red, green or yellow peppers; small broccoli florets; mangetout; chopped aubergine; sliced mushrooms; peas; French beans, chopped into 4 cm (1½ in) lengths
1 tbsp chopped fresh basil or 1 tsp dried basil
25 g (1 oz) Parmesan, grated

1 Cook the pasta in plenty of boiling water according to the directions on the packet.
2 Meanwhile, heat the oil in a large pan. Add the onion and garlic and cook over a moderate heat for 5 minutes. Add the tomatoes, tomato puree, prepared vegetables and basil.
3 Cook for 4 minutes, or until the vegetables are tender but still firm.
4 Drain the pasa and return to the pan. Add the sauce and stir in the Parmesan.

Vegetarian pasta bolognese

Packed with protein, fibre and iron, this delicious pasta sauce goes well with spaghetti and tagliatelle.

SERVES 4

Per serving: 508 calories, 7 g fat, of which 1 g saturates, 83 g carbohydrate, of which 11 g sugars, 28 g protein, 11 g fibre, 0.3 g salt

350 g (12 oz) dried spaghetti or tagliatelle
1 tbsp olive oil
1 onion, chopped
2 carrots, peeled and finely chopped
1 large courgette, finely chopped
400 g (14 oz) tinned chopped tomatoes
250 g (9 oz) ready-cooked brown or green lentils (e.g. Merchant Gourmet, or 400 g (14 oz) tinned lentils)
1 tsp mixed herbs
1 tbsp Parmesan, grated

1 Cook the pasta in plenty of boiling water according to the directions on the packet.
2 Heat the oil in a large frying pan. Add the vegetables and cook, stirring often until softened (approximately 5 minutes). Add the tomatoes, lentils and herbs. Cook until the sauce thickens slightly. Stir in the cheese and heat through.
3 Drain the pasta and return to the pan. Add the lentil mixture to the drained pasta. Mix well to combine, then serve.

Macaroni cheese with vegetables

Not only is this healthy version of the classic dish high in protein, it also includes extra vegetables to boost the fibre and vitamin content.

SERVES 4

Per serving: 528 calories, 15 g fat, of which 8 g saturates, 77 g carbohydrate, of which 12 g sugars, 22 g protein, 6 g fibre, 0.5 g salt

350 g (12 oz) wholegrain macaroni (or other pasta shapes)
1 tsp olive oil
1 large onion, sliced
225 g (8 oz) sliced vegetables of your choice (e.g. mushrooms, peppers, tomatoes, courgettes)
25 g (1 oz) butter
25 g (1 oz) cornflour
600 ml (1 pint) milk
50 g (2 oz) mature Cheddar cheese

1 *Heat the oven to 180°C/160°C fan/Gas 4.*
2 *Cook the pasta in plenty of boiling water according to the directions on the packet. Drain.*
3 *In a non-stick pan, sauté the vegetables in the olive oil over a high heat until browned.*
4 *Whisk together the butter, cornflour and milk in a saucepan over a medium heat until thickened. Stir in the cheese.*
5 *In a large baking dish, layer half the pasta, vegetables and sauce. Repeat, finishing with a layer of sauce.*
6 *Bake for approximately 20 minutes or until the top is slightly brown.*

Vegetable paella

This is a vegetarian version of the classic Spanish paella that uses vegetables instead of the fish. The nuts and peas add protein to the dish.

SERVES 4

Per serving: 543 calories, 15 g fat, of which 2 g saturates, 88 g carbohydrate, of which 12 g sugars, 15 g protein, 9 g fibre, 0.9 g salt

2 tbsp olive oil
1 onion, chopped
2 garlic cloves, crushed
4 celery sticks, chopped
1 red, yellow and green pepper, sliced
1 tsp paprika
350 g (12 oz) rice
400 g (14 oz) tinned chopped tomatoes
900 ml (1 ½ pints) vegetable stock (or water plus 2 vegetable stock cubes)
225 g (8 oz) frozen peas
2 tbsp chopped parsley
50 g (2 oz) almonds or cashew nuts
Salt and pepper, to taste

1 *Heat the oil in a large pan and sauté the onion, garlic, celery and peppers for 5 minutes.*
2 *Add the paprika and rice and stir for another 2–3 minutes. Add the tomatoes and stock, bring to the boil, then simmer for 15–20 minutes until the liquid has been absorbed.*
3 *Add the peas, season to taste, and continue cooking for 5 minutes. Stir in the parsley and nuts, then serve.*

Chickpea and spinach pilaf

This dish makes an ideal pre-workout meal as it contains basmati rice and chickpeas, which both have a low GI. It also delivers good amounts of protein, fibre and iron.

SERVES 4

Per serving: 459 calories, 11 g fat, of which 1 g saturates, 75 g carbohydrate, of which 3 g sugars, 16 g protein, 8 g fibre, 2.2 g salt

2 tbsp olive oil
1 onion, chopped
2 garlic cloves, crushed
300 g (10 oz) basmati rice
Zest of 1 unwaxed lemon
900 ml (1 ½ pints) vegetable stock
425 g (15 oz) tin chickpeas, drained
125 g (4 oz) baby spinach leaves
50 g (2 oz) black olives (pitted)
Salt and pepper

1 Heat the oil in a large saucepan and saute the onion over a gentle heat for 2 minutes. Add the garlic and basmati rice and continue cooking while continuously stirring, for a further 2 minutes until the grains become translucent.

2 Add the lemon zest and the vegetable stock, bring to the boil then simmer for 20–25 minutes until the liquid has been absorbed and the rice is cooked.

3 Add the chickpeas and continue cooking over a gentle heat for a further 3 minutes. Add the spinach and leave the pan to stand for another couple of minutes to wilt.

4 Stir in the olives, season with salt and pepper and serve.

Butternut squash risotto

Butternut squash is rich in beta-carotene, which has powerful antioxidant properties, helping neutralise free radicals and protect against heart disease and cancer. It also benefits the skin and can be converted into vitamin A in the body.

SERVES 4

Per serving: 468 calories, 13 g fat, of which 2 g saturates, 76 g carbohydrate, of which 9 g sugars, 11 g protein, 7 g fibre, 0.8 g salt

3 tbsp olive oil
1 large onion, chopped
1 tsp ground cumin
1 tsp ground coriander
300 g (10 oz) risotto rice
1 litre (1¾ pints) hot vegetable stock (or water plus 2 vegetable stock cubes)
350 g (12 oz) butternut squash, peeled, deseeded and cut into 12 mm (½ in) pieces
1 medium courgette, diced
125 g (4 oz) fresh or frozen peas
1 tbsp fresh chopped parsley
25 g (1 oz) flaked toasted almonds
Salt and pepper

1 Heat the olive oil in a large pan. Add the onion and cook for 2 minutes until translucent. Stir in the spices and continue cooking for a further minute.

2 Add the rice and stir until the grains are coated with the oil. Add the hot vegetable stock one ladle at a time; stir and simmer for approximately 10 minutes.

3 Add the butternut squash and courgette; continue cooking for a further 15 minutes.

4 Add the peas and continue cooking for a further
cont.

5 minutes until all the liquid has been absorbed and the rice is tender but firm in the centre. Perfect risotto is creamy but not solid, and the rice should still have a little bite.

5 _Stir in the parsley and season to taste. Scatter over the almonds and serve immediately._

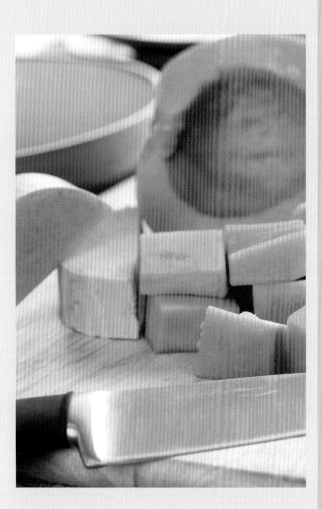

Beans 'n' rice

This is a vegetarian adaptation of the traditional West Indian dish. The combination of beans and rice increases the overall protein value of the dish. It can be made as spicy, hot or mild as you wish.

SERVES 4

Per serving: 559 calories, 14 g fat, of which 8 g saturates, 93 g carbohydrate, of which 9 g sugars, 15 g protein, 11 g fibre, 1.8 g salt

1 tbsp oil
1 onion, chopped
1 green chilli, deseeded and finely chopped
350 g (12 oz) white rice
900 ml (1½ pints) vegetable stock (or water plus
2 vegetable stock cubes)
2 large tomatoes, sliced
420 g (15 oz) tinned red kidney beans, or any other
beans of your choice
50 g (2 oz) coconut cream
2 tbsp fresh chopped coriander or parsley

1 _Heat the oil in a pan and fry the onion for approximately 5 minutes. Add the chilli and rice and fry for a further 2 minutes._

2 _Add the stock and tomatoes, bring to the boil, and simmer for 10 minutes._

3 _Add the beans and a little extra water if the mixture looks dry. Cover and cook for a further 5 minutes until the rice is cooked._

4 _Stir in the coconut cream and then stir in the coriander or parsley._

Couscous with roasted vegetables and cashew nuts

SERVES 4

Per serving: 172 calories, 13 g fat, of which 3 g saturates, 8 g carbohydrate, of which 5 g sugars, 7 g protein, 3 g fibre, 0.4 salt

½ red pepper
½ yellow pepper
200 g (7 oz) cherry tomatoes, halved
1 courgette, sliced
2 tbsp olive oil
250 g (9 oz) couscous
400 ml (14 fl oz) hot vegetable stock or water
100 g (3½ oz) cashew nuts
A small handful of fresh coriander, chopped
Salt and pepper

1 Heat the oven to 200°C/180°C fan/Gas 6.
2 Remove the seeds from the peppers and cut them into wide strips. Place in a large roasting tin with the cherry tomatoes and courgettes. Drizzle over the olive oil and toss lightly so that the vegetables are well coated in the oil.
3 Roast in the oven for approximately 30 minutes until the peppers are slightly charred on the outside and tender in the middle. Allow to cool, then roughly chop the peppers.
4 Put the couscous in a large bowl and cover with the hot stock or water. Stir briefly, cover, and allow to stand for 5 minutes until the stock has been absorbed. Fluff up with a fork.
5 Add the roasted vegetables, nuts and coriander. Season to taste with salt and black pepper. Serve.

Quinoa with vegetables and almonds

Quinoa is a seed (although it looks like a grain) and has a delicate slightly nutty flavour. It has a higher protein and iron content than grains. This dish is also a good source of vitamins A and E.

SERVES 4

Per serving: 451 calories, 15 g fat, of which 2 g saturates, 63 g carbohydrate, of which 21 g sugars, 17 g protein, 4 g fibre, 0.2 g salt

1 tbsp oil
1 large onion, chopped
2 carrots, peeled and diced
1 garlic clove, crushed
350 g (12 oz) quinoa
900 ml (1½ pints) water
50 g (2 oz) raisins
50 g (2 oz) toasted flaked almonds
Salt and pepper

1 Heat the oil in a heavy-based saucepan and cook the onion for 5 minutes. Add the carrots and garlic and cook for a further 5 minutes.
2 Add the quinoa and water and season to taste with the salt and pepper. Bring to the boil, cover and simmer for 15–20 minutes until the water has been absorbed. Stir in the raisins and almonds, then serve.

16 SPORTS SNACKS

Nutty flapjacks

Oats have a low GI and are also a great source of iron, B vitamins and fibre. The walnuts provide omega-3 oils for improved post-workout recovery and heart-health. What better excuse, then, to indulge in these tasty treats?

MAKES 12 FLAPJACKS

Per flapjack: 254 calories, 16 g fat, of which 7 g saturates, 23 g carbohydrate, of which 11 g sugars, 4 g protein, 2 g fibre, 0.3 g salt

150 g (5 oz) butter
50 g (2 oz) light brown sugar
100 g (3½ oz) golden syrup
225 g (8 oz) porridge oats
75 g (3 oz) chopped walnuts

1 Heat the oven to 180°C/160°C fan/Gas 4.
2 Lightly oil a 23-cm square baking tin.
3 Put the butter or margarine, sugar and syrup in a heavy-based saucepan and heat together, stirring occasionally, until the butter has melted.
4 Remove from the heat and mix in the oats and walnuts until thoroughly combined.
6 Transfer the mixture into the prepared tin, level the surface, and bake in the oven for 20–25 minutes until golden brown around the edges but still soft.
7 Remove from the oven and leave in the tin to cool. While still warm, score into 12 bars with a sharp knife.

Options:

Date and walnut: Add 50 g chopped dates
Almond and walnut: Add 50 g flaked toasted almonds
Apricot and almond: Substitute 100 g flaked toasted almonds for the walnuts, and add 50 g chopped dried apricots

Honey flapjacks

MAKES 12 FLAPJACKS

Per flapjack: 263 calories, 15 g fat, of which 6 g saturates, 27 g carbohydrate, of which 14 g sugars, 5 g protein, 0.2 g salt, 2 g fibre

125 g (4 oz) butter
100 g (3½ oz) brown sugar
50 g (2 oz) honey
225 g (8 oz) porridge oats
50 g (2 oz) chopped nuts (e.g. walnuts, almonds, hazelnuts)
50 g (2 oz) seeds, e.g. any combination of pumpkin, sunflower, hemp, linseeds or sesame seeds
50 g (2 oz) raisins

1 Heat the oven to 180°C/160°C fan/Gas 4.
2 Line an 18-cm square shallow tin with baking parchment.
3 Place the butter, sugar and honey in a pan and heat until the butter has melted. Stir in the oats, nuts and dried fruit.
4 Spread the mixture in the tin and press down well. Bake for 20–25 minutes until just golden brown around the edges. Remove from the oven and leave to cool in the tin before turning out and cutting into slices.

Coconut energy bars

MAKES 12 BARS

Per bar: 221 calories, 15 g fat, of which 8 g saturates, 18 g carbohydrate, of which 9 g sugars, 4 g protein, 3 g fibre, 0.1 g salt

150 g (5 oz) porridge oats
75 g (3 oz) flaked almonds
100 g (3½ oz) desiccated coconut
75 g (3 oz) unsalted butter
225 g (8 oz) honey
50 g (2 oz) light brown sugar
1 tsp vanilla extract
50 g (2 oz) chopped ready-to-eat dates
50 g (2 oz) chopped ready-to-eat dried apricots

1 *Heat the oven to 180°C/160°C fan/Gas 4.*
2 *Line an 18-cm square shallow tin with baking parchment.*
3 *Mix the oats, almonds and coconut together on a baking tray and bake for 10–12 minutes, stirring occasionally, until lightly browned. Reduce the oven temperature to 150°C/130°C fan/Gas 3.*
4 *Place the butter, honey, sugar and vanilla in a small saucepan over medium heat. Heat until melted, then pour over the granola mixture. Add the dates and apricots and stir well.*
5 *Spread the mixture into the prepared tin and lightly press down the mixture. Bake for 25–30 minutes, until lightly golden brown. Cool before cutting into squares.*

Granola bars

MAKES 12 BARS

Per bar: 252 calories, 15 g fat, of which 6 g saturates, 24 g carbohydrate, of which 11 g sugars, 6 g protein, 3 g fibre, 0.2 g salt

125 g (4 oz) porridge oats
50 g (2 oz) chopped nuts (almonds, walnuts or pecans)
50 g (2 oz) sunflower or pumpkin seeds
50 g (2 oz) wheatgerm
75 g (3 oz) wholewheat flour
½ tsp baking powder
½ tsp ground cinnamon
125 g (4 oz) butter
75 g (3 oz) dark brown sugar
1 large egg, lightly beaten
1 tsp vanilla extract
75 g (3 oz) dried fruit of your choice (raisins, chopped dates, chopped apricots, cranberries)

1 *Heat the oven to 180°C/160°C fan/Gas 4.*
2 *Line an 18-cm square shallow tin with baking parchment that overhangs the tin on all sides by at least 2 cm.*
3 *Spread the oats, nuts and seeds on a baking sheet and bake them for about 10 minutes, or until they are lightly toasted, stirring once or twice to ensure even cooking. Remove from the oven and allow the mixture to cool.*
4 *In a large mixing bowl, combine the wheatgerm, flour, baking powder and cinnamon.*
5 *Melt the butter and sugar in a small saucepan. Remove from the heat and mix in the egg and vanilla. Add to the flour mixture until just combined, then stir in the oat mixture and dried fruit until well combined.*

cont.

6 Pour the mixture into the prepared baking pan, spreading evenly. Bake the bars until they are set, about 25–30 minutes. Allow to cool then lift the slab of granola bars from the tin using the overhanging parchment as handles and place on a cutting board. Cut into 12 bars.

Apricot energy bars

These bars deliver slow- and fast-release carbohydrate, along with protein and unsaturated fats, which makes them ideal for fuelling long intense workouts. Apricots are rich in beta-carotene, a powerful antioxidant that helps protect cell membranes, DNA and body proteins from free radical damage.

MAKES 12 BARS

Per bar: 221 calories, 10 g fat, of which 3 g saturates, 30 g carbohydrate, of which 19 g sugars, 4 g protein, 3 g fibre, 0.1 g salt

125 g (4 oz) ready-to-eat dried apricots, roughly chopped
150 ml water
50 g (2 oz) butter
75 g (3 oz) runny honey
150 g (5 oz) brown sugar
175 g (6 oz) porridge oats
50 g (2 oz) raisins
50 g (2 oz) pecan nuts
50 g (2 oz) pumpkin seeds

1 Heat the oven to 190°C/170°C fan/Gas 4.
2 Line an 18 x 18 cm cake tin with baking parchment.
3 Put the apricots and water in a saucepan, bring to the boil and simmer gently, uncovered, for 10 minutes or until the apricots have softened. Transfer to a food processor and process to a thick smooth puree.

4 Spoon the puree back into the pan and add butter, honey and sugar. Warm over a low heat, stirring occasionally, for 5 minutes or until the sugar has dissolved.
5 Stir in the remaining ingredients. Spoon into the prepared tin and bake for 15 minutes. When cool, remove from the tin and discard the baking parchment. Cut into 12 bars.

Fruit and nut energy bars

These energy bars made from dried fruit, nuts and seeds are packed with fibre, B vitamins, vitamin E, iron and zinc – and are more nutritious than commercial energy bars.

MAKES 16 BARS

Per bar: 314 calories, 18 g fat, of which 6 g saturates, 32 g carbohydrate, of which 25 g sugars, 6 g protein, 3 g fibre 0.2 g salt

75 g (3 oz) almonds
75 g (3 oz) cashew nuts
75 g (3 oz) blanched hazelnuts (without skins)
50 g (2 oz) mixed seeds (e.g. pumpkin, flax, hemp, sunflower)
150 g (5 oz) porridge oats
150 g (5 oz) dried figs
150 g (5 oz) dried dates
125 g (4 oz) sultanas
150 g (5 oz) butter
75 g (3 oz) runny honey
75 g (3 oz) light brown sugar

1 *Heat the oven to 180°C/160°C fan/Gas 4.*
2 *Line a 29 x 21 cm baking tin with baking parchment.*
3 *Place the nuts, seeds and oats in a food processor, pulse briefly, and then add the dried fruit. Pulse again until the fruit is roughly chopped.*
4 *Melt the butter, honey and sugar in a saucepan over a medium heat. Pour over the fruit and nut mixture, and stir.*
5 *Spoon into the prepared baking tin, press down lightly, and bake for 15–20 minutes. Cool before cutting into bars.*

Coconut balls

Perfect for fuelling before and during long training sessions and ideal for those preferring a low-carbo-hydrate diet and, thus, looking for an alternative to high-carbohydrate energy bars! The fat in coconut oil, once labelled as unhealthy, is now considered good for you. It consists of medium chain triglycerides (MCTs), which are readily converted into energy by the liver, and have a beneficial effect on blood choles-terol levels.

MAKES 12 BALLS

Per ball: 108 calories, 10g fat, of which 9 g saturates, 3 g carbohydrate, of which 3 g sugars, 1 g protein, 3 g fibre, 0.1 g salt

175 g (6 oz) desiccated coconut
2 tsp coconut oil, melted
3 tbsp maple syrup
2 tbsp unsweetened coconut milk
½ tsp vanilla extract
½ tsp ground cinnamon
⅛ tsp sea salt

1 *Place 125 g (4 oz) of the desiccated coconut, along with the coconut oil, in a food processor. Process on high speed, until it reaches a paste-like consistency but is not completely smooth.*
2 *Add the maple syrup, coconut milk, vanilla, cinnamon and salt, and process until well combined. Add the remaining desiccated coconut and pulse until just combined.*
3 *Shape the mixture into 12 (1-inch) balls and refrigerate for at least an hour and for up to 5 days.*

Anzac cookies

These cookies are one of the tastiest ways of using coconut, and make a great refuelling snack. A rich source of medium chain fatty acids, which are digested and absorbed more readily than other fats, coconut is also high in lauric acid, which has anti-bacterial and antiviral properties.

MAKES 15

Per cookie: 199 calories, 12 g fat, of which 8 g saturates, 20 g carbohydrate, of which 10 g sugars, 3 g protein, 2 g fibre, 0.2 g salt

125 g (4 oz) butter, melted
1 tbsp golden syrup
100 g (3½ oz) self-raising flour
125 g (4 oz) sugar
125 g porridge oats
100 g (3½ oz) desiccated coconut
1 egg, beaten

1 *Heat the oven to 170°C/150°C fan/Gas 3.*
2 *Line a baking sheet with baking parchment.*
3 *Melt the butter and syrup in a small saucepan.*
4 *Mix the dry ingredients in a bowl. Add the melted butter and syrup, and the egg. Mix well.*
5 *Form into small balls with your hands (2.5 to 5 cm/1 to 2 inches in diameter) and place on the baking sheet. Flatten slightly.*
6 *Bake for 10–15 minutes until light golden coloured. Remove from the oven and cool on a wire rack.*

Oat cookies

These simple oat cookies are ideal for eating on the move and can be carried in a kit bag/jersey pocket for a tasty post-workout treat.

MAKES 20 COOKIES

Per cookie: 126 calories, 6 g fat, of which 3 g saturates, 16 g carbohydrate, of which 8 g sugars, 2 g protein, 1 g fibre, 0.1 g salt

125 g (4 oz) butter
125 g (4 oz) brown sugar
1 egg
1 tsp vanilla extract
1 tbsp golden syrup
150 g (5 oz) porridge oats
75 g (3 oz) plain flour
¼ tsp baking powder
¼ tsp ground cinnamon
50 g (2 oz) raisins

1 *Heat the oven to 180°C/160°C fan/Gas 4.*
2 *Line a baking sheet with baking parchment.*
3 *Using a hand-held beater, mix together the butter and sugar until light and fluffy. Beat in the eggs and vanilla.*
4 *Add the remaining ingredients and mix until just combined. You should have a fairly stiff mixture.*
5 *Form into small balls and place on the prepared baking sheet. Use a fork to flatten them slightly. Bake for approximately 10 minutes until golden, then remove from the oven to cool on a wire rack..*

Blueberry and walnut muffins

This recipe is a delicious way of adding antioxidant-rich blueberries to your diet. These muffins provide fibre and vitamin E.

MAKES 12 MUFFINS

Per muffin: 161 calories, 8 g fat, of which 3 g saturates, 19 g carbohydrate, of which 6 g sugars, 5 g protein, 2 g fibre, 0.2 g salt

125 g (4 oz) self-raising white flour
125 g (4 oz) self-raising wholemeal flour
50 g (2 oz) sugar
50 g (2 oz) butter, melted
1 large egg
1 tsp vanilla extract
200 ml (7 fl oz) milk
125 g (4 oz) fresh blueberries or 85 g (3 oz) dried blueberries
50 g (2 oz) walnuts, chopped

1 *Heat the oven to 200°C/180°C fan/Gas 6.*
2 *Line 12 muffin tins with paper muffin cases.*
3 *In a bowl, mix together the flours and sugar. In a separate bowl, mix together the melted butter, egg, vanilla and milk, then pour into the flour mixture. Stir until just combined.*
4 *Gently fold in the blueberries and walnuts.*
5 *Spoon the mixture into the prepared muffin tins to about two-thirds full and bake for approximately 20 minutes until the muffins have risen and are golden.*

Apple and oat muffins

Oats provide slow release complex carbohydrate thanks to their soluble fibre content.

MAKES 12 MUFFINS

Per muffin: 184 calories, 6 g fat, of which 1 g saturates, 29 g carbohydrate, of which 12 g sugars, 4 g protein, 2 g fibre, 0.4 g salt

175 g (6 oz) self-raising flour
125 g (4 oz) oats
125 g (4 oz) light brown sugar
½ tsp salt
4 tbsp rapeseed oil
1 tsp vanilla extract
1 large egg
250 ml (9 fl oz) milk or buttermilk
125 g (4 oz) grated apples

1 *Heat the oven to 190°C/170°C fan/Gas 5.*
2 *Line 12 muffin tins with paper muffin cases.*
3 *Mix together the flour, oats, sugar, baking powder and salt in a large bowl.*
4 *Combine the oil, vanilla, egg and milk in a separate bowl, then stir into the flour mixture. Fold in the grated apple.*
5 *Spoon the mixture into the muffin cases, filling them two-thirds full.*
6 *Bake for approximately 20 minutes until firm to the touch and light brown.*

Raisin muffins

The perfect refuelling snack that no athlete should be without! I find that a half and half mixture of white and wholemeal flour gives a good result, but you may use just wholemeal flour if you prefer.

MAKES 12 MUFFINS

Per muffin: 143 calories, 5 g fat, of which 1 g saturates, 22 g carbohydrate, of which 9 g sugars, 4 g protein, 0.2 g salt, 2 g fibre

125 g (4 oz) self-raising flour
125 g (4 oz) wholemeal self-raising flour
Pinch of salt
4 tbsp rapeseed oil
40 g (1½ oz) soft brown sugar
1 egg
200 ml (7 fl oz) milk
75 g (3 oz) raisins

1 *Heat the oven to 200°C/180°C fan/Gas 6.*
2 *Line 12 muffin tins with paper muffin cases.*
3 *Mix the flours and salt together in a bowl. Add the oil, sugar, egg and milk. Mix well. Stir in the raisins.*
4 *Spoon into the muffin cases and bake for approximately 20 minutes until golden brown.*

Banana and walnut muffins

These healthy muffins contain plenty of vitamin B6 (from the bananas), potassium and also omega-3 oils from the walnuts, making them one of the most delicious yet nutritious ways of refuelling after training!

MAKES 12

Per muffin: 169 calories, 7 g fat, of which 3 g saturates, 23 g carbohydrate, of which 11 g sugars, 4 g protein, 1 g fibre, 0.2 g salt

2 large ripe bananas, mashed
85 g (3 oz) sugar
50 g (2 oz) butter, softened
1 egg
125 ml (4 fl oz) milk
200 g (7 oz) self-raising flour
50 g (2 oz) chopped walnuts
½ tsp ground nutmeg

1 *Heat the oven to 200°C/180°C fan/Gas 6.*
2 *Line 12 muffin tins with paper muffin cases.*
3 *Mix together the bananas, sugar and butter. Beat in the egg and milk. Fold in the flour, walnuts, salt and nutmeg.*
4 *Spoon into the muffin cases and bake for 20 minutes until firm to the touch and golden brown.*

Banana cake

Bananas are a good source of fibre, vitamin B6, vitamin C, potassium and manganese. They also contain prebiotics, which promote friendly bacteria (probiotics) in the intestines. This easy-to-make recipe is a delicious way of refuelling after exercise.

MAKES 12 SLICES

Per slice: 203 calories, 6 g fat, of which 4 g saturates, 33 g carbohydrate, of which 16 g sugars, 4 g protein, 1 g fibre, 0.5 g salt

2 large ripe bananas
250 ml (9 fl oz) milk
300 g (10 oz) self-raising flour (or half wholemeal, half white)
125 g (4 oz) brown sugar
Pinch of salt
½ tsp each of mixed spice and ground cinnamon
1 egg
75 g (3 oz) butter, melted

1 *Heat the oven to 170°C/150°C fan/Gas 5.*
2 *Mash the bananas with the milk.*
3 *Mix together the flour, sugar, salt and spices in a bowl. Add the banana mixture, together with the egg and oil. Mix until well combined.*
4 *Spoon into a lightly oiled 900 g (2 lb) loaf tin. Bake for about 1 hour. Check the cake is cooked by inserting a skewer or knife into the centre. It should come out clean.*

Apple cake

Tasty enough to serve non-athletic guests for tea, as well as refuelling your muscles between workouts, this recipe is a good way of smuggling extra fruit into your diet. It is lower in sugar than conventional cakes and the grated apple and the oil make the cake deliciously moist.

MAKES 12 SLICES

Per slice: 180 calories, 5 g fat, of which 1 g saturates, 30 g carbohydrate, of which 13 g sugars, 4 g protein, 2 g fibre, 0.3 g salt

300 g (10 oz) self-raising flour (half wholemeal, half white)
125 g (4 oz) brown sugar
1 tsp ground cinnamon
2 cooking apples, peeled and grated
4 tbsp rapeseed oil
2 eggs
125 ml (4 fl oz) milk

1 *Heat the oven to 170°C/150°C fan/Gas 4.*
2 *Mix together the flour, sugar and cinnamon in a bowl. Add the grated apple, oil, eggs and milk and combine well.*
3 *Spoon into a lightly oiled 2lb loaf tin and bake for about 1–1½ hours. Check the cake is cooked by inserting a skewer or knife into the centre. It should come out clean.*

REFERENCES AND FURTHER READING

Chapter one

Allender, S., Scarborough, P., Peto, V., *et al.*, *European Cardio-vascular Disease Statistics* (British Heart Foundation Health Promotion Research Group, Department of Public Health, University of Oxford and Health Economics Research Centre, Department of Public Health, University of Oxford, 2008)

American Dietetic Association, Dieticians of Canada, American College of Sports Medicine, *et al.*, 'American College of Sports Medicine position stand: nutrition and athletic performance', *Medical Science Sports Exercise*, 41 (3), (2009) pp. 709–731.

Arefhosseini, S. R., Edwards, C. A., Malkova, D., *et al.*, 'Effect of advice to increase carbohydrate and reduce fat intake on dietary profile and plasma lipid concentrations in healthy post-menopausal women', *Annals of Nutrition and Metabolism*, 54(2), (2009), pp. 138–44.

Ascherio, A. and Willett, W. C., 'Health effects of trans fatty acids', *American Journal of Clinical Nutrition*, 66 (4), (1997), pp. 1006–1010.

Astrup, A., Dyerberg, J., Elwood, P., *et al.*, 'The role of reducing intakes of saturated fat in the prevention of cardiovascular disease: where does the evidence stand in 2010?', *The American Journal of Clinical Nutrition*, 93(4), (2011), pp. 684–688.

Basu, S., Yoffe, P., Hills, N., *et al.*, 'The relationship of sugar to population-level diabetes prevalence: an economic analysis of repeated cross-sectional data', *PLOS One*, 8(2), (2013).

Beis, L. Y., Willkomm, L., Ross, R., Bekele, Z., *et al.* Food and macronutrient intake of elite Ethiopian distance runners', *J. Int. Soc. Sports Nutr.*, 2011, May 19;8:7.

Benton, D. 'The plausibility of sugar addiction and its role in obesity and eating disorders', *Clinical Nutrition*, 29 (3) (2009), pp 288–303.

Boisseau, N., Vermorel, M., Rance, M., *et al.* 'Protein requirements in male adolescent soccer players', *European Journal of Applied Physiology*, 100 (2007), pp. 27–33.

Bonthuis, M., Hughes, M. C., Ibiebele, T. I., *et al.*, 'Dairy consumption and patterns of mortality of Australian adults', *European Journal of Clinical Nutrition*, 64 (2010), pp. 569–577.

Burke, D. G., Collier, G. R., Hargreaves, M., *et al.*, 'Glycaemic index – a new tool in sports nutrition', *International Journal of Sports Nutrition*, 8 (1998), pp. 401–15.

Burke, L. M., Hawley, J. A., Wong, S. H., *et al.*, 'Carbohydrate for training and competition', *Journal of Sports Science*, 29 (2011), pp. 17–27.

Burke, L., *Practical Sports Nutrition*. (Human Kinetics, 2007)

Chowdhury R. *et al.*, 'Association of Dietary, Circulating, and Supplement Fatty Acids With Coronary Risk: A Systematic Review and Meta-analysis', *Ann Intern Med*, 160 (6) (2014) pp. 398–406.

Davidenko, O., Darcel, N., Fromentin, G., *et al.*, 'Control of protein and energy intake – brain mechanisms', *European Journal of Clinical Nutrition*, 67 (2013), pp. 455–461.

de Oliveira Otto, M. C., Mozaffarian D, Kromhout D, *et al.*, 'Dietary intake of saturated fat by food source and incident cardiovascular disease: the multi-ethnic study of athero-sclerosis', *American Journal of Clinical Nutrition*, 96(2), (2012), pp. 397–404.

Dreon, D. M., Fernstrom, H. A., Campos, H., *et al.*, 'Change in dietary saturated fat intake is correlated with change in mass of large low-density-lipoprotein particles in men' *American Journal of Clinical Nutrition*, 67 (5), (1998), pp 828–836.

Elwood, P. C., Givens, D. I., Beswick, A. D., *et al.*, 'The survival advantage of milk and dairy consumption: an overview of evidence from cohort studies of vascular diseases, diabetes and cancer', *Journal of The American College of Nutrition*, 27(6), (2008), pp.723–734.

Elwood, P. C., Pickering, J. E., Givens, *et al.*, 'The consumption of milk and dairy foods and the incidence of vascular disease and diabetes: an overview of the evidence', *Lipids*, 45(10), (2010), pp. 925–939.

Estruch, R., Emilio, R., Salas–Salvadó, J., *et al.*, 'Primary prevention of cardiovascular disease with a Mediterranean diet', *The New England Journal of Medicine*, 368(14), (2013), pp. 1279–1290.

Fallaize, R., Wilson, L., Gray, J., *et al.*, 'Variation in the effects of three different breakfast meals on subjective satiety and subsequent intake of energy at lunch and evening meal', *European Journal of Nutrition*, 52(4), (2012).

Foster-Powell, K., Holt, S., Brand-Miller, J. C., 'International table of glycaemic index and glycaemic load values: 2002', *American Journal Clinical Nutrition*, 76 (2002), pp. 5–56.

German, J. B., Gibson, R. G., Krauss, R. M., *et al.*, 'A reappraisal of the impact of dairy foods and milk fat on cardiovascular disease risk', *European Journal of Nutrition*, 48(4), (2009), pp. 191–203.

Gillman, M. W., Cupples, L. A., Gagnon, D., *et al.*, 'Margarine intake and subsequent coronary heart disease in men', *Epidemiology*, 8 (2), (1997), pp. 144–149.

Halliday, T., Peterson, N. J., Thomas, J. J., *et al.*, 'Vitamin D status relative to diet, lifestyle, injury and illness in college athletes', *Medical Science Sports Exercise*, 43 (2011), pp. 335–43.

Hamilton, B., 'Vitamin D and athletic performance: the potential role of muscle', *Asian Journal of Sports Medicine*, 2 (4), (2011), pp. 211– 219.

Hooper, L., et al., 'Reduced or modified dietary fat for preventing cardiovascular disease' *Cochrane Database Syst Rev.* (2012) May 16;5.

Howard, B.V., Van Horn, L., Hsia, J., *et al.*, 'Low-fat dietary pattern and risk of cardiovascular disease: the women's health initiative randomized controlled dietary modification trial', *Journal of the American Medical Association*, 95(6), (2006), pp. 655–666.

Hu T, Mills K.T., Yao L., Demanelis K., *et al.*, 'Effects of low-carbohydrate diets versus low-fat diets on metabolic risk factors: a meta-analysis of randomized controlled clinical trials.' *Am J. Epidemiol*, 2012 Oct 1; 176 Suppl 7: S44–54.

International Olympic Committee (IOC), 'Consensus statement on sports nutrition 2010' *Journal of Sports Science*, 4 (29) Suppl (2011), 1:S3–4.

Jequier, E., and Constant. F., 'Water as an essential nutrient: the physiology basis of hydration', *European Journal of Clinical Nutrition*, 64 (2010) pp. 115–123.

Johnson, R. K., Appel, L. J., Brands, M., *et al.*, 'Dietary sugars intake and cardiovascular health: a scientific statement from the American Heart Association'. *Circulation* 120 (2009), pp. 1011–1020.

Johnston, C. S., Tjonn, S. L., Swan, P. D., *et al.*, Ketogenic low-carbohydrate diets have no metabolic advantage over nonketogenic low-carbohydrate diets, *Am. J. Clin. Nutr.*, 2006 May; 83(5):1055–61.

Keys A. B., *Seven Countries: A Multivariate Analysis of Death and Coronary Heart Disease* (Harvard University Press,1980).

Larson-Meyer, D. E., and Willis, K. S., 'Vitamin D and athletes', *Current Sports Medicine Reports*, 9 (2010), pp. 220–226.

Leidy, H. J., Tang, M., Armstrong, C. L., *et al.*, 'The effects of consuming frequent, higher protein meals on appetite and satiety during weight loss in overweight/obese men', *Obesity*, 19 (2011), pp. 818–824.

Lopez-Garcia, E., Schulze, M. B., Meigs, J. B., *et al.*, 'Consumption of trans fatty acids is related to plasma biomarkers of inflammation and endothelial dysfunction', *The Journal of Nutrition*, 135 (2005), pp. 562–566.

Lustig, R., *Fat Chance: The Bitter Truth About Sugar*, (Fourth Estate, 2013)

Mensink R. P., Zock, P. L., Kester, A. D., *et al.*, 'Effects of dietary fatty acids and carbohydrate on the ratio of serum total to HDL cholesterol and on serum lipids and apolipoproteins: a meta-analysis of 60 controlled trials', *American Journal of Clinical Nutrition*, 77 (5), (2003), pp. 1146–1155.

Mensink, R. P. and Katan, M. B., 'Effect of dietary trans fatty acids on high-density and low-density lipoprotein cholesterol levels in healthy subjects' *The New England Journal of Medicine*, 323 (1990), pp. 439–44.

Morenga L. T., Mallard, S., Mann, J., 'Dietary sugars and body weight: systematic review and meta-analyses of randomised controlled trials and cohort studies', *British Medical Journal*, 346 (2013), e7492.

Needleman I. *et al.*, 'Oral health and elite sport performance', *Br J Sports Med*, 49 (2015) pp 3-6.

Neurofast (2013) 'NeuroFAST consensus opinion on food addiction'. www.neurofast.eu/consensus

Noakes, T., 'Chapter 4: Salt Balance in the body' in *Waterlogged: The Serious Problem of Overhydration in Endurance Sports* (Human Kinetics, 2012).

Onywera, V. O., Kiplamai, F. K., Boit, M. K. *et al.*, Food and macronutrient intake of elite Kenyan distance runners. *Int. J. Sport Nutr. Exerc. Metab.*, 2004 Dec; 14(6):709–19.

Phillips, S. M. and Van Loon, L. J., 'Dietary protein for athletes: from requirements to optimum adaptation', *Journal Sports Science*, 29 (2011), Suppl 1: S29–38.

Phillips, S. M., Moore, D. R., Tang, J. E., *et al.*, 'A critical examination of dietary protein requirements, benefits and excesses in athletes', *International Journal of Sports Nutrition and Exercise Metabolism*, 17 (2007), pp. 58–78.

Ramsden, C. E., Zamora, D., Leelarthaepin, B., *et al.*, 'Use of dietary linoleic acid for secondary prevention of coronary heart disease and death: evaluation of recovered data from the Sydney Diet Heart Study and updated meta-analysis', *British Medical Journal*, 346 (2013).

Rodriguez, N. R., Di Marco, N. M., Langley, S., *et al.*, 'American College of Sports Medicine position stand: Nutrition and athletic performance', *Medical Science Sports Exercise* (2009), 41(3), pp. 709–731.

Siri-Tarino, P. W., Sun, Q., Hu, F. B., *et al.*, 'Meta-analysis of prospective cohort studies evaluating the association of saturated fat with cardiovascular disease', *American Journal of Clinical Nutrition*, 91 (3), (2010), pp. 535–546.

Sloth, B., Krog–Mikkelsen, I., Flint, A., *et al.*, 'No difference in body weight decrease between a low-glycaemic-index and a high-glycaemic-index diet but reduced LDL cholesterol after 10-wk ad libitum intake of the low-glycaemic-index diet', *American Journal of Clinical Nutrition*, 80 (2004), pp. 337–47.

Taylor, R. S., Ashton, K. E., Moxham, T., *et al.*, 'Reduced dietary salt for the prevention of cardiovascular disease: a meta–analysis of randomized controlled trials (Cochrane Review)', *American Journal of Hypertension*, 24 (8), (2011), pp. 834–853.

Toth, P. P., (2005) 'The "good cholesterol": High-density lipoprotein', *Circulation*, 111(5), (2005), pp. 89–91.

Troesch, B., Hoeft, B., McBurney M., *et al.*, 'Dietary surveys indicate vitamin intakes below recommendations are common in representative Western countries', *British Journal of Nutrition*, 108:4 (2012), pp. 692–698.

US Department of Agriculture, 'Oxygen radical absorbance capacity of selected foods', (Nutrient Data Laboratory, Agricultural Research Service, 2007)

Volek, J. S. and Forsythe, C. E., 'The case for not restricting saturated fat on a low carbohydrate diet', *Nutrition Metabolism*, 2 (2005).

Wu, C. L., and Williams, C., 'A low glycaemic index meal before exercise improves endurance running capacity in men', *International Journal of Sports Nutrition and Exercise Metabolism*, 16 (2006), pp. 510–527.

Chapter two

Achten, T., Halson, S. L., Moseley, L., *et al.*, 'Higher dietary carbohydrate content during intensified running training results in better maintenance of performance and mood state', *Journal of Applied Physiology*, 96(4), (2004), pp. 1331–1340.

Beelen, M., Koopman, R., Gijsen, A. P., *et al.*, 'Protein coingestion stimulates muscle protein synthesis during resistance-type exercise', *American Journal of Physiology*, 295 (2008), pp. 70–77.

Beelen, M., Zorenc, A., Pennings B., *et al.*, 'Impact of protein coingestion on muscle protein synthesis during continuous endurance type exercise', *American Journal of Physiology*, 300 (2011), pp. 945–954.

Bloomer, R. J., Sforzo, G. A., Keller, B. A., *et al.*, 'Effects of meal form and composition on plasma testosterone, cortisol and insulin following resistance exercise', *International Journal of Sports Nutrition*, 10 (2000), pp. 415–24.

Bowtell, J. L., Sumners, D. P., Dyer, A., *et al.*, 'Montmorency cherry juice reduces muscle damage caused by intensive strength exercise', *Medicine and Science in Sports Exercise*, 43(8) (2011), pp. 1544–1551.

Burke, L. M., Hawley, J.A., Wong, S. H., *et al*,. 'Carbohydrate for training and competition', *Journal of Sports Science*, 29 (2011), pp. 17–27.

Burke L.M. 'Fueling strategies to optimize performance: training high or training low?' *Scand J Med Sci Sports.* (2010) Oct;20 Suppl 2:48-58.

Churchward-Venne, T. A., *et al.*, 'Nutritional regulation of muscle protein synthesis with resistance exercise: strategies to enhance anabolism', *Nutrition and Metabolism* (2012) 9:40.

Chryssanthopoulos, C., William, C., Nowitz, A., *et al.*, 'The effect of a high carbohydrate meal on endurance running capacity', *International Journal of Sports Nutrition*, 12 (2002), pp. 157–171.

Cockburn, E., Hayes, R. P., French, D. N., *et al.*, 'Acute milk-based protein-CHO supplementation attenuates exercise-induced muscle damage', *Applied Physiology, Nutrition, and Metabolism*, 33 (4), (2008), pp. 775–783.

Cockburn, E., Robson–Ansley, P., Hayes, P. R., *et al*, 'Effect of volume of milk consumed on the attenuation of exercise-induced muscle damage', *European Journal of Applied Physiology*, 112(9), (2012), pp. 3187–3194.

Coggan, A. R. and Coyle, E. F., 'Carbohydrate ingestion during prolonged exercise: effects on metabolism and performance', *Exercise and Sports Science Reviews* (1991) 19, pp. 1–40.

Elliot, T. A., Cree, M. G., Sanford, A. P., *et al.*, 'Milk ingestion stimulates net muscle protein synthesis following resistance exercise', *Medicine and Science in Sports Exercise*, 38 (4), (2006), pp. 667–74.

Febbraio, M. A., Chui, A., Angus, D. J., *et al.*, 'Effects of carbohydrate ingestion before and during exercise on glucose kinetics and performance', *Journal of Applied Physiology*, 89 (2000), pp. 2220–2226.

Febbraio, M. A., Keenan, J., Angus, D. J., *et al.*, 'Pre-exercise carbohydrate ingestion, glucose kinetics and muscle glycogen use: effect of glycaemic index', *Journal of Applied Physiology*, 89 (2000), pp. 1845–1851.

Ferguson-Stegall, L., McCleave, E., Ding, Z., *et al.*, 'Aerobic exercise training adaptations are increased by postexercise carbohydrate-protein supplementation', *Journal of Nutrition and Metabolism,* (2011), Jun 9 Article ID 623182, 11 pages.

Gilson, S. F., Saunders, M. J., Moran, C. W., *et al.*, 'Effects of chocolate milk consumption on markers of muscle recovery during intensified soccer training', *Medicine & Science in Sports & Exercise*, 7 (19), (2009), 18; 7:19.

Gonzalez, J. T., Veasey, R. C., Rumbold, P. L., 'Breakfast and exercise contingently affect postprandial metabolism and energy balance in physically active males', *British Journal of Nutrition,* 23 (2013), pp. 721–732.

Halson S. L. *et al.*, 'Effects of carbohydrate supplementation on performance and carbohydrate oxidation after intensified cycling training', *Journal of Applied Physiology*, 94(4), (2004), pp. 1245–53.

Hartman, J. W., Tang, J. E., Wilkinson, S. B., *et al.*, 'Consumption of fat-free fluid milk after resistance exercise promotes greater lean mass accretion than does consumption of soy or carbohydrate in young, novice, male weightlifters', *American Journal of Nutrition*, 86(2), (2007), pp. 373–81.

Hawley, J. A. and Burke, L. M., 'Carbohydrate availability and training adaptation: effects on cell metabolism', *Exercise and Sports Sciences Reviews*, 38 (2010), pp. 152–160.

Hawley, J. A., Burke, L. M., Philips, S. M., 'Nutritional modulation of training–induced skeletal muscle adaptations', *Journal of Applied Physiology*, 100 (2011), pp. 834–45.

Howatson, G., McHugh, M. P., Hill, J. A., *et al.*, 'Influence of tart cherry juice on indices of recovery following marathon running', *Scandinavian Journal of Medicine and Science in Sports*, 20(6), (2010), pp. 843–52.

International Olympic Committee (IOC) 'Consensus Statement on Sports Nutrition 2010', *Journal of Sports Science,* 29 (2011) Suppl 1:S3–4.

Jamurtas, A. Z., Tofas, T., Fatouros, I. *et al.*, 'The effects of low and high glycemic index foods on exercise performance and beta-endorphin responses', *Journal of the International Society of Sports Nutrition*, 8 (2011).

Josse, A. R., Tang, J. E., Tarnopolsky, M. A., *et al.*, 'Body composition and strength changes in women with milk and resistance exercise', *Medicine and Science in Sports Exercise*, 42(6), (2010), pp. 1122–1130.

Karp, J. R., Johnston, J. D., Tecklenburg, S., *et al.*, 'Chocolate milk as a post-exercise recovery aid', *International Journal of Sports Nutrition Exercise Metabolism*, 16(1), (2006) pp. 78–91.

Luden, N. D., Saunders, M. J., Todd, M. K., *et al.*, 'Post-exercise carbohydrate-protein-antioxidant ingestion increase CK and muscle soreness in cross-country runner', *International Journal of Sports Nutrition Exercise Metabolism*, 17 (2007), pp. 109–122.

Maffucci, D. M. and McMurray, R. G. 'Towards optimising the timing of the pre-exercise meal', *International Journal of Sports Nutrition*, 10 (2000), pp. 103–13.

Maughan, R. J. and Shireffs, S. M. 'Nutrition for sports performance: issues and opportunities', *Proceedings of the Nutrition Society*, 71 (1), (2012), pp. 112–119.

Moore, D. R., Areta, J., Coffey, V. J., *et al.*, 'Daytime pattern of post-exercise protein intake affects whole-body protein turnover in resistance-trained males', *Nutrition & Metabolism*, 9 (91), (2012) Oct 16; 9(1):91.

Moore, D. R., Robinson, M. J., Fry, J. L., *et al.*, 'Ingested protein dose response of muscle and albumin protein synthesis after resistance exercise in young men', *American Journal of Clinical Nutrition*, 89 (2009), pp. 161–168.

Neufer, P. D., Costill, D. L., Flynn, M. G., *et al.*, 'Improvements in exercise performance: effects of carbohydrate feedings and diet', *Journal of Applied Physiology*, 62 (1987), pp. 983–988.

Pagoto S. L. and Appelhans B.M., 'A call for an end to the diet debates *JAMA*. (2013) 310(7): 687–688.

Paoli, A., Moro, T., Bianco, A., *et al.*, 'Exercising fasting or fed to enhance fat loss? Influence of food intake on respiratory ratio and excess postexercise oxygen consumption after a bout of endurance training', *International Journal of Nutritional Exercise Metabolism*, 21 (1), (2011), pp. 48–54.

Phillips, S. M. and Van Loon, L. J. 'Dietary protein for athletes: from requirements to optimum adaptation', *Journal of Sports Science*, 29 (2011), Suppl 1:S29–38.

Phillips, S. M., Moore, D. R., Tang, J. E., *et al.*, 'A critical examination of dietary protein requirements, benefits and excesses in

athletes', *International Journal of Sports Nutrition and Exercise Metabolism*, 17 (2007), pp. 58–78.

Res, P. T., Groen, B., Pennings, B., *et al.*, 'Protein ingestion prior to sleep improves post-exercise overnight recovery', *Medicine and Science in Sports Exercise*, 44 (2012), pp. 1560–1569.

Rodriguez, N. R., Di Marco, N. M., Langley, S., *et al.*, 'American College of Sports Medicine position stand: Nutrition and athletic performance', *Medical Science Sports Exercise*, (2009), 41(3), pp. 709–731.

Rollo, I. and Williams, C. 'Effect of mouth-rinsing carbohydrate solutions on endurance performance', *Sports Medicine*, 41(6), (2011), pp. 449–61.

Sherman, W. M., Pedan, M. C. and Wright, D. A. 'Carbohydrate feedings 1 hour before exercise improve cycling performance', *American Journal of Clinical Nutrition*, 54 (1991), pp. 866–870.

Shirreffs, S. M., Watson, P. and Maughan, R. J., 'Milk as an effective post-exercise rehydration drink', *British Journal of Nutrition*, 98 (1), (2007), pp. 173–180.

Smith, J. W., Pascoe, D. D., Passe, D. H., *et al.*, 'Curvilinear dose-response relationship of carbohydrate (0–120 g·h(−1)) and performance', *Medicine and Science in Sports Exercise,* 45 (2), (2013), pp. 336–41.

Stannard, S. R., Constantini, N. W. and Miller, J. C., 'The effect of glycaemic index on plasma glucose and lactate levels during incremental exercise', *International Journal of Sports Nutrition and Exercise Metabolism*, 10 (2000), pp. 51–61.

Tarnopolsky, M. A., Gibala, M., Jeukendrup, A. E., *et al.*, 'Nutritional needs of elite endurance athletes. Part I. Carbohydrate and fluid requirements', *European Journal of Sports Science*, 5 (2005), pp. 9–14.

Thomas, D. E., Brotherhood, J. R. and Brand, J. C. 'Carbohydrate feeding before exercise: effect of glycaemic index', *International Journal of Sports Medicine*, 12 (1991), pp. 180–6.

Van Loon L. J. 'Application of protein or protein hydrolysates to improve postexercise recovery', *International Journal of Sports Nutrition and Exercise Metabolism*, 17 (2007), S104–117.

Van Proeyen, K., Szlufcik, K., Nielens, H., *et al.*, 'Beneficial metabolic adaptations due to endurance exercise training in the fasted state', *Journal of Applied Physiology*, 110(1), (2011), pp. 236–245.

Wilkinson, S. B., Tarnopolsky, M. A., MacDonald, M. J., *et al.*, 'Consumption of fluid skim milk promotes greater protein accretion after resistance exercise than does consumption of an isonitrogenous and isoenergetic soy-protein beverage', *American Journal of Clinical Nutrition*, 85 (4), (2007), pp. 1031–1040.

Wu, C. L. and Williams, C. 'A low glycaemic index meal before exercise improves endurance running capacity in men', *International Journal of Sports Nutrition and Exercise Metabolism*, 16 (2006), pp. 510–527.

Wu, C. L., Nicholas, C., Williams, C., *et al.*, 'The influence of high carbohydrate meals with different glycaemic indices on

substrate utilisation during subsequent exercise', *British Journal of Nutrition*, 90 (6), (2003), pp. 1049–1056.

Zaja A., *et al.*, 'The Effects of a Ketogenic Diet on Exercise Metabolism and Physical Performance in Off-Road Cyclists' *Nutrients*. (2014) Jul; 6(7): 2493–2508.

Zawadzki, K. M., Yaspelkis, B. B., Ivy, J. L., *et al.*, 'Carbohydrate-protein complex increases the rate of muscle glycogen storage after exercise', *Journal of Applied Physiology*, 72 (1992), pp. 1854–1859.

Chapter three

Almond, C. S., Shin, A. Y., Fortescue, E. B., *et al.*, 'Hyponatremia among runners in the Boston Marathon', *The New England Journal of Medicine*, 352 (2005), pp. 1550–1556.

Armstrong, L. E. 'Caffeine, body fluid-electrolyte balance and exercise performance', *International Journal of Sports Nutrition*, 12 (2002), pp. 189–206.

Armstrong, L. E., Costill, D. L., Fink W. J., *et al.*, 'Influence of diuretic-induced dehydration on competitive running performance', *Medicine and Science in Sports and Exercise*, 17 (1985), pp. 456–61.

Armstrong, L. E., Pumerantz, A. C., Roti, M. W., *et al.*, 'Fluid, electrolyte and renal indices of hydration during 11 days of controlled caffeine consumption', *International Journal of Sport Nutrition and Exercise Metabolism*, 15 (2005), pp. 252–265.

Below, P. R., Mora-Rodriguez, R., Gonzalez-Alonso, J., *et al.*, 'Fluid and carbohydrate ingestion independently improve performance during one hour of intense exercise', *Medicine and Science in Sports and Exercise*, 27 (1995), pp. 200–10.

Cheuvront, S. N., Carter, R., Castellani, J. W., *et al.*, 'Hypohydration impairs endurance exercise performance in temperate but not cold air', *Journal of Applied Physiology*, 99 (2005), pp. 1972–1976.

Cheuvront, S. N., Carter, R., and Sawka, M. N. 'Fluid balance and endurance exercise performance', *Current Sports Medicine Reports,* 2 (2003), pp. 202–208.

Churchward-Venne, T. A., Burd, N. A., Phillips, S. M., *et al.*, 'Nutritional regulation of muscle protein synthesis with resistance exercise: strategies to enhance anabolism', *Nutrition & Metabolism*, 9 (2012) 9:40.

Cosgrove, S. D. and Black, K. E., 'Sodium supplementation has no effect on endurance performance during a cycling time-trial in cool conditions: a randomized cross-over trial', *Journal of the International Society of Sports Nutrition*, 10 (2013) 10:30.

Currell, K., and Jeukendrup, A. E., 'Superior endurance performance with ingestion of multiple transportable carbohydrate', *Medicine and Science in Sports and Exercise* 40 (2008), pp. 275–81.

Gigou, P. Y., Lamontagne-Lacasse, M. and Goulet, E. D. B. 'Meta-analysis of the effects of pre-exercise hypohydration on endurance performance, lactate threshold and [Vdot] O2max', *Medicine and Science in Sports and Exercise* 42 (2010), pp. 361–362.

Goulet, E. D., 'Dehydration and endurance performance in competitive athletes', *Nutrition Reviews*, 70 (2012), pp. 32–136.

Goulet, E. D., 'Effect of exercise-induced dehydration on endurance performance: evaluating the impact of exercise protocols on outcomes using a meta-analytic procedure' *British Journal of Sports Medicine*, 47 (2013), pp. 679–686.

James, L. J., Evans, G. H., Madin, J., *et al.*, 'Effect of varying the concentrations of carbohydrate and milk protein in rehydration solutions ingested after exercise in the heat', *British Journal of Nutrition*, 31 (2013), pp 1–7.

Jentjens, R. L., Underwood, K., Achten, J., *et al.*, 'Exogenous carbohydrate oxidation rates are elevated after combined ingestion of glucose and fructose during exercise in the heat', *Journal of Applied Physiology* 100 (2006), pp. 807–81.

Jequier, E. and Constant, F., 'Water as an essential nutrient', *European Journal of Clinical Nutrition*, 8(3), (2010), pp. 115–123.

Kennerly, K. M., Nieman, D. C., Henson, D. A., *et al.*, 'Influence of banana versus sports beverage ingestion on 75 km cycling performance and exercise-induced inflammation', *Medicine and Science in Sports and Exercise*, 43(5), (2011), pp. 340–341.

Lee, J. K., Shirreffs, F. M., Maughan, R. J., *et al.*, 'Cold drink ingestion improves exercise endurance capacity in the heat', *Medicine and Science in Sports and Exercise*, 40(9), (2008), pp. 1637–1644.

Logan-Sprenger, H. M., Heigenhauser, G. J., Jones, G. L., *et al.*, 'Increase in skeletal-muscle glycogenolysis and perceived exertion with progressive dehydration during cycling in hydrated men', *International Journal of Sports Nutrition and Exercise Metabolism* 23(3), (2013) pp. 220–229.

Minetto, M. A., Holobar, A., Botter, A., *et al.*, 'Origin and development of muscle cramps.' *Exercise and Sports Science Reviews*, 41(1), (2013), pp. 3–10.

Moore, D. R., Robinson, M. J., Fry, J. L., *et al.*, 'Ingested protein dose response of muscle and albumin protein synthesis after resistance exercise in young men', *American Journal of Clinical Nutrition*, 89 (2009), pp. 161–168.

Noakes, T. D., 'Is drinking to thirst optimum?' *Annals of Nutrition and Metabolism*, 57 (2010), pp. 9–17.

Noakes, T., 'Chapter 4: Salt Balance In the body' In *Waterlogged: The serious problem of overhydration in endurance sports* (Human Kinetics, 2012).

Phillips, S. M., Moore, D. R., Tang, J. E., *et al.*, 'A critical examination of dietary protein requirements, benefits and excesses in athletes', *International Journal of Sports Nutrition and Exercise Metabolism*, 17 (2007), pp. 58–78.

Rodriguez, N. R., Di Marco, N. M., Langley, S., *et al.*, 'American College of Sports Medicine position stand: Nutrition and athletic performance', *Medical Science Sports Exercise* (2009), 41(3), pp. 709–731.

Sawka, M. N. *et al.* 'American College of Sports Medicine Position stand. Exercise and fluid replacement', *Medicine and Science in Sports Exercise*, 39 (2007), pp. 377–390.

Sawka, M. N., 'Physiological consequences of hypohydration: exercise performance and thermoregulation', *Medicine and Science in Sports Exercise*, 24 (1992), pp. 657–670.

Schoffstall, J. E., Branch J. D., Leutholtz, B. C., 'Effects of dehydration and rehydration on the one-repetition maximum bench press of weight-trained males', *The Journal of Strength and Conditioning Research*, 15(1), (2001), pp.102–8.

Schwellnus, M. P., Drew, N., Collins, M., 'Increased running speed and previous cramps rather than dehydration or serum sodium changes predict exercise-associated muscle cramping: a prospective cohort study in 210 Ironman triathletes', *British Journal of Sports Medicine* 45(8), (2011), pp. 650–656.

Shirreffs, S. M. and Sawka, M. N. 'Fluid and electrolyte needs for training, competition, and recovery', *Journal of Sports Science*, 29 (2011), pp. 39–46.

Shirreffs, S. M., Watson, P. and Maughan, R. J., 'Milk as an effective post-exercise rehydration drink', *British Journal of Nutrition*, 98(1), (2007), pp. 173–180.

Siegel, A. J., d'Hemecourt, P., Adner, M. M., *et al.*, 'Exertional dysnatremia in collapsed marathon runners: a critical role for point-of-care testing to guide appropriate therapy', *American Journal of Clinical Pathology*, 132 (2009), pp. 336–340.

Smith, J. W., Passe, D. D., Passe, D. H., *et al.*, 'Curvilinear dose-response relationship of carbohydrate (0–120 g·h⁻¹) and performance', *Medicine and Science in Sports Exercise* 45(2), (2013) pp. 336–41.

Tang, J. E., Moore, D. R., Kujbida G. W., *et al.*, (2009), 'Ingestion of whey hydrolysate, casein, or soy protein isolate: effects on mixed muscle protein synthesis at rest and following resistance exercise in young men', *Journal of Applied Physiology*, 107(3), (2009), pp. 987–992.

Tsintzas, O. K., Williams, C., Singh, R., *et al.*, 'Influence of carbohydrate electrolyte drinks on marathon running performance', *European Journal of Applied Physiology*, 70 (1995), pp. 154–60.

Wallis, G. A., Rowlands, D. S., Shaw, C., *et al.*, 'Oxidation of Combined Ingestion of Maltodextrins and Fructose during Exercise', *Medicine & Science in Sports & Exercise*, 37(3), (2005), pp. 426–432.

Zachwieja, J. J., Costill, D. L., Beard, G. C., *et al.*, 'The effects of a carbonated carbohydrate drink on gastric emptying, gastro-intestinal distress, and exercise performance', *International Journal of Sports Nutrition*, 2(3), (1992), pp. 239–50.

Chapter four

Belza, A., Ritz, C., Sørensen, M. Q., *et al.*, 'Contribution of gastroenteropancreatic appetite hormones to protein-induced satiety', *American Journal of Clinical Nutrition*, 97(5), (2013), pp. 980–989.

Benardot D., *et al.*, (2005). 'Between-meal energy intake effects on body composition, performance and total caloric consumption in athletes', *Medicine and Science in Sports and Exercise*, 37(5), (2005), S 339.

Betts, J., *et al.*, 'The causal role of breakfast in energy balance and health: randomized controlled trial in lean adults'. *Am J Clin Nutr* (2014) vol. 100 (2) pp 539–47.

Brunstrom, J. M. and Mitchell, G. L., 'Effects of distraction on the development of satiety' *British Journal of Nutrition*, 96 (2006), pp. 761–769.

Cameron, J. D., Cyr, M. J. and Doucet, E., 'Increased meal frequency does not promote greater weight loss in subjects who were prescribed an 8-week equi-energetic energy-restricted diet', *British Journal of Nutrition*, 103(8), (2010), pp. 1098–101.

Cavanagh, K., Vartanian, L. R., Herman, C. P., *et al.*, 'The Effect of Portion Size on Food Intake is Robust to Brief Education and Mindfulness Exercises', *Journal of Health Psychology*, (2013) [Epub ahead of print].

Clayton, D.J. *et al.*, 'Effect of Breakfast Omission on Energy Intake and Evening Exercise Performance'. *Med Sci Sports Exerc.* (2015) vol 47(12) pp. 2645–52.

Clayton, D.J. & James, L. 'The effect of breakfast on appetite regulation, energy balance and exercise performance'., *Proc Nutr Soc* (2015) Dec 14:1–9. (Epub ahead of print).

Deighton, K., Zahra J. C. and Stensel, D. J., 'Appetite, energy intake and resting metabolic responses to 60 min treadmill running performed in a fasted versus a postprandial state', *Appetite*, 58 (2012), pp. 946–954.

Donnelly, J. E., Blair, S. N., Jakicic, J. M., *et al.*, 'American College of Sports Medicine Position Stand. Appropriate physical activity intervention strategies for weight loss and prevention of weight regain for adults', *Medicine and Science in Sports Exercise*, 41 (2), (2009), pp. 459–71.

Flood, J. E. and Rolls, B. J., 'Soup preloads in a variety of forms reduce meal energy intake', *Appetite*, 49 (3), (2007), pp. 626–634.

Fowler, S. P., Williams, K., Resendez, R. G., *et al.*, 'Fueling the obesity epidemic? Artificially sweetened beverage use and long-term weight gain', *Obesity*, 16 (2008), pp. 1894–1900.

Garber, C. E., Blissmer, B., Deschenes, M. R., *et al.*, 'American College of Sports Medicine position stand. Quantity and quality of exercise for developing and maintaining cardiorespiratory, musculoskeletal, and neuromotor fitness in apparently healthy adults: guidance for prescribing exercise', *Medicine and Science in Sports Exercise*, 43(7), (2009), pp. 1334–1359.

Gonzalez, J. T., Veasey, R. C., Rumbold, P. L., 'Breakfast and exercise contingently affect postprandial metabolism and energy balance in physically active males', *British Journal of Nutrition*, 23 (2013), pp. 721–32.

Heilbronn, L. K., de Jonge, L., Frisard, M. I., *et al.*, 'Effect of 6-month calorie restriction on biomarkers of longevity, metabolic adaptation, and oxidative stress in overweight individuals: a randomized controlled trial', *The Journal of the American Medical Association*, 295 (13), (2006), pp.1539–1348.

Janssen, I., Heymsfield, S. B., Allison, D. B., *et al.*, 'Body mass index and waist circumference independently contribute to the prediction of nonabdominal, abdominal subcutaneous, and visceral fat', *American Journal of Clinical Nutrition April,* 75, no. 4 pp. 683–88, (2002).

Jequier, E., 'Pathways to Obesity', *International Journal of Obesity*, 2 (2002), pp. 12–17

La Bounty, P. M., Campbell, B. I., Antonio, J., *et al.*, 'International Society of Sports Nutrition position stand: meal frequency', *Journal of the International Society of Sports Nutrition*, 8 (2011) Mar 16, 8:4.

Leidy, H. J., Ortinau, L. C., Douglas, S. M., *et al.*, 'Beneficial effects of a higher-protein breakfast on the appetitive, hormonal, and neural signals controlling energy intake regulation in overweight/obese, "breakfast-skipping", late-adolescent girls', *American Journal of Clinical Nutrition*, 97(4), (2013), pp. 677–88.

Leproult, R. and Van Cauter, E., 'Role of sleep and sleep loss in hormonal release and metabolism', *Endocrine Development*, 17 (2010), pp. 11–21.

Mattes, R. D., 'Hunger and thirst: issues in measurement and prediction of eating and drinking', *Physiology & Behavior,* 100(1), (2010), pp. 22–32.

McCrory, M. A., Fuss, P. J., McCallum, J. E., *et al.*, 'Dietary variety within food groups: association with energy intake and body fatness in men and women', *American Journal of Clinical Nutrition*, 69 (1999), pp. 440–7.

Nedeltcheva, A. V., Kilkus, J. M., Imperial, J., *et al.*, 'Sleep curtailment is accompanied by increased intake of calories from snacks', *American Journal of Clinical Nutrition*, 89 (1), (2009), pp. 126–133.

Pagoto S., Appelhans, B. M., 'A call for an end to the diet debates', *Journal of the American Medical Association*, 310(7), (2013), p.68.

Palmer, M. A., Capra, S. and Baines, S. K., 'Association between eating frequency, weight, and health', *Nutritional Reviews*, 67 (7), (2009), pp. 379–90.

Pasiakos, S. M., Cao, J. J., Margolis, L. M., *et al.*, 'Effects of high protein diets on fat-free mass and muscle protein synthesis following weight loss: a randomized controlled trial', *FASEB Journal*, 27 (9), (2013), pp. 3837–3847.

Patel, S. R., Malhotra, A., White, D. P., *et al.*, 'Association between Reduced Sleep and Weight Gain in Women', *American Journal of Epidemiology*, 164 (10), (2006), pp. 947–954.

Phillips, S. M. and Van Loon, L. J., 'Dietary protein for athletes: from requirements to optimum adaptation', *Journal of Sports Science*, 29 (2011), pp. 29–38.

Rolls, B. J., Roe, L. S. and Meeng, J. S., 'Salad and satiety: energy density and portion size of a first-course salad affect energy intake at lunch', *Journal of American Dietetic Association*, 104 (10), (2004), pp. 1570–1576.

Rosenbaum, M. & Leibel, R. L., 'Adaotive thermogenesis in humans,' *International Journal of Obesity*, 34 (2010), pp. 47–55.

Santos, F. L., Esteves, S. S., da Costa Peraira, A., *et al.*, 'Systematic review and meta-analysis of clinical trials of the effects of low carbohydrate diets on cardiovascular risk factors', *Obesity Reviews*, 13 (2012), pp. 1048–1066.

Shai, I., Schwarzfuchs, M. D., Henkin, Y., *et al.*, 'Weight Loss with a Low-Carbohydrate, Mediterranean, or Low-Fat Diet', *New England Journal of Medicine*, 359 (2008), pp. 229–241.

Spiegel, K., Tasali, E., Penev, P., *et al.*, 'Sleep curtailment in healthy young men is associated with decreased leptin levels, elevated ghrelin levels, and increased hunger and appetite', *Annals of Internal Medicine*, 141(11), (2004), pp. 846–850.

St-Onge, M. P., O'Keeffe, M., Laferrère, B., *et al.*, 'Short sleep duration, glucose dysregulation and hormonal regulation of appetite in men and women', *Sleep*, 35 (11), (2012), pp. 1503–1510.

Stote, K. S., Baer, D. J., Spears, K., *et al.*, 'A controlled trial of reduced meal frequency without caloric restriction in healthy, normal-weight, middle-aged adults', *American Journal of Clinical Nutrition*, 85 (4), (2007), pp. 981–988.

Tal, A., and Wansink, B., 'Fattening fasting: hungry grocery shoppers buy more calories, not more food', *JAMA Internal Medicine*, 173 (12), (2013), pp. 1146–1148.

Taylor, M. A., and Garrow, J. S., 'Compared with nibbling, neither gorging nor a morning fast affect short term energy balance in obese patients in a chamber calorimeter', *International Journal of Obesity Relating Metabolic Disorders*, 5(4), (2001), pp. 519–28.

Tremblay, A., Royer, M. M., Chaput, J. P., *et al.*, 'Adaptive thermogenesis can make a difference in the ability of obese individuals to lose body weight', *International Journal of Obesity*, 37 (2013), pp. 759–764.

Tremblay, A., Simoneau, J. And Bouchard, C., *et al.*, 'Impact of exercise intensity on body fatness and skeletal muscle metabolism', *Metabolism*, 43 (7), (1994), pp. 814–8.

Tucker, L. A. and Thomas, K. S., 'Increasing total fiber intake reduces risk of weight and fat gains in women', *Journal of Nutrition*, 139 (2009), pp. 576–581.

Van Proeyen, K., Szlufcik, K., Nielens, H., *et al.*, 'Beneficial metabolic adaptations due to endurance exercise training in the fasted state', *Journal of Applied Physiology*, 110(1), (2011), pp. 236–245.

Volek, J. S., Phinney, S. D., Forsythe, C. E., *et al.*, 'Carbohydrate restriction has a more favorable impact on the metabolic syndrome than a low fat diet', *Lipids*, 44 (2009), pp. 297–309.

Wansink, B. and Kim, J., 'Bad Popcorn in Big Buckets: Portion Size Can Influence Intake as Much as Taste', *Journal of Nutrition Education and Behavior*, 37 (2005), pp. 242–5.

Chapter five

American Dietetic Association, Dietitions of Canada, American College of Sports Medicine, *et al.*, 'American College of Sports Medicine position stand: Nutrition and athletic performance', *Medicine and Science in Sports and Exercise*, 41(3) (2009), pp. 709–31.

Buford, T. W., Kreider R. B., Stout, J. R., *et al.*, 'International Society of Sports Nutrition position stand: creatine supplementation and exercise', *Journal of International Society of Sports Nutrition*, 4 (2007).

Campbell, B., Kreider, R. B., Ziegenfuss, T., *et al.*, 'International Society of Sports Nutrition position stand: protein and exercise', *Journal of International Society of Sports Nutrition*, 4:8 (2007).

Cockburn, E., Robson-Ansley, P., Hayes, P. R., *et al.*, 'Effect of volume of milk consumed on the attenuation of exercise-induced muscle damage', *European Journal of Applied Physiology*, 112 (2012), pp. 3187–3194.

Dorgan, J. F., Judd, J. T., Longcope C., *et al.*, 'Effects of dietary fat and fiber on plasma and urine androgens and estrogens in men: a controlled feeding study', *American Journal of Clinical Nutrition*, 64(6), (1996), pp. 850–5.

Elliot, T. A., Cree, M. G., Sanford, A. P., *et al.*, 'Milk ingestion stimulates net muscle protein synthesis following resistance exercise', *Medicine and Science in Sports and Exercise*, 38(4), (2006), pp. 667–74.

Gualano, B., Roschel, H., Lancha-Jr, A. H., *et al.*, 'In sickness and in health: The widespread application of creatine supplementation'. *Amino Acids*, (2012) 43:519–29

Halton, T. L. and Hu, F. B., 'The effects of high protein diets on thermogenesis, satiety and weight loss: a critical review', *Journal of the American College of Nutrition*, 23(5), (2004), pp. 373–85.

Hämäläinen, E. K., Adlercreutz, H., Puska, P., *et al.*, 'Decrease of serum total and free testosterone during a low-fat high-fibre diet', *Journal of Steroid Biochemistry*, 18(3), (1983), pp. 369–70.

Hartman, J. W., Tang, J. E., Wilkinson, S. B., *et al.*, 'Consumption of fat-free fluid milk after resistance exercise promotes greater lean mass accretion than does consumption of soy or carbohydrate in young, novice, male weightlifters', *American Journal of Clinical Nutrition*, 86(2), (2007), pp. 373–81.

Houston, M. E., 'Gaining weight: The scientific basis of increasing skeletal muscle mass', *Canadian Journal of Applied Physiology*, 24 (1999), pp. 305– 316.

International Olympic Committee (IOC), 'Consensus Statement on Sports Nutrition 2010' *Journal of Sports Science*, 4(29) Suppl (2011), 1:S3–4.

Weigle, D. S., Breen, P. A., Matthys, C. C., *et al.*, 'A high-protein diet induces sustained reductions in appetite, ad libitum caloric intake, and body weight despite compensatory changes in diurnal plasma leptin and ghrelin concentrations', *American Journal of Clinical Nutrition*, 82, (2005), pp. 41–48.

Westerterp-Plantenga, M. S., Lemmens, S. G. and Westerterp, K. R., *et al.*, 'Dietary protein – its role in satiety, energetics, weight loss and health', *British Journal of Nutrition*, 108 (2012), pp. 105–12.

Willis, L. H., Slentz, C. A., Bateman, L. A., *et al.*, 'Effects of aerobic and/or resistance training on body mass and fat mass in overweight or obese adults', *Journal of Applied Physiology*, 113 (12), (2012), pp. 1831–1837.

Karp, J. R., Johnston, J. D., Tecklenburg, S., *et al.*, 'Chocolate milk as a post-exercise recovery aid' *International Journal of Sports Nutrition Exercise Metabolism*, 16(1), (2006) pp. 78–91.

Koopman, R., Wagenmakers, A. J., Manders, R. J., *et al.*, 'Combined ingestion of protein and free leucine with carbohydrate increases postexercise muscle protein synthesis in vivo in male subjects', *American Journal of Physiology: Endocrinology and Metabolism* 288(4), (2005), pp. 645–653.

Kraemer, W. J., Adams, K., Cafarelli, E., (2009) 'American College of Sports Medicine position stand. Progression models in resistance training for healthy adults', *Medical Science Sports Exercise*, 41 (2009), pp. 687–708.

Lemon, P. W., Tarnopolsky, M. A., MacDougall, J. D., *et al.*, 'Protein requirements and muscle mass/strength changes during intensive training in novice bodybuilders', *Journal of Applied Physiology*, 73 (1992), pp. 767–775.

Moore, D. R., Robinson, M. J., Fry, T. L., *et al.*, 'Ingested protein dose response of muscle and albumin protein synthesis after resistance exercise in young men', *American Journal of Clinical Nutrition*, 89 (2009), pp. 161–168.

Ngo, T. H., Barnard, R. J., Tymchuk, C. M., *et al.*, 'Effect of diet and exercise on serum insulin, IGF–I, and IGFBP–1 levels and growth of LNCaP cells in vitro (United States)', *Cancer Causes & Control*, 13 (2002), pp. 929–935.

Norton L. E. and Layman D. K (2006) 'Leucine Regulates Translation Initiation of Protein Synthesis in Skeletal Muscle after Exercise'. *Journal of Nutrition*, 36(2), 533S–537S.

Phillips, S. M. and Van Loon, L. J. 'Dietary protein for athletes: from requirements to optimum adaptation', *Journal of Sports Science*, 29 (2011), pp. 29–38

Phillips, S. M., Moore, D. R., Tang, J. E., *et al.* 'A critical examination of dietary protein requirements, benefits and excesses in athletes', *International Journal of Sports Nutrition and Exercise Metabolism*, 17 (2007), pp. 58–78.

Rennie, M. J. and Tipton, K. D., 'Protein and amino acid metabolism during and after exercise and the effects of nutrition', *Annual Review of Nutrition*, 20 (2000), pp. 457–83.

Rodriguez, N. R., Di Marco, N. M., Langley, S., *et al.*, 'American College of Sports Medicine position stand: Nutrition and athletic performance', *Medical Science Sports Exercise* (2009), 41(3), pp. 709–731.

Rozenek, R., Ward, P., Long, S., *et al.*, 'Effects of high-calorie supplements on body composition and muscular strength following resistance training', *The Journal of Sports Medicine and Physical Fitness*, 42(3), (2002), pp340–147.

Tipton K. D. and Wolfe R. R., 'Protein needs and amino acids for athletes', *Journal of Sports Science*, 22 (1), (2007), pp. 65–79.

Tipton, K. D., Borsheim, E., Wolf, S. E., *et al.*, 'Acute response of net muscle protein balance reflects 24-h balance after exercise and amino acid ingestion', *American Journal of Physiology: Endocrinology Metabolsim*, 284(1), (2003), pp. 76–89.

Tipton, K. D., Ferrando, A. A., Phillips, S. M., *et al.*, 'Postexercise net protein synthesis in human muscle from orally administered amino acids', *American Journal of Physiology*, 276 (1999), pp. 628–634.

Van Proeyen, K., Szlufcik, K., Nielens, H., *et al.*, 'Beneficial metabolic adaptations due to endurance exercise training in the fasted state', *Journal of Applied Physiology*, 110(1), (2011), pp. 236–245.

Weisgarber, K. D., Candow, D. G. and Vogt, E. S., 'Whey Protein Before and During Resistance Exercise Has No Effect on Muscle Mass and Strength in Untrained Young Adults', *International Journal of Sports Nutrition and Exercise Metabolism*, 22 (2012), pp. 463–469.

Wilkinson, S. B., Tarnopolsky, M. A., Macdonald, M. J., *et al.*, 'Consumption of fluid skim milk promotes greater protein accretion after resistance exercise than does consumption of an isonitrogenous and isoenergetic soy-protein beverage', *American Journal of Clinical Nutrition*, 85 (2007), pp. 1031–1040.

Willoughby, D. S., Stout, J. R. and Wilborn, C. D., 'Effects of resistance training and protein plus amino acid supplementation on muscle anabolism, mass, and strength', *Amino Acids*, 32(4), (2007), pp. 467–477.

Chapter six

Armstrong, L. E., Pumerantz, A. C., Roti, M. W., *et al.*, 'Fluid, electrolyte and renal indices of hydration during 11 days of controlled caffeine consumption,' *International Journal of Sports Nutrition and Exercise Metabolism*, 15 (2005), pp. 252–265.

Buford, T. W., Kreider, R. B., Stout, J. R., *et al.*, 'International Society of Sports Nutrition position stand: creatine supplementation and exercise', *Journal of International Society of Sports Nutrition*, 4 (2007).

Burke, L. M. 'Caffeine and sports performance', *Applied Physiology, Nutrition, and Metabolism*, 33(6), (2008), pp. 1319–1334.

Calder, P. C., 'n–3 polyunsaturated fatty acids, inflammation, and inflammatory diseases', *American Journal of Clinical Nutrition*, 83(6), (2006), pp. 1505–1519.

Campbell, C., Prince, D., Braun, M., *et al.*, 'Carbohydrate-supplement form and exercise performance', *International Journal of Sports Nutrition and Exercise Metabolsim*, 18(2), (2008), pp. 179–190.

Candow, D. G., Chilibeck, P. D., Burke, D. G., *et al.*, 'Effect of glutamine supplementation combined with resistance training in young adults', *European Journal of Applied Physiology*, 86 (2), (2001), pp. 142–149.

Carr, A. J., Hopkins, W. G. and Gore, C. J., 'Effects of acute alkalosis and acidosis on performance: a meta-analysis', *Sports Medicine*, 41(10), (2011), pp. 801–14.

Castell, L. M. and Newsholme, E. A., 'The effects of oral glutamine supplementation on athletes after prolonged exhaustive exercise', *Nutrition*, 13 (1997), pp. 738–42.

Cermak, N. M., Gibala, M. J. and van Loon L. J., 'Nitrate supplementation's improvement of 10 km time trial performance in trained cyclists', *International Journal of Sports Nutrition and Exercise Metabolism*, 1 (2012), pp. 64– 71.

Cooper, R., Neclerio, F., Allgrove, J., *et al*, 'Creatine supplementation with specific view to exercise/sports performance: an update', *Journal of the International Society of Sports Nutrition*, 9:33 (2012).

Derave, W., Ozdemir, M. S., Harris, R. C., *et al*,. 'Beta-alanine supplementation augments muscle carnosine content and attenuates fatigue during repeated isokinetic contraction bouts in trained sprinters', *Journal of Applied Physiology*, 103 (2007), pp 1736–1743.

Dodd, S. L., Herb, R. A. and Powers, S. K., 'Caffeine and exercise performance', *Sports Medicine*, 15 (1993), pp. 14–23.

Doherty, M. and Smith, P. M., 'Effects of caffeine ingestion on exercise testing: a meta-analysis', *International Journal of Sports Nutrition and Exercise Metabolism,* 14 (2004), pp. 626–646.

Forbes, S. C., Candow, D. G., Little, J. P., *et al.*, 'Effect of Red Bull energy drink on repeated Wingate cycle performance and bench-press muscle endurance', *International Journal of Sports Nutrition and Exercise Metabolism*, 17(5), (2007), pp. 433–444.

Gebauer, S. K., Psota, T. L., Harris, W. S., *et al.*, 'n-3 fatty acid dietary recommendations and food sources to achieve essentiality and cardiovascular benefits', *American Journal of Clinical Nutrition*, 83 (2006), pp. 1526–1535.

Geyer, H., Parr. M. K., Mareck, U., *et al.*, 'Analysis of non-hormonal nutritional supplements for anabolic – androgenic steroids – results of an international study', *International Journal of Sports Medicine*, 25(2), (2004), pp. 124–129.

Gleeson, M., 'Dosing and Efficacy of Glutamine Supplementation in Human Exercise and Sport Training', *Journal of Nutrition*, 138 (10), (2008), pp. 2045–2049.

Graham, T. E. and Spriet, L. L., 'Performance and metabolic responses to a high caffeine dose during prolonged exercise', *Journal of Applied Physiology*, 71(6), (1991), pp. 2292–2298.

Graham, T. E. and Spriet, L. L., 'Metabolic, catecholamine and exercise performance responses to various doses of caffeine', *Journal of Applied Physiology*, 78 (1995), pp. 867–874.

Greer, B. K., Woodard, J. L., White, J. P., *et al.*, 'Branched chain amino acid supplementation and indicators of muscle damage after endurance exercise', *International Journal of Sports Nutrition of Exercise Metabolism*, 17, (2007), pp. 595–607.

Gualano, B., Roschel, H., Lancha-Jr, A. H., *et al.*, 'In sickness and in health: The widespread application of creatine supplementation', *Amino Acids*, 43 (2012), pp. 519–529.

Halliday, T. M., Peterson, N. J., Thomas, J. J., *et al.*, 'Vitamin D status relative to diet, lifestyle, injury and illness in college athletes', *Medicine and Science in Sports and Exercise*, 43 (2011), pp. 335–343.

Hamilton, B., 'Vitamin D and athletic performance: the potential role of muscle', *Asian Journal of Sports Medicine*, 2(4), (2011), pp. 211–219.

Hill, A. M., Buckley, J. D., Murphy, K. J. *et al.*, 'Combining fish-oil supplements with regular aerobic exercise improves body composition and cardiovascular disease risk factors', *American Journal of Clinical Nutrition*, 85(5), (2007), pp. 1267–1274.

Hoffman, J. R., Ratamess, N. A., Tranchina, C. P., *et al.*, 'Effect of a proprietary protein supplement on recovery indices following resistance exercise in strength/power athletes', *Amino Acids*, 38(3), (2010), pp. 771–778.

Hoffman, J. R., Ratamess, N. A., Faigenbaum, A. D., *et al.*, 'Short-duration beta-alanine supplementation increases training volume and reduces subjective feelings of fatigue in college football players', *Nutrition Research*, 28 (2008), pp. 31–35.

Informed Sport http://informed-sport.com/.

Kennerly, K. M., Nieman, D. C., Henson, D. A., *et al.*, 'Influence of banana versus sports beverage ingestion on 75 km cycling performance and exercise-induced inflammation' *Medicine and Science in Sports and Exercise*, 43(5), (2011), pp. 340–341.

Kim H. J. *et al.*, 'Studies on the safety of creatine supplementation.' *Amino Acids*, 40 (2011), pp. 1409–1418.

Lansley, K. E., Winyard, P. G., Fulford, J., *et al.*, 'Dietary nitrate supplementation reduces the O_2 cost of walking and running: a placebo-controlled study', *Journal of Applied Physiology*, 110 (2011a), pp. 591–600.

Lansley, K. E., Winyard, P. G., Bailey, S. J., *et al.*, 'Acute dietary nitrate supplementation improves cycling time trial performance', *Medical Science and Sports Exercise*, 43 (2011b), pp. 1125–1131.

Larson-Meyer, D. E. and Willis, K. S., 'Vitamin D and athletes', *Current Sports Medicine Reports*, 9(4), (2010), pp. 220–226.

Lenn, J., Uhl, T., Mattacola, C., *et al.*, 'The effects of fish oil and isoflavones on delayed onset muscle soreness', *Medicine and Science in Sports and Exercise*, 34(10), (2002), pp. 1605–1613.

Lugaresi, R., Leme, M., Painelli, V. S., *et al.*, 'Does long-term creatine supplementation impair kidney function in resistance trained individuals consuming a high protein diet', *Journal of the International Society of Sports Nutrition*, 10 (2013).

Madsen, K., MacLean, D. A., Kiens, B., *et al.*, 'Effects of glucose and glucose plus branched chain amino acids or placebo on bike performance over 100 km', *Journal of Applied Physiology*, 81 (1996), pp. 2644–2650.

Mason, W. L., McConell, G. and Hargreaves, M., 'Carbohydrate ingestion during exercise: liquid vs solid feedings', *Medicine and Science in Sports and Exercise*, 25(8), (1993), pp. 966–969.

MHRA (2012) www.mhra.gov.uk

Middleton, N., Jelen, P. and Bell, P. G., 'Whole blood and mononuclear cell glutathione response to dietary whey protein supplementation in sedentary and trained male human subjects', *International Journal of Food Sciences and Nutrition*, 55(2), (2004), pp. 131–141.

Murphy, M., Eliot, K., Heuertz, R. M., *et al.*, 'Whole Beetroot Consumption Acutely Improves Running Performance', *Journal of the Academy of Nutrition Dietetics*, 112 (2012), pp. 548–552.

Noreen, E. E., Sass, M. J., Crowe, M. L., *et al.*, 'Effects of supplemental fish oil on resting metabolic rate, body composition, and salivary cortisol in healthy adults', *Journal of the International Society of Sports Nutrition*, 7 (2010).

Phillips, T., Childs, A. C., Dreon, D. M., *et al.*, 'A dietary supplement attenuates IL–6 and CRP after eccentric exercise in untrained males', *Medicine and Science in Sports and Exercise*, 35(12), (2003), pp. 2032–2037.

Rawson, E. S. and Volek, J. S., 'Effects of creatine supplementation and resistance training on muscle strength and weightlifting performance', *Journal of Strength and Conditioning Research*, 17 (2003), pp. 822–831.

Slater, G., Jenkins, D., Logan, P., *et al.*, 'HMB supplementation does not affect changes in strength or body composition during resistance training in trained men', *International Journal of Sports Nutrition*, 11 (2001), pp. 383–96.

Tang, J. E., Moore, D. R., Kujbida, G. W., *et al.*, (2009) 'Ingestion of whey hydrolysate, casein, or soy protein isolate: effects on mixed muscle protein synthesis at rest and following resistance exercise in young men', *Journal of Applied Physiology*, 107(3), (2009), pp. 987–992.

Tipton, K. D., Elliot, T. A., Cree, M. G., *et al.*, 'Ingestion of casein and whey proteins result in muscle anabolism after resistance exercise', *Medicine and Science in Sports and Exercise*, 36(12), (2004), pp. 2073–1081.

Tipton, K. D., Elliot, T. A., Cree, M. G., *et al.*, 'Stimulation of net muscle protein synthesis by whey protein ingestion before and after exercise', *American Journal of Physiology, Endocrinology and Metabolism*, 292(1), (2007), pp. 71–76.

Too, B. W., Cicai, S., Hockett, K. R., *et al.*, 'Natural versus commercial carbohydrate supplementation and endurance running performance', *Journal of the International Society of Sports Nutrition*, 9:27 (2012).

WADA (2013) The 2013 Prohibited list, www.wada-ama.org

Walser, B., Giordano, R. M. and Stebbins, C. L., *et al.*, 'Dietary supplementation with DHA and EPA augments skeletal muscle blood flow during rhythmic contraction', Federation of American Societies for Experimental Biology (2005).

Willoughby, D. S., Stout, J. R., Wilborn, C. D., *et al.*, 'Effects of resistance training and protein plus amino acid supplementation on muscle anabolism, mass, and strength', *Amino Acids*, 32(4), (2007), pp. 467–77.

Wilson, J. M., Fitschen, P. J., Campbell, B., *et al.*, 'International Society of Sports Nutrition Position Stand: beta-hydroxy-beta-methylbutyrate(HMB)', *J. Int. Sports Nutr.*, (2013) Feb 2;10(1):6

Wylie, L. J., Kelly, J., Bailey, S. J., *et al.*, 'Beetroot juice and exercise: pharmacodynamic and dose-response relationships', *Journal of Applied Physiology*, 115 (2013), pp. 325–336.

Yaspelkis, B. B., Patterson, J. G., Anderla, P. A., *et al.*, 'Carbohydrate supplementation spares muscle glycogen during variable-intensity exercise', *Journal of Applied Physiology*, 75(4), (1993), pp. 1477–85.

Chapter twelve

Barr, S. I. and Rideout, C. A., 'Nutritional considerations for vegetarian athletes', *Nutrition*, 20 (2004), pp. 696–703.

Craig, W. J., Mangels, A. R., American Dietetic Association, 'Position of the American Dietetic Association: vegetarian diets', *Journal of the American Dietetic Association*, 109(7), (2009), pp. 1266–1282.

Crowe, F. L., Appleby, P. N., Travis, R. C., *et al.*, 'Risk of hospitalization or death from ischemic heart disease among British vegetarians and non-vegetarians: results from the EPIC-Oxford cohort study', *American Journal of Clinical Nutrition*, 97 (2013), pp. 597–603.

Eisinger, M. and Ernahrungswiss, Z., 'Nutrient intake of endurance runners with lacto-ovo vegetarian diet and regular Western diet', (1994) vol. 33, pp. 217–29

Rodriguez, N. R., DiMarco, N. M., Langley, S., *et al.*, 'Position of the American Dietetic Association, Dietitians of Canada, and the American College of Sports Medicine: Nutrition and athletic performance', *Journal of the American Dietetic Association*, 100 (2009), pp. 1543–1556.

Williams, M. H. *Nutritional aspects of human physical and athletic performance* (Charles C Thomas Publisher, 1985), pp. 415–416.

INDEX

General index

Index of recipes